Ergogenic Aids in SPORT

Ergogenic Aids in SPORT

Edited by
Melvin H. Williams, Ph.D.
Old Dominion University

Human Kinetics Publishers
Champaign, IL 61820

Publications Director
Richard Howell

Production Director
Margery Brandfon

Editorial Staff
Joyce Tikalsky, Copyeditor
Peg Goyette, Proofreader

Typesetters
Carol McCarty
Sandra Meier

Text Layout
Lezli Harris

Cover Design and Layout
Jack Davis

Library of Congress Catalog Number: 82-84695

ISBN: 0-931250-39-0

9 8 7 6 5 4 3 2 1

Human Kinetics Publishers, Inc.
Box 5076
Champaign, Illinois 61820

M
2-1-85

Contents

Preface   **vii**

Part 1. Nutritional Ergogenic Aids   **1**

Chapter 1. Carbohydrates, Muscle Glycogen,   3
and Muscle Glycogen Supercompensation
    William M. Sherman

Chapter 2. Proteins, Vitamins, and Iron   27
    Emily M. Haymes

Chapter 3. Water and Electrolytes   56
    William G. Herbert

Part 2. Pharmacological Ergogenic Aids   **99**

Chapter 4. Amphetamines   101
    John L. Ivy

Chapter 5. Caffeine   128
    Peter Van Handel

Chapter 6. Anabolic Steroids   164
    David R. Lamb

Part 3. Physiological Ergogenic Aids   **183**

Chapter 7. Oxygen   185
    Alfred F. Morris

Chapter 8. Blood Doping   202
    Melvin H. Williams

Part 4. Psychological Ergogenic Aids   **221**

Chapter 9. Hypnosis   223
  William P. Morgan and David R. Brown

Chapter 10. Covert Rehearsal Strategies   253
  John M. Silva III

Chapter 11. Stress Management Procedures   275
  Rod K. Dishman

Part 5. Mechanical Ergogenic Aids   **321**

Chapter 12. Extrinsic Biomechanical Aids   323
  Edward C. Frederick

Chapter 13. Physical Warm-up   340
  B. Don Franks

Preface

It was a special event, the tenth running of the New York City Marathon. Fred Lebow, initiator and director of the marathon, had national coverage on all three major television networks, and the Comsat Corporation arranged to have the race televised via satellite throughout the world. Lebow secured commitments from a variety of national corporations to guarantee a one million dollar prize to the winner.

Alberto Roe, the American record holder, had trained 8 to 10 hours per day over the past year in preparation for this event. He knew he was in peak condition and would shatter his current record. However, he also knew there would be serious challenges from the Japanese, Finns, East Germans, and New Zealanders. He was leaving nothing to chance.

In the past year, Alberto had trained at altitude for several months and had had three pints of blood removed and frozen. He had also used a new type of anabolic steroid that would maximize his red blood cell (RBCs) production and had consumed a special nutritional compound with iron, vitamin B_{12}, and folic acid to ensure optimal development of the RBCs.

During this time, the biomechanists working at Off Balance, the running-gear company that sponsored Roe, had developed a poly-ethylene racing suit that would cut air resistance markedly at his racing speed and would permit an increase in heat dissipation. Moreover, they had developed a special racing shoe for him, weighing less than an ounce per pair and composed of a new elas-tomer that would double the rebounding force from the pavement.

During the last few days before the marathon, Roe began final preparations. The stored blood was infused into his veins and he initiated his carbohydrate-loading regimen with a new product de-signed to maximize the glycogen content in both the fast- and slow-twitch fibers. His personal sports psychologist was with him to help manage any stress at this crucial time that could disrupt his preparation for the race. He was given numerous posthypnotic suggestions to help him cruise through the race without fatigue, and he practiced the mental image of breaking the tape every hour.

About an hour before the race, Roe consumed a pint of water de-signed to maximize body water supplies for optimal temperature regulation. He also consumed a special amphetamine-caffeine mix-ture to provide an optimal anxiety level, carefully prescribed by his physician and sports psychologist. This mixture was also designed to optimize the free fatty acid levels in the blood in order to provide a glycogen-sparing effect. Every 2 miles during the race a handler would give him special fluid solutions and some concentrated ox-ygen through a specially designed breathing apparatus.

A far-fetched scenario? Possibly. However, although all of these mechanisms to increase sports performance capacity may not have been used collectively, some have been used individually in at-tempts to provide a competitive edge in certain sports.

Throughout history, sports have played an important role in most societies, and their importance has accelerated rapidly in the last 30 years. Athletes have always been searching for a magical in-gredient or technique to give them a competitive advantage over opponents. Athletes, particularly winning athletes, are esteemed in their societies. In some countries they are considered national treasures and are treated accordingly by their governments. Else-where, particularly in the United States, the financial rewards may be rather lucrative, totaling millions of dollars per year. In the Olympic Games, a victory is often construed to indicate the superi-ority of one country's political system over another's. Additional examples may be traced from our recent history back to the Gre-cian Olympic Games.

Accompanying the sports explosion in the past 20 years has been a phenomenal increase in research on all aspects of sports perfor-mance. Exercise physiologists, sports psychologists, biomechanists and other sports medicine professionals have conducted thousands of experiments in attempts to discover the limitations, or barriers, to maximal human physical performance potential. Many investigators have conducted research in attempts to remove or lower physiological, psychological, and mechanical barriers to maximal performance. When special substances or techniques beyond training regimens are employed to improve performance, the term *ergogenic aids* has been used to categorize these diverse methods. The term *ergogenic* means "tending to increase work," or "work producing"; thus, any method that could elicit an ergogenic effect might prove to be beneficial in sports, for it might increase an athlete's physical or mental capacity. Many substances or treatments have been used in attempts to increase performance capacity in the following ways: (a) to improve physiological capacity directly, (b) to remove psychological restraints to physiological capacity, or (c) to provide a mechanical advantage specific to the sport.

In *Ergogenic Aids in Sport*, these aids are grouped into five categories: In the nutritional aids section, William M. Sherman details the relation of carbohydrate loading to endurance performance, Emily M. Haymes reviews the research on vitamin and iron supplements, and William G. Herbert explores the role of water consumption. In the pharmacological aids section, John L. Ivy and Peter Van Handel analyze the roles of two stimulants, amphetamines and caffeine, respectively. David R. Lamb provides a new interpretation of the research on anabolic steriods. Two physiological aids alleged to benefit the gas transport system in the body, oxygen and blood doping, are analyzed by Alfred F. Morris and Melvin H. Williams, respectively. For the psychological aids, William P. Morgan and David R. Brown provide a contemporary review of hypnosis, John M. Silva synthesizes the research on covert rehearsal strategies, and Rod K. Dishman provides a comprehensive review of stress management procedures. Several topics relative to mechanical ergogenic aids are analyzed. E.C. Frederick presents an overview of extrinsic biomechanical aids that might be used to improve efficiency in sports, and B. Don Franks discusses methods of physical warm-up.

Before beginning each chapter, the reader should be aware of the methodological problems associated with ergogenic aids research. Most of the authors address the methodological problems specific to their topics, but a broad overview here may be helpful. A major problem in interpreting the research is that different methodological approaches are used among studies on a single aid. For example, in pharmacological research, different dosages of drugs may have been used, or highly trained subjects may have been used in one study and untrained subjects in another. Many of these methodological irregularities are highlighted in the two chapters dealing with amphetamines and blood doping, but most of the other chapters also give some emphasis to this point.

Another problem is the placebo effect, that is, psychological benefits incurred when the subjects believe they have received an ergogenic aid when they have received placebos, or inert treatments. Other ramifications of the psychological effects associated with ergogenic aid research are discussed thoroughly by Morgan and Brown in the chapter on hypnosis. Lamb also presents an interesting analysis of the placebo effect with experienced weightlifters using anabolic steroids.

One last point involves medical, or health-related, and ethical considerations. In the use of some ergogenic aids there appear to be, in general, no ethical or medical problems associated with their use. In this category would be included water, carbohydrate loading, vitamin and iron supplements, covert rehearsal strategies, stress management procedures, warm-up techniques, and mechanical aids within the rules. On the other hand, certain agents, particularly amphetamines and anabolic steroids, have been condemned on both ethical and medical grounds. Moreover, others, such as hypnosis, caffeine and blood doping, may be in a gray zone of ethics. For example, blood doping may be an inexpensive means to achieve the effect of altitude training but may be in violation of International Olympic Committee doping regulations.

The purpose of *Ergogenic Aids in Sport* is not to address these ethical or medical issues at great length, but simply to present the facts relative to the efficacy of each ergogenic aid. However, it is to be hoped that whenever an ergogenic aid is associated with a medical risk (such as the amphetamines and anabolic steroids discussed in this book) or other aids not covered here (such as vitamin B_{15} and tranquilizers), those associated with the conduct of sports will make such risks known to athletes.

Not all possible ergogenic aids have been included in this monograph, but those addressed cover the broad spectrum of substances and treatments that have been used in attempts to improve sports performance. It is hoped that this presentation will give the reader an awareness of ergogenic aid mechanisms, their use by athletes, and a thorough review of the available research on their effectiveness.

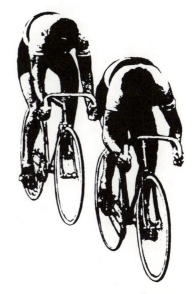

Part 1
Nutritional
Ergogenic Aids

1

Carbohydrates, Muscle Glycogen, and Muscle Glycogen Supercompensation

William M. Sherman

The muscle's use of metabolic fuels for muscular contraction during exercise has always been an important topic of investigation, because intramuscular fuel sources play a dominant role in the capacity for maintaining the muscle's force production. In 1939, Christensen and Hansen performed several investigations which demonstrated the effect of exercise intensity on the relative degree of muscular combustion of fat and carbohydrate (CHO) and the effect of preceding high fat and high CHO diets on the capacity to

William M. Sherman, M.S., is with the Exercise Physiology Laboratory, Department of Physical and Health Education, at the University of Texas in Austin.

Appreciation is extended to Dr. David L. Costill, Mr. William J. Fink, and Mr. Rich L. Sharp for helpful comments during the preparation of this chapter.

Information regarding muscle glycogen stores in marathon runners was collected in collaboration with Mr. Larry Armstrong, Dr. David L. Costill, and Mr. William J. Fink at Ball State University, and Mr. Tom Murray, Dr. Fredrick C. Hagerman, Mr. Robert Staron, and Dr. Robert Hikida at Ohio University, Athens, Ohio.

I would like to extend my thanks to the subjects who have participated in investigations at our laboratory and to Dr. David L. Costill for his endless support. Research conducted at Ball State University, 1977-1981, has been supported by the National Dairy Council, the Graduate Student Research Fund and Sigma Xi, The Scientific Research Foundation.

perform prolonged aerobic exercise (Christensen & Hansen, 1939). They found that, in general, as the intensity of exercise increased, the relative contribution of CHO as muscular fuel increased (based on expired respiratory gas measurements). In addition, 3 days of a low CHO diet significantly reduced exercise time to exhaustion, whereas 3 days of a high CHO diet significantly increased exercise time to exhaustion (80 min vs. 210 min). They based these differing capacities to perform the exercise task on the effect of the preceding diets on the body's CHO stores: that is, a low CHO diet reduced body CHO stores while a high CHO diet increased body CHO stores. They felt the primary influence of these diets was through alterations in liver glycogen stores, because at that time it was thought that muscle CHO stores were only accessible during anaerobic exercise.

The development of the biopsy needle and the reintroduction of the "punch-biopsy" technique by Bergström (1962) allowed the extension of experiments concerning the use of metabolic fuels directly to the skeletal muscle. Work in the late 1960s by several Scandinavian investigators pointed out the importance of muscle glycogen as a fuel for the capacity to perform intense, prolonged aerobic exercise. They demonstrated that the capacity to exercise at intensities between 70 and 80% $\dot{V}O_2$max was related to the preexercise level of muscle glycogen (Bergström, Hermansen, Hultman, & Saltin, 1967; Bergström & Hultman, 1967a; Hermansen, Hultman, & Saltin, 1967; Hultman, 1967; Saltin & Hermansen, 1967). On this basis, many investigators have examined the relationship between exercise and CHO ingestion on muscle glycogen synthesis during various conditions, for example, high CHO diet, low CHO diet, and fasting. In addition, many investigators have attempted to design the best regimen to elevate the muscle's glycogen stores to higher-than-normal levels—that is, supercompensated, overloaded—for the possible benefit of enhancing subsequent performance. This chapter will review our current knowledge of the interrelationships of CHO ingestion, exercise, and muscle glycogen synthesis as they relate to the ergogenic and/or nonergogenic effect of muscle glycogen supercompensation on exercise performance.

Theoretical Benefits

Factors Affecting the Use of Muscle Glycogen

The relative contribution of CHO sources to exercise metabolism has been thoroughly examined and has been shown to occur over a wide range of exercise intensities (Saltin & Karlsson, 1971). At intensities less than 40-50% $\dot{V}O_2$max, muscle glycogen degradation is only minimal and, based on respiratory gas measurements, the primary metabolic fuel is fat. As the exercise intensity increases, the relative contribution of fuel shifts toward the predominant utilization of muscle glycogen. At 90-95% $\dot{V}O_2$max, CHO provides as much as 95% of the total energy output (see Figure 1).

It has been shown repeatedly during cycling exercise that at 70-75% $\dot{V}O_2$max glycogen utilization follows an exponential pattern of degradation (Figure 1). This workload apparently could not be maintained when the glycogen depots (measured in the vastus lateralis) were depleted to less than 25 mmoles glucosyl units/kg wet muscle weight (mmol gu/kg ww) (Bergström et al., 1967; Hultman, 1967; Saltin & Hermansen, 1967), because the perception of fatigue (inability to continue exercise at the same intensity) appears to be related to these low muscle glycogen levels (Borg, 1973; Costill, Coyle, Dalsky, Evans, Fink, & Hooper, 1977). Unfortunately, it has not been directly determined that the same pattern of muscle glycogen breakdown occurs in the gastrocnemius (Costill, Jansson, Gollnick, & Saltin, 1974) during running. Such verification would seem feasible to ascertain, because running involves a much larger muscle mass and a less specific recruitment pattern, and runners must carry their weight. It is known, however, that running up to 30 km at 75% $\dot{V}O_2$max (Costill, Gollnick, Jansson, Saltin, & Stein, 1973) and running 16 km at 80% $\dot{V}O_2$max followed by five 1-minute sprints at 130% $\dot{V}O_2$max (Costill, Sherman, Fink, Maresh, Witten, & Miller, 1981) does not reduce the muscle's glycogen stores to levels as low as those measured following cycling to exhaustion (49 and 55 vs. less than 25 mmol gu/kg ww, respectively). We recently measured muscle glycogen levels in 10 male runners following a marathon performance, and only then was muscle glycogen depleted to levels commonly observed after cycling to exhaustion, 25 mmol gu/kg ww (Sherman, Costill, Fink, Hagerman, Armstrong, & Murray, Note 1). This points out the marked differences in the two exercise modalities, a factor that should be considered in studies examining the etiology of fatigue.

Not only is muscle glycogen degradation exponential during cycling, but the *rate* of glycogen utilization is directly proportional to the intensity of the exercise (% $\dot{V}O_2$max); it must be pointed out that this relationship has been demonstrated for cycling exercise (Hermansen et al., 1967). This observation supports the so-called "preferred fuel" status of muscle glycogen and might be explained by three factors: (a) Aerobic metabolism does not exclude the glycolytic pathway but affects flux through glycolysis. Thus, CHO de-

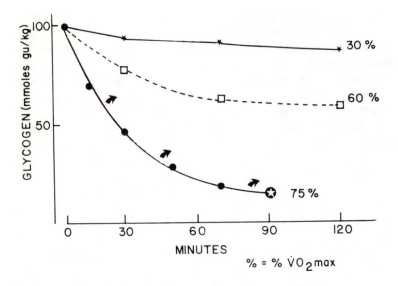

Figure 1—Depicts the pattern of muscle glycogen depletion (vastus lateralis) during cycling exercise at various exercise intensities (% $\dot{V}O_2$max). The arrows indicate the direction in which the pattern of muscle glycogen depletion shifts during exercise following muscle glycogen supercompensation. (Adapted from "Muscle Glycogen Utilization During Work of Different Intensities" by B. Saltin and J. Karlsson, *Advances in Experimental Medicine and Biology,* 1971, 11, 289-299.)

gradation provides necessary glycolytic intermediates and occurs to some extent even when the primary fuel is fat (Keul, Doll, & Keppler, 1972). (b) There is greater efficiency of ATP production relative to the amount of oxygen consumed when CHO is the energy source compared to fat (Holloszy & Booth, 1976). (c) Phosphorylase is a flux-generating step such that when the enzyme is saturated, provides the continued breakdown of muscle glycogen (Newsholme & Crabtree, 1979).

Muscle fiber recruitment patterns during aerobic exercise have been described as indicated by the relative use of muscle glycogen in PAS-stained fast-twitch (FT) and slow-twitch (ST) muscle fibers. Various studies have shown that the ST fibers are the first to become glycogen depleted, and, as the exercise task continues, the FT fibers are recruited to provide additional muscular force. However, at exhaustion, the FT fibers are still adequately supplied with glycogen (Costill et al., 1973; Gollnick, Piehl, Saubert, Armstrong, & Saltin, 1972). Thus, the idea that exhaustion is simultaneous with absolute low levels of muscle glycogen is an oversimplification, because exhaustion may be related to the biochemical factors that predominate as a result of the prevailing recruitment pattern. It is possible that the FT fibers that remain glycogen filled are not within the previously trained FT fiber pool and are less capable of being recruited. It is more likely, however, that the uptake of glucose and fat by the depleted fibers is not sufficient to supply the necessary tension for force production because of insufficient (ATP) generation (Essen, Pernow, Gollnick, & Saltin, 1975). This would increase the ADP/ATP ratio that would stimulate glycolysis (Newsholme & Start, 1973). Because the glucose uptake is inadequate and the glycogen stores in the primarily recruited fibers are insufficient, those fibers are eliminated from the usable muscle fiber pool. As a result, the required work intensity cannot be maintained, and, if exercise is to be continued, the exercise intensity must be reduced (Pernow & Saltin, 1971). It must be pointed out that both fiber types were depleted of muscle glycogen stores (PAS staining) in the biopsy samples of marathoners following the race (Sherman et al., Note 1). In addition, exhaustion can, under various conditions, be related not only to lactate accumulation, hyperthermia, and dehydration, but also to disrupted electromechanical coupling within the fibers, synaptical fatigue, and central nervous system and related psychological factors. Indeed, Fitts and colleagues (Fitts, Kim, & Witzmann, 1979) have demonstrated fatigue (as measured by a decline in Po) in rat muscle consisting predominantly of ST and FTa fibers, which was not correlated with muscle glycogen depletion.

Muscle Glycogen Stores

Muscle glycogen stores are variable depending on previous diet and exercise patterns. In untrained, nontraining individuals on an uncontrolled diet, muscle glycogen stores are roughly 80-90 mmol gu/kg ww (Bergström & Hultman, 1967a; Hultman, 1967). Training individuals, however, consuming a mixed diet during 3 days of tapering running exercise (90, 40, and 40 minutes at 73% $\dot{V}O_2$max), have muscle glycogen stores of about 130-135 mmol gu/kg ww 24 hours following their last run (Sherman, Costill, Fink, & Miller, 1981; Sherman, 1980). Similarly, trained runners resting 2 days after their last training run (40 minutes at 70% $\dot{V}O_2$max) and consuming a mixed diet have muscle glycogen stores of about 180 mmol gu/kg ww (Costill, Blom, & Hermansen, 1981). It is presently unknown, however, whether these differences in glycogen levels are the result of chronic training or simply of the last exercise bout, a difference that should be considered in studies examining muscle glycogen synthesis (Gorski, Palka, Puch, & Kiczka, 1976). Work by

Piehl and colleagues (Piehl, Adolfsson, & Nazar, 1974), however, supports the conclusion that the higher muscle glycogen levels in one-leg trained cyclists occurred as a result of chronic training. Work by Costill and colleagues with runners (Costill, Blom, & Hermansen, 1981) also supports this conclusion. Furthermore, the muscle glycogen stores of single FT and ST fibers in humans are no different either in their levels of muscle glycogen or in glycogen synthase activity (Essen & Hendricksson, 1974; Piehl & Karlsson, 1977). Thus, muscle glycogen levels in ST and FT muscle fiber should be similar in trained and untrained muscle, respectively.

The Effect of Diet and Exercise on Muscle Glycogen Stores

In an effort to assess the effect of exercise-induced glycogen depletion on the subsequent resynthesis of muscle glycogen, Bergström and Hultman (1967b) performed one-legged cycling activity at 75% $\dot{V}O_2$max until the exercising leg was exhausted. Thereafter, they consumed a high CHO diet for 3 days, rested, and biopsied the vastus lateralis at exhaustion and at 24-hr intervals for 3 days. They demonstrated that the depletion of muscle glycogen was localized to the exercised muscle and the subsequent glycogen synthesis resulted in muscle glycogen stores above the preexercise level. After 3 days, the exercised leg had more than doubled its glycogen content while the unexercised leg's glycogen content fluctuated only minimally (see Figure 2). This was the first published report of human muscle glycogen supercompensation, although Embden and Habs (1927) were the first to observe the phenomenon, and Yampolskaya (1950) coined the term *supercompensation*. From this early experiment, it was summarized that glycogen synthesis is localized to the muscle and muscle fibers that have been previously exercised, and some form of "depleting" exercise must be employed to supercompensate muscle glycogen stores.

Subsequent studies have demonstrated that the pattern of resynthesis of muscle glycogen stores following exercise-induced depletion is a biphasic response (Kochan, Lamb, Lutz, Perrill, Reimann, & Schlender, 1979; Yakovlev, 1968). Following the cessation of exercise and dependent on ingestion of CHO, muscle glycogen is rapidly resynthesized to preexercise levels, provided there has not been prior muscle glycogen supercompensation. Muscle glycogen then increases very gradually to above-normal levels, implying that two separate mechanisms of glycogen resynthesis exist: a rapid resynthesis related to the acute depletion of the muscle's glycogen depot and a slow resynthesis dependent on the intake of di-

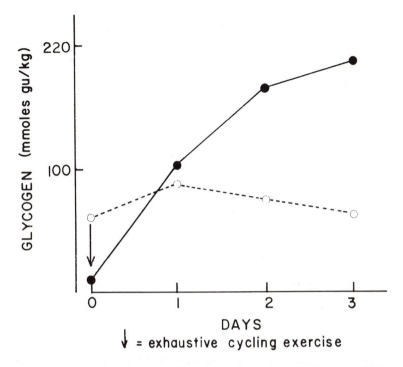

Figure 2—Muscle glycogen resynthesis in a glycogen depleted leg (filled circle) during 3 days of a high CHO diet versus muscle glycogen levels in the nonexercised leg (open circle) during the same time period. Arrow indicates cycling exercise to exhaustion. From "Muscle Glycogen Synthase After Exercise: An Enhancing Factor Localized to the Muscle Cells in Man" by J. Bergström and E. Hultman, *Nature*, 1967, 210, 309-310. Copyright 1967 by Nature. Reprinted by permission.

etary CHO (Hultman, 1967; Kochan, 1978; Saltin & Hermansen, 1967).

It is well established that the amount of CHO consumed following exercise plays an important role in the subsequent resynthesis of muscle glycogen after its degradation. Unless sufficient CHO is ingested, muscle glycogen stores will not be normalized on a day-to-day basis between training bouts, nor will efforts to supercompensate muscle glycogen stores be successful. In general, there is an increasing glycogen storage that is in proportion to the amount of dietary CHO consumed. This was previously demonstrated following cycling exercise (Hultman, 1967; Saltin & Hermansen, 1967) and was recently shown during recovery of glycogen stores following running exercise (Costill, Sherman, Fink, Maresh, Witten, & Miller, 1981). Consuming between 150 and 650 g CHO/day

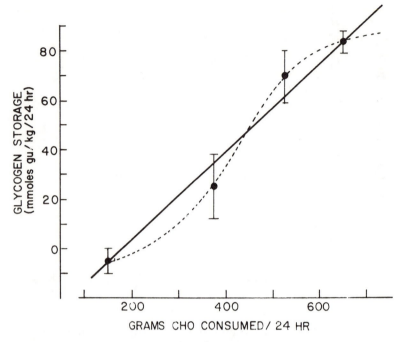

Figure 3—The relationship of the amount of CHO ingested versus the storage of muscle glycogen following depleting running exercise, $r = .84$ (Costill, Sherman, Fink, Maresh, Witten, & Miller, 1981). More recent work suggests that a plateau exists for CHO ingestion exceeding 500-600 g CHO/day. From "The Role of Dietary Carbohydrate in Muscle Glycogen Resynthesis After Strenuous Running" by K.L. Costill, W.M. Sherman, W.J. Fink, C. Maresh, M. Witten, and J.M. Miller, *American Journal of Clinical Nutrition*, 1981, 34, 1831-1836. Copyright 1981 by *American Journal of Clinical Nutrition*. Reprinted by permission.

resulted in proportionately larger increases in muscle glycogen storage (see Figure 3). More recent work, however, suggests that CHO consumption in excess of 600 g CHO/day will not result in proportionately larger amounts of muscle glycogen synthesized (Costill, Blom, & Hermansen, 1981). This is also supported by Blom and colleagues (Blom, Vaage, Kardel, & Hermansen, 1980), who demonstrated that when 1.4 to 2.0 g glucose/kg body weight were consumed every 2 hours following exhausting cycling exercise, the rate of muscle glycogen resynthesis reached a plateau. Thus, it appears that an upper limit exists in the amount of CHO that can be effectively synthesized into glycogen by the muscle, and unless the liver is storing liver glycogen, it would be reasonable to assume that excess CHO intake above that used to synthesize liver and muscle glycogen and support other body functions would be converted to fat. Recently, it has been emphasized that muscle glycogen depletion is a very potent stimulus for its resynthesis, so strong in fact, that muscle glycogen storage predominates over liver glycogen storage (Fell, McLane, Winder, & Holloszy, 1980; Maehlum, Felig, & Wahren, 1978) and can occur in animals (Fell et al., 1980) and in humans (Maehlum & Hermansen, 1978) in the absence of dietary CHO (but at a slower rate).

The type of dietary CHO also appears to play a role in the amount of glycogen stored in skeletal muscle (Costill, Sherman, Fink, Maresh, Witten, & Miller, 1981). Six male runners depleted their muscle glycogen stores during a 16-km run (80% $\dot{V}O_2max$) followed by five 1-minute sprints (130% $\dot{V}O_2max$) and consumed either a starch or glucose diet (650 g CHO/day) during the 2 days following the exercise. During the first 24 hours there was no difference in the synthesis of muscle glycogen between the two types of dietary CHO. At 48 hours, however, the starch diet resulted in significantly greater glycogen synthesis than the glucose diet. Because starches result in maintained elevation of serum insulin compared to glucose (Hodges & Krehl, 1965), and because insulin activates glycogen synthase (Cohen, Nimmo, & Proud, 1979), it was proposed that the differences in the levels of serum insulin between the two types of CHO resulted in the different amounts of glycogen synthesized. Therefore, consuming starch-based diets in the time period following the initial 24 hours after exercise should result in relatively larger amounts of muscle glycogen synthesis when compared to equivalent glucose-based diets. From this study it was also concluded that athletes training heavily on a day-to-day basis should consume a diet that derives approximately 70% of its calories from CHO to ensure "normalized" muscle glycogen stores prior to the next training session (Costill, Sherman, Fink, Maresh, Witten, & Miller, 1981).

An Analysis of the Proposed Regimens to Supercompensate Muscle Glycogen Stores

After the landmark study by Bergström and Hultman (1967b), a series of investigations were conducted in an attempt to identify the regimen of exercise and diet that would best elevate muscle glycogen stores to supercompensated levels prior to performance tasks. The main purpose of elevating muscle glycogen stores to supercompensated levels is to shift the exponential curve of muscle glycogen degradation up and to the right (Figure 1). Theoretically, this would extend, in time, the point at which low levels of muscle glycogen would impair performance compared to a nonglycogen supercompensated state at the same relative work intensity (70-80% $\dot{V}O_2$max).

Several review articles have depicted the possible regimens to supercompensate muscle glycogen stores (Astrand & Rohdal, 1977, p. 496; Saltin & Hermansen, 1967), although the most classic experiment that directly manipulated depleting exercise and high CHO and low CHO diets was conducted by Ahlborg and colleagues (Ahlborg, Bergström, Brohult, Ekelund, Hultman, & Maschio, 1967). In one trial, subjects cycled to exhaustion and consumed a high CHO diet for 3 days. In two other trials, subjects cycled to exhaustion and consumed a low CHO diet for either 1 or 3 days followed by another bout of exhaustive cycling and then consumed a high CHO diet for 3 days. These trials elevated muscle glycogen stores 164, 182, and 192% above preexercise levels, respectively, or to 135, 150, and 165 mmol gu/kg ww, respectively. Based on this experiment and others (Bergström et al., 1967; Bergström & Hultman, 1967a; Saltin & Hermansen, 1967), it has been generally concluded that muscle glycogen stores can be elevated to about 220 mmol gu/kg ww. The best regimen involved two bouts of exhaustive cycling exercise, between which 3 days of a low CHO diet was consumed (less than 5% calories derived from CHO), and after which the subject rested and consumed a high CHO diet (greater than 95% of the calories derived from CHO).

There may be, however, severe consequences associated with this regimen: (a) The 3 days of low CHO diet lead to hypoglycemia and associated nausea, fatigue, dizziness, and irritability; (b) Two bouts of exhaustive exercise during the week prior to an important competition might result in injury and disrupt tapering for the event; (c) A diet containing 95% CHO is not a practical diet. In addition, the known differences of glycogen degradation between cycling and running might also be reflected in the muscle's response to CHO loading, because all prior regimens used cycling as the exercise modality. With these points in mind, we evaluated three types of muscle glycogen supercompensation regimens in six well-trained runners (mean $\dot{V}O_2$max 63 ml/kg/min). The regimens utilized a standardized depletion-taper sequence of running exercise on the treadmill at 73% $\dot{V}O_2$max and also used realistic diets—15, 50, and 70% of the calories were derived from CHO during low, mixed, and high CHO phases, respectively. The results indicated that muscle glycogen stores could be elevated to high levels using a "modified" regimen of diet and exercise (Sherman, 1980; Sherman, Costill, Fink, & Miller, 1981). The specific sequence of depletion-tapering exercise and dietary CHO intake appears in

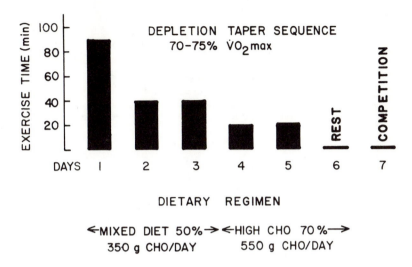

Figure 4—A modified sequence of depletion-tapering exercise and dietary manipulation that results in supercompensated levels of muscle glycogen.

Figure 4. In addition, a comparison of the "modified" regimen to the classical regimen appears in Figure 5. We recently measured muscle glycogen levels in runners preparing for a marathon who undertook the modified supercompensation regimen voluntarily. Levels comparable to our previous investigation were obtained (mean 195, range 170-230 mmol gu/kg ww), supporting the use of this modified regimen by athletes to maximize muscle glycogen levels.

The Mechanism of Muscle Glycogen Supercompensation

Although muscle glycogen supercompensation has been investigated for a number of years, until recently little progress had been made in determining the mechanism of muscle glycogen supercompensation. The rate-limiting enzyme for glycogen synthesis is glycogen synthase (Danforth, 1965), which is known to exist in two interconvertible forms. The I-form (nonphosphorylated) is independent of glucose-6-phosphate (G6P) for its activation, whereas the D-form (phosphorylated) is dependent on G6P for its activation. It has been thought that under physiological conditions only the I-form of the enzyme is active (Bergström, Hultman, & Roch-Norlund, 1972). This was based on the fact that after depleting exercise, the percentage of the enzyme in the I-form (I-form/I + D − form = activity ratio) increased and, as glycogen

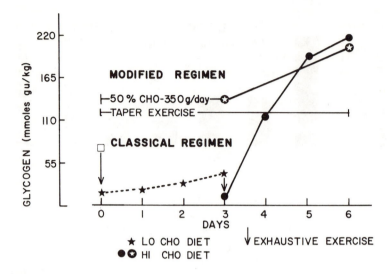

Figure 5—A comparison of the results of the modified glycogen loading regimen depicted in Figure 4 with the results of the "classical" method of glycogen loading developed by Scandinavian investigators.

stores were "normalized," the percentage of the enzyme in the I-form decreased back to predepletion levels in a negative feedback manner (fast phase of the biphasic response). In spite of this "inactive" enzyme, during a muscle glycogen supercompensation regimen, muscle glycogen levels continue to increase (slow phase of the biphasic response), which indicated that the enzyme was still active and the measurement of activity ratio was not sensitive enough to detail changes in the enzyme that occurred independently of the activity ratio.

Following exhaustive exercise, metabolites that affect glycogen synthase, namely, ATP and G6P, do not fluctuate appreciably (Hultman, Bergström, & Roch-Norlund, 1971; Maehlum, Host-mark, & Hermansen, 1978). Recently, it has been shown that the glycogen synthase subunit can be phosphorylated at any of one to six sites which produces different enzyme kinetics dependent on the phosphorylation state (Brown, Thompson, & Mayer, 1977). The different forms of the enzyme can be determined because they differ in their sensitivity to activation by G6P.

With this in mind, Kochan and colleagues (Kochan et al., 1979) replicated the classical regimen of muscle glycogen supercompensation utilizing one-legged cycling exercise. Muscle glycogen supercompensation occurred and the activity ratio followed the previously described pattern. During the actual supercompensa-

tion phase, however, they identified intermediate forms of glycogen synthase (between the I-form and D-form) which had depressed activity ratios but had enhanced sensitivity to activation by
G6P. They proposed that after 24 hours postdepletion the intermediate forms of the enzyme remained with enhanced sensitivity;
this occurred as a result of serum insulin levels exerting their effect
on the enzyme (Rochan et al., 1979) secondary to high CHO ingestion. It is important to note that the intermediate forms of glycogen
synthase, with enhanced sensitivity to activation by G6P, gradually lost this kinetic property over the 3-day loading period, probably
as the acute effect of the exhaustive exercise diminished.

We recently sampled the gastrocnemius of six trained runners
after either 2 days of rest or 24 hours following a previous 2 days of
running for 40 minutes at 70-75% $\dot{V}O_2$max. Analysis of glycogen
synthase in a fashion similar to that of Kochan et al. (1979) indicated that the sensitivity of the enzyme to activation by G6P was
significantly depressed in the 2-day rest period trial (see Figure 6).
This would indicate that daily exercise maintains an increased sensitivity of glycogen synthase to activation and may explain, in part,
why trained runners have higher levels of muscle glycogen and
why the modified regimen of muscle glycogen supercompensation, without exhaustive exercise but with daily running activity,
resulted in muscle glycogen levels similar to those reported following the classical regimen. The chronic effect of exercise and its influence on glycogen synthase may also explain why trained runners, rested 2 days and consuming a mixed diet, have muscle glycogen levels approaching 180 mmol gu/kg ww (Costill et al., 1981).

In light of these observations, it appears that an absolute low
level of muscle glycogen is not the prerequisite for muscle glycogen
supercompensation. Rather, exercise which is sufficient to maintain the intermediate forms of the enzyme with their enhanced
sensitivity to activation may be all that is necessary to maximize
muscle glycogen synthesis, providing sufficient CHO is consumed. It is feasible, therefore, that no "special" regimen of muscle glycogen supercompensation is necessary in well trained runners, and it may be necessary to think of muscle glycogen levels as
being "some degree of full" rather than as supercompensated or
nonsupercompensated.

In addition to manipulating exercise and diet to induce muscle
glycogen supercompensation, trained individuals not only have
higher levels of muscle glycogen than untrained individuals, but
also use muscle glycogen at a reduced rate during aerobic exercise.
The muscle glycogen "sparing" effect of training is related to the
muscle's increased capacity to oxidize fat as fuel (Holloszy &

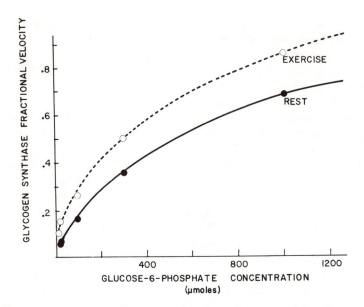

Figure 6—The effect of 2 days of rest and 2 days of exercise (40 min @ 70% $\dot{V}O_2$max, muscle sampled 24 hr after exercise) on the relative sensitivity of glycogen synthase to its activator G6P. Fractional velocity = enzyme activity at subsaturating levels of G6P/enzyme activity at saturating levels of G6P.

Booth, 1976). This has been demonstrated both in animals (Baldwin, Fitts, Booth, Winder, & Holloszy, 1975) and in humans (Piehl, Adolfsson, & Nazar, 1974) and may occur partly as a result of the inhibition of citrate on phosphofructokinase (Jansson, 1980). Therefore, trained individuals should be able to utilize the trained state of their muscle (increased capacity to oxidize fat) in addition to inducing high muscle glycogen levels (increased sensitivity of glycogen synthase to activation) to enhance their endurance capacity.

Research Findings of Increased Performance

Laboratory Investigations

Many investigations have documented that supercompensated muscle glycogen stores improve performance during cycling activity (70-85% $\dot{V}O_2$max) in the laboratory setting (Ahlborg et al., 1967; Bergström et al., 1967; Bergström et al., 1972; Saltin & Hermansen, 1967). The same documentation, however, has not appeared describing running performance in a laboratory setting. Galbo and colleagues (Galbo, Holst, & Christensen, 1980), however, used both running and cycling exercise in a recent study that documented the advantage of elevated muscle glycogen stores for improved endurance (by vastus lateralis biopsy).

Actual Competitive Performance Investigations

Perusal of the literature reveals no documentation of the advantage of muscle glycogen supercompensation for cycling competition, and only one study exists for actual running competition (Karlsson & Saltin, 1971). In a study employing repeated measures and a 30-km race, subjects underwent dietary modifications in two trials that resulted in precompetition glycogen levels of 94 and 193 mmol gu/kg ww (vastus lateralis biopsy). All subjects finished the race in their best time when they began the race with elevated muscle glycogen stores. Examination of split times at 2-km intervals for the two trials indicated that the elevated muscle glycogen stores did not permit subjects to run faster initially, but rather allowed them to maintain their optimal pace for a longer period of time. The investigators indirectly calculated that muscle glycogen lowered to 16.5-27.5 mmol gu/kg ww were the levels that began to interfere with pace. Recall that muscle glycogen levels in other running studies have rarely reached this low level, and work by Costill and colleagues (Costill et al., 1974) has indicated that the gastrocnemius muscle is used predominantly during running. Karlsson and Saltin's study appears to be the only investigation that has directly attempted to evaluate the effect of muscle glycogen supercompensation during running competition. It would, perhaps, be advantageous for other investigators to replicate this experiment employing a marathon or longer ultramarathon event.

Other Possible Benefits of Muscle Glycogen Supercompensation

It has been previously reported that 3.0 to 5.0 g of water are associated with each gram of muscle glycogen (Olsson & Saltin, 1970, 1969), and it has been proposed that the water liberated as muscle glycogen is degraded can be utilized to regulate body temperature and offset dehydration. Not only would this association affect body weight, which could be detrimental to running efficiency (Cureton, Sparling, Evans, Johnson, King, & Purvis, 1978), but there has not been consistency in reports of changes in body weight with muscle glycogen supercompensation (Galbo et al., 1980; Plyley, Costill, & Fink, 1980; Sherman, 1980). In fact, evidence exists which suggests the reported ratio of glycogen to glycogen-bound water of 1.0:3.0-5.0 does not hold (Sherman, Plyley, Sharp, Van Handel, McAllister, Fink, & Costill, 1982), and the water that may be associated with glycogen stores has no positive benefit on regulation of body temperature or in offsetting dehydration (Plyley et al., 1980).

Research Findings of Detrimental or Indefinite Effects

Applicability of Muscle Glycogen Supercompensation to Athletic Events

It is generally agreed that carbohydrate loading is of no benefit for endurance events shorter than 60 minutes because athletes working at 70-80% $\dot{V}O_2$max for 60 minutes do not reach critically depleted levels of muscle glycogen which would impair performance. It is during the next 30 minutes and beyond that muscle glycogen stores become critically low and fatigue occurs. Not until recently, however, has the applicability of muscle glycogen stores and their supercompensation been of interest in anaerobic events.

Suitability of Muscle Glycogen Supercompensation to Anaerobic Exercise

Several studies have shown that the amount of lactate produced during intense aerobic and anaerobic exercise is related to the glycogen content of the muscle (Asmussen, Klausen, Nielson, Techow, & Tonder, 1974; Kelman, Maughan, & Williams, 1975; Klausen, Piehl, & Saltin, 1975). Phosphorylase is a flux-generating step for the breakdown of muscle glycogen (Newsholme & Crabtree, 1979), and lactate is the end product of glycolysis whose production is essential for continued glycolysis (provides reducing equivalents, i.e., NAD) during anaerobic exercise. Therefore, recent studies have set out to determine the critical lower limit of muscle glycogen content which inhibits lactate production and reduces anaerobic work capacity. Recent work by Jacobs (1981) suggests that muscle glycogen levels at about 40 mmol gu/kg ww is the level at which anaerobic exercise is hindered by impaired lactate production. In addition, work by Klausen and Sjogaard (1980) supports the hypothesis that performance of 400 m dash to 1500 m events can be adversely affected when lactate production is impaired due to low levels of muscle glycogen. On this basis, it would be advisable for athletes competing in anaerobic events to ensure sufficient muscle glycogen stores on a day-to-day basis, and, in situations where multiple anaerobic performances are required in 1 day, to practice muscle glycogen supercompensation.

Suitability for Aerobic Exercise

The magnitude of muscle glycogen stores has also been shown to affect its utilization during aerobic exercise. Gollnick and colleagues (Gollnick, Pernow, Essen, Jansson, & Saltin, 1980) recently demonstrated that the relative contribution of substrate oxidized during exercise is related to, and may be controlled by, the intracellular availability of muscle glycogen. This is consistent with other investigations that have observed a greater reliance on muscle glycogen when glycogen levels are higher than when they are lower at the same relative work load (Galbo et al., 1980; Gollnick et al., 1972). In a recent study, three separate 21-km performance runs were performed by trained runners who started the runs with muscle glycogen levels of 207, 203, and 159 mmol gu/kg ww. There was no difference among the trials in performance run times or % $\dot{V}O_2$max between the first and fourth miles and every 3 miles thereafter. In spite of this, muscle glycogen levels following all three trials were not different and averaged 102, 96, and 95.6 mmol gu/kg ww which represented changes in muscle glycogen of 105, 107, and 63 mmol gu/kg ww, respectively. These observations suggest, therefore, that muscle glycogen utilization occurred in excess of that necessary to complete the task and was related to the level of muscle glycogen at the beginning of the run. This is supported by a significant correlation between initial muscle glycogen levels and their magnitude of use during the 21-km performances, $r = .69$ (Sherman, 1980; Sherman et al., 1981). In this light, it would be interesting to know if the glycogen "sparing" effect of caffeine ingestion persists when muscle glycogen stores are elevated prior to endurance performance (Essig, Costill, & Van Handel, 1980).

The fact that there was no difference in performances among the trials mentioned above (21-km runs) is not surprising and is in agreement with the work of Karlsson and Saltin (1971). But the fact that all three trials ended with similar muscle glycogen levels at the end of the runs raises the question of whether muscle glycogen supercompensation would have been beneficial in a longer run. Gollnick and colleagues (Gollnick, Pernow, Essen, Jansson, & Saltin, 1980) reported that the uptake of blood glucose was enhanced when absolute levels of muscle glycogen were lower when compared to higher absolute levels of muscle glycogen at the same relative work intensity. Thus, it seems that in performances where muscle glycogen levels are initially relatively lower, glucose uptake would be enhanced to meet the muscle's need for CHO. In such a case, the enhanced rate of glucose uptake would deplete the liver's glucose reserve much more quickly than during a performance where muscle glycogen reserves were relatively higher. Thus, in the situation of lower initial muscle glycogen, an athlete would suffer from exhaustion earlier as a result of hypoglycemia (Galbo et al., 1980). Therefore, because muscle glycogen supercompensation is known to enhance liver glycogen stores (Hultman & Nilsson, 1971) as well as muscle glycogen stores, the elevation of both of these CHO sources would result in increasing the length of time that high intensity (70-80% $\dot{V}O_2$max) aerobic exercise can be performed by offsetting the depletion of these CHO sources.

Summary and Conclusions

The preceding discussion has outlined current knowledge (1981) of the use of muscle glycogen during exercise and has described the interaction of diet and exercise with the intent to supercompensate muscle glycogen stores. The applicability and effect of muscle glycogen supercompensation on both anaerobic and aerobic exercise also was discussed. Based on this information, the following conclusions can be made:

1. The preexercise level of muscle glycogen influences the length of time that aerobic exercise can be performed until exhaustion, although low glycogen levels and other factors may interact to cause exhaustion.
2. Glycogen synthesis is increased in proportion to the amount of dietary CHO ingested, up to 500-600 g CHO/day, following acute exercise. A diet containing 70% of the calories derived from CHO is recommended for athletes undergoing hard training on a day-to-day basis.
3. Exercise maintains a sensitivity of glycogen synthase to activation and may be responsible in part for muscle glycogen supercompensation and the higher levels of muscle glycogen found in trained athletes.
4. Muscle glycogen supercompensation (to levels greater than 200 mmol gu/kg ww) can best be accomplished by exercise that "tapers-down" during the 6 days preceding competition and a diet that is high in CHO (525 g CHO/day) during the 3 days prior to the competition. Muscle glycogen stores can be elevated to about 180-190 mmol gu/kg ww in well trained runners resting for 2 days and consuming 400 g CHO/day.

5. Enhanced muscle glycogen stores will allow an athlete to *maintain a high work intensity longer, not work faster*, during prolonged aerobic exercise.

6. Athletes who perform regular anaerobic exercise should be concerned with maintaining levels of muscle glycogen above 40 mmol gu/kg ww so as not to hinder performance by compromising the muscle's capacity to produce lactate. This is especially important during repeated anaerobic exercise bouts.

The above points will assist the athlete to ensure at least a normal metabolic state of the muscle, and, in situations requiring prolonged endurance, to optimize the metabolic events known to enhance performance. These recommendations, however, cannot replace the beneficial effect of consistent training.

Reference Note

1. Sherman, W., Costill, D., Fink, W., Hagerman, F., Armstrong, L., & Murray, T. The prolonged effects of a 42.2 km footrace on muscle enzymes. *Journal of Applied Physiology*, submitted for publication, 1983.

References

AHLBORG, B.G., Bergström, J., Brohult, J., Ekelund, L.G., Hultman, E., & Maschio, G. Human muscle glycogen content and capacity for prolonged exercise after different diets. *Foersvarsmedicin*, 1967, **3**, 85-99.

ASMUSSEN, K., Klausen, K., Nielson, L.E., Techow, O.S.A., & Tonder, P.J. Lactate production and anaerobic work capacity after prolonged exercise. *Acta Physiologica Scandinavica*, 1974, **90**, 731-742.

ASTRAND, P.O., & Rodahl, K. *Textbook of work physiology*. New York: McGraw-Hill, 1977.

BALDWIN, K.M., Fitts, R.J., Booth, F.W., Winder, W.W., & Holloszy, J.O. Depletion of muscle and liver glycogen during exercise: Protective effect of training. *Pflugers Archives*, 1975, **354**, 203-212.

BERGSTRÖM, J. Muscle electrolytes in man: Determined by neutron activation analysis in needle biopsy specimens. A study on normal subjects, kidney patients, and patients with chronic diarrhoea. *Scandinavian Journal of Clinical and Laboratory Investigation*, 1962, **14**. (Supplement 68)

BERGSTRÖM, J., Hermansen, L., Hultman, E., & Saltin, B. Diet, muscle glycogen, and physical performance. *Acta Physiologica Scandinavica*, 1967, **71**, 140-150.

BERGSTRÖM, J., & Hultman, E. A study of the glycogen metabolism during exercise in man. *Scandinavian Journal of Clinical and Laboratory Investigation*, 1967, pp. 218-228. (a)

BERGSTRÖM, J., & Hultman, E. Muscle glycogen synthesis after exercise: An enhancing factor localized to the muscle cells in man. *Nature*, 1967, **210**, 309-310. (b)

BERGSTRÖM, J., Hultman, E., & Roch-Norlund, A.E. Muscle glycogen synthase in normal subjects. Basal values, and effect of glycogen depletion by exercise and of a carbohydrate-rich diet following exercise. *Scandinavian Journal of Clinical and Laboratory Investigation*, 1972, **29**, 231-236.

BLOM, P., Vaage, O., Kardel, D., & Hermansen, L. Effect of increasing glucose loads on the rate of muscle glycogen resynthesis after prolonged exercise. *Acta Physiologica Scandinavica*, 1980, **108**, C11. (Abstract)

BORG, G.A. Perceived exertion: A note on history and methods. *Medicine and Science in Sports*, 1973, **5**, 90-93.

BROWN, J.H., Thompson, B., & Mayer, S.E. Conversion of skeletal muscle glycogen synthase to multiple glucose-6-phosphate dependent forms by cyclic adenosine monophosphate dependent and independent protein kinases. *Biochemistry*, 1977, **16**, 5501-5508.

CHRISTENSEN, E.H., & Hansen, O. Respiratorischer Quotient and O_2-Aufnahme. *Scandinavian Archives of Physiology*, 1939, **81**, 180-189.

COHEN, P., Nimmo, H.G., & Proud, C.G. How does insulin stimulate glycogen synthesis? *Biochemical Society Symposia*, 1979, **43**, 69-95.

COSTILL, D.L., Blom, P., & Hermansen, L. Influence of acute exercise and endurance training on muscle glycogen storage. *Medicine and Science in Sports and Exercise*, 1981, **13**, 90. (Abstract)

COSTILL, D.L., Coyle, E.F., Dalsky, W., Evans, W., Fink, W.J., & Hooper, D. Effects of elevated plasma FFA and insulin in muscle glycogen usage during exercise. *Journal of Applied Physiology*, 1977, **43**, 695-699.

COSTILL, D.L., Gollnick, P.D., Jansson, E., Saltin, B., & Stein, B. Glycogen depletion in human muscle fibers during distance running. *Acta Physiologica Scandinavica*, 1973, **89**, 374-383.

COSTILL, D.L., Jansson, E., Gollnick, P.D., & Saltin, B. Glycogen utilization in leg muscle of men during level and uphill running. *Acta Physiologica Scandinavica*, 1974, **94**, 475-481.

COSTILL, K.L., Sherman, W.M., Fink, W.J., Maresh, C., Witten, M., & Miller, J.M. The role of dietary carbohydrate in muscle glycogen resynthesis after strenuous running. *American Journal of Clinical Nutrition*, 1981, **34**, 1831-1836.

CURETON, K.G., Sparling, P.B., Evans, B.W., Johnson, S.M., King, O.D., & Purvis, J.W. Effect of experimental alterations in excess weight on aerobic capacity and distance running performance. *Medicine and Science in Sports*, 1978, **10**, 194-199.

DANFORTH, W.H. Glycogen synthase activation in skeletal muscle. Inter-conversion of two forms and control of glycogen synthesis. *Journal of Biological Chemistry*, 1965, **240**, 588-593.

EMBDEN, G., & Habs, H. Ueber chemische und biologische Veraenderunger der Muskulator nach oefters wiederholter faradischer Reizung. I. Mitteilung. *Zeitschrift für Physiologische Chemie*, 1927, **171**, 16-39.

ESSEN, B., & Hendriksson, J. Glycogen content of individual muscle fibers in man. *Acta Physiologica Scandinavica*, 1974, **90**, 645-647.

ESSEN, B., Pernow, B., Gollnick, P.D., & Saltin, B. Muscle glycogen content and lactate uptake in exercising muscles. In H. Howald & J.R. Poortmans (Eds.), *Metabolic adaptation to prolonged physical exercise*. Basel: Birkhauser Verlag, 1975.

ESSIG, D., Costill, D.L., & Van Handel, P.J. Effects of caffeine ingestion on utilization of muscle glycogen and lipids during leg ergometer cycling. *International Journal of Sports Medicine*, 1980, **1**, 86-90.

FELL, R.D., McLane, J.A., Winder, W.W., & Holloszy, J.O. Preferential resynthesis of muscle glycogen in fasting rats after exhausting exercise. *American Journal of Physiology*, 1980, **238**, 328-332.

FITTS, R.J., Kim, D.H., & Witzmann, F.A. The development of fatigue during high intensity and endurance exercise. In F.J. Nagle & H.J. Montoye (Eds.), Madison: University of Wisconsin Press, 1979.

GALBO, H., Holst, H.H., & Christensen, N.J. The effect of different diets and insulin on the hormonal response to prolonged exercise. *Acta Physiologica Scandinavica*, 1980, **107**, 19-32.

GOLLNICK, P.D., Pernow, B., Essen, B., Jansson, E., & Saltin, B. Availability of glycogen and plasma FFA for substrate utilization in leg muscle of man during exercise. *Clinical Physiology*, 1980, **1**, 1-22.

GOLLNICK, P.D., Piehl, K., Saubert, C.W., Armstrong, R.B., & Saltin, B. Diet, exercise, and glycogen changes in human muscle fibers. *Journal of Applied Physiology*, 1972, **33**, 421-425.

GORSKI, J., Palka, P., Puch, P., & Kiczka, K. The post-exercise glycogen recovery in tissues of trained rats. *Acta Physiologica Polonica*, 1976, **27**, 47-53.

HERMANSEN, L., Hultman, E., & Saltin, B. Muscle glycogen during prolonged severe exercise. *Acta Physiologica Scandinavica*, 1967, **71**, 129-139.

HODGES, R.E., & Krehl, W.A. The role of carbohydrates in lipid metabolism. *American Journal of Clinical Nutrition*, 1965, **17**, 334-346.

HOLLOSZY, J.O., & Booth, F.A. Biochemical adaptations to endurance exercise. *Annual Review of Physiology*, 1976, **18**, 273; 291.

HULTMAN, E. Studies on muscle metabolism of glycogen and active phosphate in man with special reference to exercise and diet. *Scandinavian Journal of Clinical and Laboratory Investigation*, 1967, **19**. (Supplement 94)

HULTMAN, E., Bergström, J., & Roch-Norlund, A.E. Glycogen storage in human skeletal muscle. *Advances in Experimental Medicine and Biology*, 1971, **11**, 273-288.

HULTMAN, E., & Nilsson, L.H. Liver glycogen in man. Effect of different diets and muscular exercise. *Advances in Experimental Medicine and Biology*, 1971, **11**, 143-154.

INTERNATIONAL *Journal of Sports Medicine*, 1982, **3**, 22-24.

JACOBS, I. Lactate, muscle glycogen and exercise performance in man. *Acta Physiologica Scandinavica*, 1981. (Supplement 495)

JANSSON, E. Diet and muscle metabolism in man with special reference to fat and carbohydrate utilization and its regulation. *Acta Physiologica Scandinavica*, 1980. (Supplement 487)

KARLSSON, J., & Saltin, B. Diet, muscle glycogen and endurance performance. *Journal of Applied Physiology*, 1971, **31**, 203-206.

KELMAN, G.R., Maughan, R.J., & Williams, C. The effect of dietary modifications on blood lactate during exercise. *Journal of Physiology*, 1975, **251**, 34-35P.

KEUL, J., Doll, E., & Keppler, D. *Energy metabolism of human muscle.* Baltimore: University Park Press, 1972.

KLAUSEN, K., Piehl, K., & Saltin, B. Muscle glycogen stores and capacity for anaerobic work. In H. Howald & J.R. Poortmans (Eds.), *Metabolic adaptation to prolonged physical exercise.* Basel: Birkhauser Verlag, 1975.

KLAUSEN, K., & Sjogaard, G. Glycogen stores and lactate accumulation in skeletal muscle of man during intense bicycle exercise. *Scandinavian Journal of Sports Sciences*, 1980, **2**, 7-12.

KOCHAN, R.G. *Glycogen synthase control of skeletal muscle glycogen resynthesis following exercise in humans.* Unpublished doctoral dissertation, University of Toledo, 1978.

KOCHAN, R.G., Lamb, D.R., Lutz, S.A., Perrill, C.V., Reimann, E.M., & Schlender, K.K. Glycogen synthase activation in human skeletal muscle: Effect of diet and exercise. *American Journal of Physiology*, 1979, **236**, E660-666.

MAEHLUM, S., Felig, P., & Wahren, J. Splanchnic glucose and muscle glycogen metabolism after glucose feeding during postexercise recovery. *American Journal of Physiology*, 1978, **235**, E255-260.

MAEHLUM, S., & Hermansen, L. Muscle glycogen concentration during recovery after prolonged severe exercise in fasting subjects. *Scandinavian Journal of Clinical and Laboratory Investigation*, 1978, **38**, 557-560.

MAEHLUM, S. Hostmark, A.T., & Hermansen, L. Synthesis of muscle glycogen during recovery after prolonged severe exercise in diabetic subjects. Effect of insulin deprivation. *Scandinavian Journal of Clinical and Laboratory Investigation*, 1978, **37**, 309-316.

NEWSHOLME, E.A., & Crabtree, B. Theoretical approaches to control of metabolic pathways and their application to glycolysis in muscle. *Journal of Molecular Cellular Cardiology*, 1979, **11**, 839-856.

NEWSHOLME, E.A., & Start, C. *Regulation in metabolism.* New York: John Wiley & Sons, 1973.

OLSSON, K.E., & Saltin, B. Variations in total body water with muscle glycogen changes in man. *Biochemistry of Exercise, Medicine and Sports*, 1969, **5**, 159-162.

OLSSON, K.E., & Saltin, B. Variations in total body water with muscle glycogen changes in man. *Acta Physiologica Scandinavica*, 1970, **80**, 11-18.

PERNOW, B., & Saltin, B. Availability of substrates and capacity for prolonged heavy exercise. *Journal of Applied Physiology*, 1971, **31**, 416-422.

PIEHL, K., Adolfsson, S., & Nazar, K. Glycogen storage and glycogen synthase activity in trained and untrained muscle of man. *Acta Physiologica Scandinavica*, 1974, **90**, 779-788.

PIEHL, K., & Karlsson, J. Glycogen synthase and phosphorylase activity in slow and fast-twitch skeletal muscle fibers in man. *Acta Physiologica Scandinavica*, 1977, **100**, 210-214.

PLYLEY, M.J., Costill, D.L., & Fink, W.J. Influence of glycogen "bound" water on temperature regulation during exercise. *Canadian Journal of Applied Sport Sciences*, 1980, **5**, 5. (Abstract)

SALTIN, B., & Hermansen, L. Glycogen stores and prolonged severe exercise. In G. Blix (Ed.), *Nutrition and physical activity.* Uppsala, Sweden: Almqvist & Wiksells, 1967.

SALTIN, B., & Karlsson, J. Muscle glycogen utilization during work of different intensities. *Advances in Experimental Medicine and Biology*, 1971, **11**, 289-299.

SHERMAN, W.M. *Dietary manipulation to induce muscle glycogen supercompensation: Effect on endurance performance.* Unpublished master's thesis, Ball State University, 1980.

SHERMAN, W.M., Costill, D.L., Fink, W.J., & Miller, J.M. The effect of exercise and diet manipulation on muscle glycogen and its subsequent utilization during performance. *International Journal of Sports Medicine*, 1981, **2**, 114-118.

SHERMAN, W.M., Plyley, M.J., Sharp, R.L., Van Handel, P.J., McAllister, R.M., Fink, W.J., & Costill, D.L. Muscle glycogen storage and its relationship with water.

YAKOVLEV, N.N. The effect of regular muscle activity on enzymes of glycogen, and glucose-6-phosphate in muscles and liver. *Biochemistry*, 1968, **33**, 602-607.

YAMPOLSKAYA, L.I. Supercompensation of the glycogen content of muscles in the recovery period after work of different rates and duration. *Physiologica SSSR*, 1950, **36**, 749-754.

2

Proteins, Vitamins, and Iron

Emily M. Haymes

In their search for substances that will improve competitive performance, athletes have speculated about the ergogenic effects of many nutrients, including protein, most vitamins, and iron. One recent study of coaches and trainers reported that 68% recommended that their athletes take vitamin supplements and "51% believed that protein was the most important factor" in increasing muscle mass (Bentivegna, Kelley, & Kalenak, 1979, p. 101). Another study reported 36% of the female athletes surveyed took B complex vitamins, 26% took iron, and 19% took vitamin C supplements during training (Werblow, Fox, & Henneman, 1978).

Why is there so much interest in protein, vitamins, and iron as potential ergogenic aids? The theories behind the use of each of the nutrients as ergogenic substances and the scientific evidence supporting or refuting their use are examined in this chapter.

Emily M. Haymes, Ph.D, F.A.C.S.M., is with the Department of Movement Science and Physical Education at the Florida State University in Tallahassee.

Protein

Proteins are large, complex molecules composed of some 20 different amino acids. The body uses amino acids to build and repair cells and tissues; to form enzymes, hemoglobin, and plasma proteins; to form hormones like insulin and epinephrine; and, under certain circumstances, for energy. When an amino acid is used for energy, the nitrogen-containing amino group is removed and forms ammonia or urea. Most of the urea is excreted from the body in the urine and sweat. The remains of the amino acid, the carbon skeleton, can be used to synthesize glucose (gluconeogenesis), fatty acids (lipogenesis), or be used directly for energy.

The recommended dietary allowance (RDA) of protein for the adult is 0.8 g/kg body w. For a 75-kg (165-lb) male this would be 60 g protein or slightly more than 2 oz/day. A female weighing 55 kg (121 lb) needs only 44 g (1.5 oz) of protein. Children actually have a greater proportional need for protein to support growth. The RDA has been set so that the requirement for protein decreases as age increases to age 18. From ages 7 to 10 the protein requirement is 1.2 g/kg; from 11 to 14 years, 1.0 g/kg; and from 15 to 18 years, 0.9 g/kg.

Theoretical Benefits

Three theories have been proposed as to why athletes and persons engaged in strenuous work or exercise may need more protein than the RDA. The first theory proposes that increases in muscle mass must be supported by greater-than-normal amounts of protein in the diet. Intensive training, strength training in particular, is frequently accompanied by increases in lean body weight and muscle mass. Strength training usually results in an increase in the myofibrillar protein, which includes both actin and myosin (Edgerton, 1973). If the increase in myofibrillar protein is due to increased protein synthesis from amino acids, then increasing the protein content of the diet could be beneficial. On the other hand, if the increase in muscle protein is due to a decrease in the rate of endogenous protein breakdown, then less exogenous (dietary) protein would be required. Goldberg, Etlinger, Goldspink, and Jablecki (1975) proposed that both an increased rate of synthesis and a decreased rate of protein destruction are responsible for increasing muscle mass.

Another theory, proposed by Yoshimura and his colleagues (Yoshimura, 1961, 1966; Yoshimura, Inoue, Yamada, & Shiraki, 1980), suggests that during the early phase of training a greater need for protein exists to support protein synthesis in skeletal muscle. In order to support this increased need for protein, erythrocytes and plasma proteins are destroyed, producing sports anemia, and the amino acids are recycled to form myoglobin and new erythrocytes. It would also seem reasonable to believe that the amino acids might be used for the increase in mitochondrial mass and enzyme formation observed during training. Yoshimura (1961) proposed that an increase in protein intake would prevent sports anemia by supplying the additional amino acids needed for protein synthesis.

The third theory concerning the increased need for protein proposes that protein is used for energy in significant amounts during exercise. This theory appears to have been proposed in 1842 by Von Liebig, but was largely discounted when no increase in nitrogen excretion was observed during exercise (Durnin, 1978). Several recent studies have, however, presented evidence supporting an increase in nitrogen turnover during exercise (Cerny, 1975; Decombaz, Reinhardt, Anantharaman, von Glutz, & Poortmans, 1979; Dohm, Puente, Smith, & Edge, 1978; Gontzea, Sutzescu, & Dumitrache, 1974, 1975; Lemon & Mullin, 1980; Mole & Johnson, 1971; Refsum & Stromme, 1974; Refsum, Gjessing, & Stromme, 1979). It appears that significant amounts of nitrogen are excreted in the sweat during exercise (Lemon & Mullin, 1980).

Much of the speculation surrounding the use of protein for energy has been focused on the glucose-alanine cycle and the possible use of the branched chain amino acids—leucine, isoleucine, and valine—for energy. The branched chain amino acids as well as aspartate and glutamate are believed to be the primary amino acids metabolized by muscle for energy (Lindsay, 1980). Because the amine group cannot be oxidized by the muscle, it is transferred out of the muscle as either alanine or glutamine. In the liver, both alanine and glutamine can be converted to glucose, whereas the amine groups will be converted to urea. Lindsay (1980) has suggested that much of the alanine and glutamine may have been derived from glucose (or glycogen) and not necessarily from protein catabolism.

Research Findings of Increased Need

Serum urea levels have been reported to increase during exercise lasting longer than an hour (Cerny, 1975; Decombaz et al., 1979; Refsum et al., 1979). Because muscle glycogen stores may be depleted during prolonged exercise, Lemon and Mullin (1980) hypothesized that protein catabolism and urea formation would be increased in a glycogen-depleted state. Significant increases in both the serum and sweat urea content during exercise in a glycogen-depleted state were found, compared to exercise following glycogen loading. Lemon and Mullin calculated that 4.4% of the total energy used following glycogen loading came from protein, whereas 10.4% of the total calories came from protein in the glycogen-depleted state. The protein source used for energy is currently unknown. Lemon and Nagle (1981) suggested the myofibrillar proteins and muscle enzymes were possible sources of the amino acids used by the muscle for energy. Because 65% of the nitrogen found in muscle is in the myofibrils (Poortmans, 1975), it would appear to be a likely source. However, no significant increase in 3-methylhistidine excretion has been observed following prolonged exercise in man (Decombaz et al., 1979; Refsum et al., 1979). An increase in 3-methylhistidine would be expected if the myofibrils are broken down. Refsum and associates (1979) reported little relationship between the amino acid changes observed during prolonged exercise and either serum albumin or muscle tissue protein composition. However, decreases in both myofibrillar and soluble protein of muscle as well as liver protein have been observed in trained rats after an exhaustive bout of exercise (Dohm et al., 1978).

The need for protein may be greater during the early phase of training than during later stages. Yoshimura (1961) observed decreases in total hemoglobin and serum protein content in all subjects receiving 1.4 g protein/kg or less per day even though all but one of the subjects was in positive nitrogen balance. The decrease in hemoglobin was observed after about 10 days of training. Increases in total hemoglobin and serum protein occurred in subjects receiving 2.3 g protein/kg or more per day, whereas little change in hemoglobin and serum protein occurred in two subjects receiving 1.9 g protein/kg. Yoshimura concluded that the protein intake needed to be 2 g/kg/day during training to prevent sports anemia.

Subsequent work by Shiraki, Yamada, and Yoshimura (1977) using three groups—a high protein group receiving 2 g/kg, a standard protein group receiving 1.25 g/kg, and a low protein group receiving 0.5 g/kg—found no significant change in total hemoglobin after 1 week of training in the high protein group, whereas total hemoglobin was reduced 11 and 12%, respectively, in the low protein and standard protein groups. Osmotic fragility of the erythrocytes increased in the low protein and standard protein groups but decreased in the high protein group during the first week of training. An increase in reticulocyte count was seen early in the first week of training in the high protein group, later during the first week in the standard protein group, but not until the third week in the low protein group. The protein intake was approximately 30% fish protein and 70% vegetable protein in both of the previous studies. Raising the animal protein intake to 57% of the total, Yoshimura et al. (1980) found that 1.2-1.3 g/kg prevented a decline in total hemoglobin during early training.

One possible explanation for sports anemia is an increase in plasma volume during training. If the plasma volume increases while the total hemoglobin content and erythrocyte number remain relatively constant, a dilution effect will occur that will result in a reduction in both hemoglobin concentration and erythrocyte count. Oscai, Williams, and Hertig (1968) reported a 6% increase in blood volume following 16 weeks of training. On the other hand, Bass, Buskirk, Iampietro, and Mager (1958) did not find a significant change in plasma volume during 3 weeks of training. It is unlikely that an increase in plasma volume could explain the difference in total hemoglobin between the high and low protein groups observed by Shiraki et al. (1977).

Gontzea et al. (1974, 1975) examined nitrogen balance in young men receiving either 1.0 or 1.5 g protein/kg as well as 10% more calories than were expended. Nitrogen balance was slightly positive during the sedentary period but became negative during 4 days of training when the protein intake was 1.0 g/kg/day. Two of six subjects were also in negative nitrogen balance with a protein intake of 1.5 g/kg. Gontzea et al. (1974) found the major increase in nitrogen excretion during exercise occurred through the sweat (22-28% of the total nitrogen excreted). In a subsequent study (Gontzea et al., 1975), 12 subjects trained for 3 weeks. Protein intake was maintained at 1.0 g/kg/day. Negative nitrogen balance was observed for the first 6 days but diminished progressively for the remainder of the 3 weeks as the nitrogen losses decreased. Gontzea et al. (1975) suggested that the decrease in protein catabolism may have been influenced by a decline in psychological stress as well as physical stress.

Negative nitrogen balance during training has been reported in several other studies. Both Celejowa and Homa (1970) and Laritcheva, Yalovaya, Shubin, and Smirnov (1978) studied weight lifters during training. Celejowa and Homa (1970) found that although mean daily protein intake was 2 g/kg, approximately 15% of the total caloric intake, 5 of the 10 athletes were in negative nitrogen balance. This suggested to the authors that 2 g/kg was inadequate for at least 50% of the competitors. The weight lifters studied by Laritcheva et al. (1978) had protein intakes ranging from 14 to 18% of the total calories. When intense preparation for important contests occurred, protein intakes below 2 g/kg resulted in negative nitrogen balance. During less intense training, nitrogen balance was maintained with protein intakes of 1.3-1.8 g/kg. Reducing the protein intake below 1.3 g/kg or the caloric intake below 2,700 kcal produced negative nitrogen balance.

Torun, Scrimshaw, and Young (1977) examined nitrogen balance in a group of young men during an isometric strength training program lasting 4 to 6 weeks. Subjects consumed meals containing either 0.5 or 1.0 g protein/kg/day. Negative nitrogen balance and a decrease in total body potassium were observed in the exercising subjects receiving 0.5 protein/kg. The decrease in total body potassium suggests a loss of lean body tissue. Decreased urinary nitrogen output has been observed during a 4-week strength training program in subjects receiving 0.8 or 2.5 g protein/kg (Marable, Hickson, Korslund, Herbert, Desjardins, & Thye, 1979). Marable and associates estimated the decrease in nitrogen excretion was sufficient to increase the lean body weight by 2 kg, but a protein intake of 0.8 g/kg was marginal for increasing muscle mass. Increasing the protein intake to 2.8 g/kg increases the amount of nitrogen excreted in the urine and sweat during training (Consolazio, Johnson, Nelson, Dramise, & Skala, 1975). Consolazio et al. found that training resulted in a significant increase in lean body mass in the subjects receiving 2.8 g protein/kg but not with a protein intake of 1.4 g/kg.

The amount of protein needed during heavy work may be related to the energy intake. Iyengar and Narasinga Rao (1979) found that 1 g protein/kg was adequate if the caloric intake equaled output, but a 20% reduction in caloric intake resulted in a negative nitrogen balance. They found an increase in urinary nitrogen output when the caloric intake was reduced. Although not measuring nitrogen balance, Rodahl, Horvath, Birkhead, and Issekutz (1962) found no decrease in physical work capacity when either the caloric intake was reduced by 50% and/or the protein intake was reduced from 70 to 4 g/day in a neutral environment. When the ambient temperature was lowered to 8° C, reductions in caloric intake and/or protein intake reduced physical work capacity.

Research Findings of Indefinite Effect

Although many of the recent studies suggest that low protein intake produces a negative nitrogen balance, most of the early studies did not find any difference in physical performance between low, normal, and high protein diets (Pitts, Consolazio, & Johnson, 1944; Darling, Johnson, Pitts, Consolazio, & Robinson, 1944). Darling et al. (1944) found no detrimental effect of a low protein diet (53 g/day) on endurance compared to diets containing a normal (95-113 g/day) or high (151-192 g/day) protein content. No significant changes in serum protein, erythrocyte count, or hemoglobin content occurred during the 2 months the subjects consumed the low protein diet while doing manual labor. Pitts et al. (1944) also failed to find significant differences in endurance between diets containing 76, 105, and 149 g protein/day. Durnin (1978) estimated the total protein intake needed by a 70 kg male exercising 4 hr/day to be 40 g/day based on the obligatory nitrogen losses. Increased muscle mass was estimated to require only an additional 6-7 g/day. The low protein intakes used by Pitts et al. and Darling et al. would have been more than adequate if Durnin's estimates are accurate.

Several studies have examined the effects of a protein-deficient diet during growth and training in rats. Rats fed diets containing 8% protein (deficient) during 12 weeks of treadmill training gained 32% less weight and had smaller hindlimb muscles than rats receiving 25% protein (normal) diets (Fuge, Crews, Pattengale, Holloszy, & Shank, 1968). However, the protein-deficient animals were able to run 62% longer than the normal protein group. This was in spite of the fact that the protein-deficient animals had lower levels of myoglobin, cytochrome c, and mitochondrial respiratory enzyme activity per gram of muscle compared to the rats with a normal protein intake. Fuge et al. suggested the low body weight of the protein-deficient animals was largely responsible for their improved endurance. Smaller muscle fibers with large surface-area-to-mass ratios may have also increased the diffusion of lactic acid out of the muscle fiber (Fuge et al., 1968).

Laritcheva et al. (1978) divided rats into three dietary groups: 6% protein (deficient), 18% protein (normal), and 30% protein (excess). Protein-deficient animals gained significantly less weight and could not swim as long as the normal-protein or protein-excess rats. Rats who received excess protein excreted 73% more nitrogen than the rats with a normal intake. The authors concluded excess protein was of little value in improving performance.

Several studies have focused on the use of protein supplements to augment the normal protein intake. Rasch and Pierson (1962) examined the effects of a 25-g protein supplement during 6 weeks of training on increases in strength and muscle hypertrophy. Significant increases in strength occurred in both protein supplement and placebo groups, but no significant change in arm girth or volume were found in either group using progressive resistance training. The protein supplement would have added 0.34 g/kg to the normal dietary protein intake which was not reported. In a subsequent study, Rasch, Hamby, and Burns (1969) used a protein supplement containing 0.69 g/kg during 4 weeks of physical training. No significant differences existed between the protein supplement and placebo groups on any of the fitness tests after 4 weeks of training. However, a significant decrease in erythrocyte count, hemoglobin concentration, and hematocrit was observed after 3 days of training in the protein supplement group. Neither study reported the dietary protein intake.

Summary

It is apparent from much of the most recent work that an increased excretion of nitrogen occurs during prolonged exercise and that this increased nitrogen excretion occurs primarily through sweating. Studies that have included sweat nitrogen losses have been almost unanimous in reporting negative nitrogen balance during training when the protein intake is 1.0 g/kg/day or below. However, it appears the body may adapt to a lower protein intake after a week of training if the caloric intake is adequate (Gontzea et al., 1975). It also appears that an increased protein intake may be more important during the early phase of training to support increases in muscle mass, myoglobin, and enzyme content, and erythrocyte formation than later during the training program. The optimal intake during this early training may be as low as 1.2 g protein/kg.

Normally, an increase in protein intake would be expected when the caloric intake increases during training. For example, a 70-kg athlete who increases the caloric intake from 3,000 to 4,000 kcal/day at the start of training would increase the protein intake from 90 to 120 g/day if 12% of the caloric intake came from protein. Protein intake relative to body weight would increase from 1.3 g/kg to 1.7 g/kg/day, which should be more than adequate in most cases.

The growing athlete has a greater need for protein relative to body weight than the adult. However, a diet that supplies 15% of the total calories as protein should meet the needs of most children training for sports.

B Complex Vitamins

Thirteen substances have been classified as vitamins. Four vitamins—A, D, E, and K—are fat soluble and are stored by the body. The remaining vitamins—those of the B complex and C—are water soluble and need to be replaced daily. The recommended dietary allowance (RDA) for adult males and females is listed in Table 1. Vitamins have a variety of different functions in the body. For the purpose of this discussion, vitamins with similar functions have been grouped together.

Vitamins belonging to the B complex group can be subdivided into two groups—those involved in the production of energy from carbohydrates and fats, and those involved in the formation of erythrocytes. Thiamine (B_1), riboflavin (B_2), niacin, and pantothenic acid all become coenzymes in the metabolic pathways for the conversion of pyruvic acid to acetyl CoA or in the electron transport system. Pyridoxine (B_6) is a coenzyme involved in protein metabolism. Folacin and cobalamin (B_{12}) are both involved in the synthesis of DNA.

Theoretical Benefits

The need for thiamine, riboflavin, and niacin should increase as energy expenditure increases. Thiamine is particularly important in carbohydrate metabolism because it becomes thiamine pyrophosphate, which is needed in the decarboxylation of pyruvate to acetyl CoA. It is also involved in the decarboxylation of alphaketo-

Table 1
Recommended Daily Dietary Allowances for Vitamins

Vitamin	Males		Females	
	19-22	23-50	19-22	23-50
Vitamin A (μg RE)[a]	1,000	1,000	800	800
Vitamin D (μg)[b]	7.5	5	7.5	5
Vitamin E (mg α TE)[c]	10	10	8	8
Vitamin C (mg)	60	60	60	60
Thiamine (mg)	1.5	1.4	1.1	1.0
Riboflavin (mg)	1.7	1.6	1.3	1.2
Niacin (mg)	18	16	14	13
Vitamin B_6 (mg)	2.2	2.2	2.0	2.0
Folacin (μg)	400	400	400	400
Vitamin B_{12} (μg)	3.0	3.0	3.0	3.0

Note: From the Food and Nutrition Board, National Academy of Sciences-National Research Council, revised 1979.

[a]1 μg RE = 1 μg retinol = 5 IU vitamin A

[b]1 μg cholecalciferol = 40 IU vitamin D

[c]1 mg α TE = 1 mg alpha tocopherol = 1 IU vitamin E

glutarate to succinate. Riboflavin is converted to the flavoprotein coenzymes, including FAD. Two coenzymes, NAD and NADP, are formed from niacin. Pantothenic acid becomes part of coenzyme A. Theoretically, when energy expenditure is large, a diet deficient in any one or all of these B vitamins could reduce performance. Because all four vitamins are water soluble, increased quantities could be excreted when sweat rates are high.

Pyridoxine becomes the coenzyme pyridoxal phosphate, which is involved in the transamination of amino acids. Theoretically, there could be a greater need for pyridoxine if the protein intake is increased above normal levels. Pyridoxal phosphate is also needed for the formation of phosphorylase A, necessary in the breakdown of glycogen, and the porphyrins, such as those found in hemoglobin. Pyridoxine deficiency could theoretically reduce the utilization of glycogen as an energy source. It could also result in less hemoglobin formation, which would reduce oxygen transport to the tissues. Both folacin and cobalamin are needed for erythrocyte maturation. Deficiency of either folacin or cobalamin can lead to megaloblastic anemia.

Research Findings of Increased Need

Interest in the effects of a deficiency of one or more B vitamins on performance reached a peak in the early 1940s. Many studies examined diets which were deficient in several B vitamins. Since many of the B complex vitamins occur in similar foods, it was often difficult to find a diet which was deficient in only one vitamin. To avoid this problem, supplements of the other B vitamins were used in several studies.

Archdeacon and Murlin (1944) examined the effect of a diet deficient in thiamine in two subjects for 4 weeks. Although endurance increased early during the deficient diet, possibly due to a training effect, it declined during the latter part of the deficiency. Supplementation of the diet with 10 mg thiamine or 10 mg pyridoxine resulted in increased endurance, but 10 mg riboflavin failed to further increase endurance. Sedentary subjects fed a diet deficient in thiamine and possibly also in niacin, pyridoxine, and pantothenic acid had lower scores on the Physical Fitness Index (PFI) after 3 to 4 weeks (Egana, Johnson, Bloomfield, Brouha, Meiklejohn, Whittenberger, Darling, Heath, Graybiel, & Consolazio, 1942). PFI scores increased in five subjects when brewers' yeast was given as a supplement. (Brewers' yeast is a rich source of thiamine, riboflavin, niacin, pantothenic acid, and pyridoxine.) However, there were no differences in oxygen debt or lactate removal following exercise.

Part of the increase in the PFI may have been due to training, because posttest scores on the control diet were greater than the predeficiency scores.

Johnson and associates (Johnson, Darling, Forbes, Brouha, Egana, & Graybiel, 1942) used a similar diet deficient in thiamine and probably in niacin, pyridoxine, and pantothenic acid for 1 week with men doing manual labor. Half of the group received a supplement containing 2 mg thiamine and the other half received a placebo. The PFI declined in both groups on the deficient diet, then increased when the diet was supplemented with 18 g of brewers' yeast. The results suggest that a deficiency in one of the other B complex vitamins may have affected endurance more than thiamine. Barborka, Foltz, and Ivy (1943) also studied trained subjects consuming a diet deficient in thiamine and riboflavin for 2 months followed by 3 weeks of yeast supplementation. Decreased work output on the bicycle ergometer, which promptly increased when the yeast supplement was used, occurred during the deficiency period. Berryman and associates (Berryman, Henderson, Wheeler, Cogswell, & Spinella, 1947) also used trained subjects to study the effects of a diet deficient in thiamine, riboflavin, niacin, and the other B complex vitamins. Subjects consumed the deficient diets for 15-18 weeks followed by 18-21 weeks of various vitamin supplements. Decreases in endurance occurred during the deficient diet phase, but the investigators observed little change in psychomotor performance. Thiamine was the first vitamin supplement added to the diet and had little effect on endurance. Addition of niacin and riboflavin resulted in improved performance.

Early and Carlson (1969) examined the effects of a multiple B vitamin supplement without first producing a deficiency state. Subjects ran for 40 minutes in a hot environment on alternate days. Fatigue was more common among the subjects receiving the placebo than the B complex vitamin supplement, which led the authors to suggest that one or more of the B vitamins, possibly thiamine and pantothenic acid, may be needed in greater amounts during training. Nijakowski (1966) reported a significant decrease in blood thiamine levels after 3 weeks of skiing training but no change in pantothenic acid or biotin levels. Skiing for 4 hours also lowered blood thiamine levels. Earlier work with rats indicated that thiamine levels decrease in the liver, kidneys, and blood but remain constant in muscle following 10 days of training (Bialecki & Nijakowski, 1964). One month of training produced significant decreases in pantothenic acid levels of skeletal and cardiac muscle, liver, kidney, and blood of rats (Bialecki & Nijakowski, 1967). Control groups were not included in any of the three studies, however.

Research Findings of Indefinite or Detrimental Effects

Although many studies have reported impaired performance during B complex vitamin deficiency, others have failed to find any reduction in performance. Keys and associates (Keys, Henschel, Mickelsen, & Brozek, 1943) found no reduction in performance when the thiamine intake was reduced to 0.23 mg/1,000 kcal for 12 weeks. Reducing the diet in riboflavin to 0.31 mg/1,000 kcal for 5 months also had no effect on performance (Keys, Henschel, Mickelsen, Brozek, & Crawford, 1944). Similar results were found when the diet was restricted to 0.16 mg thiamin, 0.15 mg riboflavin, and 1.8 mg niacin per 1,000 kcal (Keys, Henschel, Taylor, Mickelsen, & Brozek, 1944). Multiple vitamin supplements in addition to a normal dietary intake of thiamin, riboflavin, and ascorbic acid had no effect on endurance or recovery following exercise (Keys & Henschel, 1942).

Nicotinic acid (niacin) has attracted special attention because it is a potent vasodilator. Hilsendager and Karpovich (1964) found no increase in endurance or change in systolic blood pressure when 75 mg niacin was given 2 hours prior to exercise. Large doses of nicotinic acid inhibit mobilization of fatty acids and decrease the turnover rate of fat during exercise (Carlson, Havel, Ekelund, & Holmgren, 1963). Bergstrom and associates (Bergstrom, Hultman, Jorfeldt, Pernow, & Wahren, 1969) found significantly less muscle glycogen and higher blood lactate levels following 90 minutes of exercise when 1.6 g nicotinic acid was administered 2 hours before exercise. There was, however, no significant difference in the amount of work completed compared to a no-supplement condition. Pernow and Saltin (1971) found that when the leg muscles are first depleted of their glycogen stores, the administration of 1.2 g nicotinic acid 1 hour prior to exercise reduced the amount of work done. Elevated R values following nicotinic acid administration compared to no supplementation suggested that carbohydrates were the main source of energy used. The results suggest that megavitamin doses of niacin may inhibit rather than improve performance.

The less well known B complex vitamins have received much less research attention as ergogenic aids, although vitamin B_{12} (cobalamin) has been reported to be used in large quantities by some athletes (U.S. Senate, 1973). Supplementing the diet with 50 ug cobalamin/day for 7 weeks had no significant effect on performance of the Harvard Step Test or a half-mile run compared to a placebo group (Montoye, Spata, Pickney, & Barron, 1955). On the other hand, the quantities of vitamin B_{12} reportedly used by some athletes, up to 1,000 ug, are much larger than tested by Montoye et al. Lawrence and associates (Lawrence, Smith, Bower, & Riehl, 1975) supplemented the diet of swimmers with 17 mg pyridoxine and found no effect on performance compared to a placebo group.

Summary

Under conditions of prolonged deficiency of some of the B complex vitamins, deterioration in endurance has been observed. Supplementing a diet deficient in several B vitamins generally results in restoration of performance. However, if the diet contains adequate amounts of the B vitamins there appears to be little benefit from additional supplements. The effects of prolonged exercise bouts and endurance training on B complex vitamin levels need further research. Megavitamin doses of niacin inhibit mobilization of fatty acids during exercise and increase the rate of glycogen utilization.

Vitamin C

While the functions of the B vitamins are primarily to serve as co-enzymes, the functions of vitamin C are less well defined. Vitamin C (L-ascorbic acid) is involved in the formation of collagen, an important protein in many types of connective tissue, including ligaments and tendons. Ascorbic acid also plays a role in the absorption of iron. The organ with the largest concentration of ascorbic acid is the adrenal gland. Normal plasma ascorbic acid levels are 1 mg/100 ml with lower levels found during a deficiency. Low levels of leukocyte ascorbic acid are also a good indicator of deficiency (Vitale, 1976).

Theoretical Benefits

Vitamin C has been associated with the synthesis of the catecholamines (Howald, Segesser, & Korner, 1975) and with an increase in serum cortisol levels (Boddy, Hume, King, Wyers, & Rowan, 1974). Because both catecholamines and cortisol increase in response to stress, and since exercise is a form of physical stress, theoretically there could be a greater need for ascorbic acid during exercise. Boddy et al. (1974) reported an inverse relationship between the change in leukocyte ascorbic acid content and leukocyte count following 2 hours of soccer practice. The vitamin C content of the adrenal gland is reduced following exhaustive physical exercise (Van Huss, 1966).

Research Findings of Increased Need

Most of the studies which have found a beneficial effect from vitamin C supplementation on performance have used fairly large doses (0.5-1.0 g). Hoogerwerf and Hoitink (1963) found significant increases in plasma ascorbic acid content following supplementation of 1 g vitamin C for 5 days. Mechanical efficiency while riding a bicycle ergometer increased significantly only in the group receiving vitamin C. Spioch, Kobza, and Mazur (1966) also observed a significant improvement in mechanical efficiency after infusion of 0.5 g vitamin C 30 minutes prior to exercise. Significant decreases in recovery pulse rates were also observed following supplementation. Howald et al. (1975) used l g ascorbic acid/day for 14 days and an equal length of time with a placebo. Although no significant differences were noted in the total amount of work performed, pulse rates were lower at a given energy expenditure, blood glucose levels were lower, and plasma free fatty acid levels were higher after ascorbic acid supplementation. Higher levels of vanilmandelic acid, a product of catecholamine metabolism, were found in the urine after ascorbic acid was given than following the placebo. In both the Spioch et al. and Howald et al. studies, the subjects served as their own control, but the control or placebo trial always occurred first. Thus, the observed effects could have been due to a training effect.

Van Huss (1966) used four levels of vitamin C intake which were administered in a random order. Two of the drinks were orange juice with high and low levels of natural vitamin C, either 2.98 mg/kg weight or 15 mg total, respectively. The other two drinks were synthetic orange drink with or without synthetic vitamin C (2.98 mg/kg). Although no differences in performance and maximal oxygen intake were observed between trials, lower pulse rates during exercise and recovery were observed following the larger vitamin C intakes. Replication of the study with 2 mg vitamin C/kg produced the same results, but a second replication with 3 mg/kg did not (Van Huss, 1980).

Research Findings of Indefinite Effect

For every study that has reported a beneficial effect from supplementing vitamin C there appears to be at least one study that found no beneficial effects. Margaria, Aghemo, and Rovelli (1964) reported no significant change in maximal oxygen intake, time of performance, or blood lactate when subjects were given 250 mg vitamin C 90 minutes prior to exercise. Restricting the diet to 20-40 mg for 4 to 7 days and then a 500-mg supplement daily for an equal length of time had no significant effect on recovery heart rates, rectal temperature, sweat rate, or strength of subjects exposed to a hot environment (Henschel, Taylor, Brozek, Mickelsen, and Keys, 1944). The amount of vitamin C lost in the sweat was negligible even though the sweat loss ranged from 5 to 8 l/day in the hot environment.

Both Keren and Epstein (1980) and Gey, Cooper, and Bottenberg (1970) used 1,000 mg vitamin C per day. Keren and Epstein found no significant difference in maximal oxygen intake or anaerobic capacity following 21 days of training and supplementation compared to a placebo group. Gey et al. found no significant difference in the distance covered in the 12-minute-run test or frequency of injuries during 12 weeks of training between the vitamin C and placebo groups. No significant differences in oxygen intake or ventilation for three different work loads were found between groups receiving 12 g vitamin C for 5 days and a placebo (Bailey, Carron, Teece, & Wehner, 1970).

Staton (1952) examined the effects of vitamin C on muscle soreness using a supplement group who received 100 mg/day, a placebo group, and a control group. The vitamin C supplement group could do more sit-ups in the 24-hour posttest than the control group but were not significantly different from the placebo group.

Summary

While the results of the studies seem to be almost equally divided between favorable and no beneficial effect, most of the studies have simply used supplements without determining the dietary intake of vitamin C. Only Henschel et al. (1944) controlled the diet, although Hoogerwerf and Hoitink (1963) and Van Huss (1966) did determine that ascorbic acid levels of their subjects were normal prior to treatment. Because vitamin C is one of the most easily destroyed vitamins, a considerable variation in dietary intake could occur between subjects. Extreme variation within a group will tend to make small differences in performance nonsignificant. Future studies in this area should evaluate the dietary intake of the subjects if control of the diet is not possible.

Vitamin E

Four vitamins are included in the fat soluble group—vitamins A, D, E, and K. However, the only vitamin to receive much attention as a factor affecting exercise performance has been vitamin E.

Theoretical Benefits

The most active form of vitamin E is alpha tocopherol. Although vitamin E has several functions in lower animals, for example, antisterility and prevention of muscular dystrophy, its major function in humans appears to be as an antioxidant. It may prevent the unsaturated fatty acids from being oxidized and thus protect cell membranes. There is some evidence that vitamin E may protect the linings of the respiratory tract against air pollutants such as ozone (Dillard, Litov, Savin, Dumelin, & Tappel, 1978). Shephard (1980) has suggested that vitamin E may play a role in linking the electron transport system with oxidative phosphorylation. During vitamin E deficiency, less ATP is produced for each molecule of oxygen used. One of the theoretical reasons given for supplementing the diet with vitamin E is to reduce the amount of oxygen used during exercise.

Research Findings of Increased Need

Few studies have actually shown any beneficial effects on performance from supplementing the diet with vitamin E. Cureton and Pohndorf (1955) fed wheat germ oil capsules containing vitamin E to subjects in a conditioning program for 8 weeks while a matched group received placebos. Significantly greater improvements in endurance and several related tests including the brachial pulse wave and T-wave were found in the group receiving wheat germ oil than the placebo. However, Cureton (1972) has suggested that the improvements were not likely to be due to the vitamin E content, which was 21 mg/day, because the daily dietary intake usually exceeds 30 mg.

Shephard (1980) cites a study by Nagawa in which subjects were given 300 mg vitamin E or a placebo for 44 days. Lower blood lactate levels following a maximal ride on a bicycle ergometer were found at an altitude of 2,900 meters in the group that received vitamin E compared to the placebo group. Kobayashi (1974) reported increased maximal oxygen intake at 5,000 and 15,000 feet following 6 weeks of supplementation with 1,200 IU of alpha tocopherol.

Recently Dillard et al. (1978) found that pentane production increases during exercise. Since pentanes are released during peroxidation of unsaturated fatty acids, it suggests lipid peroxidation occurs during exercise. Supplementing the diet with 1,200 IU of alpha tocopherol for 2 weeks resulted in a significant reduction in pentane production during both rest and exercise. Supplementing with alpha tocopherol also increased the plasma vitamin E level from 1.0 to 2.4 mg/100 ml.

Research Findings of Indefinite or Detrimental Effects

Most of the recent studies that have examined the effects of supplementing the diet with 400-1,200 IU of vitamin E have reported no effect upon the performance of swimmers (Lawrence, Bower, Riehl, & Smith, 1975; Lawrence, Smith, Bower, & Riehl, 1975; Sharman, Down, & Sen, 1971; Shephard, Campbell, Pimm, Stuart, & Wright, 1974). Watt and associates (Watt, Romet, McFarlane, McGuey, Allen, & Goode, 1974) found no greater improvement in the maximal oxygen intake of ice hockey players receiving 1,200 IU of vitamin E compared to a placebo group.

Helgheim and associates (Helgheim, Hetland, Nilsson, Ingjer, & Stromme, 1979) examined the effects of supplementing the diet with 300 mg of vitamin E for 6 weeks on serum enzyme levels following exercise. Serum vitamin E increased from 1.3 to 2.0 mg/100 ml following supplementation. Vitamin E supplements appeared to have no significant effect on the increase in the serum enzymes creatine kinase, aspartate aminotransferase, and lactate dehydrogenase following exercise compared to the placebo group.

Summary

It would appear there is little improvement in performance to be gained from supplementing the diet with vitamin E in most situations. However, the results of Kobayashi (1974) and Dillard et al. (1978) suggest that vitamin E may play a more important role when environmental conditions are altered due to either a lower oxygen pressure (altitude) or the presence of air pollutants (especially ozone).

Iron

One of the most common nutritional deficiencies in the United States is iron deficiency. The RDA for iron is 10 mg/day for adult males and 18 mg/day for adolescent males and females and adult females. However, the average dietary intake by the female is 10-12 mg iron/day (White, 1968). One nationwide survey reported that 22% of the females 17-44 years with hemoglobin levels above 10 g/100 ml were iron deficient (Ten State Nutrition Survey, Note 1).

Theoretical Benefits

Iron has several important functions in the body. Most of the iron is found as part of the hemoglobin molecule, where it plays a major role in carrying oxygen from the lungs to the tissues. Theoretically, low iron levels will lead to low hemoglobin levels and reduce the oxygen-carrying capacity of the blood and thus limit maximal oxygen intake. Myoglobin and the cytochromes are also iron-containing proteins found in the tissues. It has recently been found that alpha glycerolphosphate oxidase is an iron-containing enzyme (Finch, 1976). A deficiency in iron could lead to lower levels in one or more of these proteins and inhibit aerobic metabolism at the tissue level.

Under normal conditions approximately 10% of the dietary iron is absorbed. However, when the iron stores are low, the amount of iron absorbed from the intestinal tract increases. Iron is excreted in the urine, feces, and sweat, and, in the female, through the menses. Males excrete approximately 1 mg iron/day while the average loss for females is 1.5 mg/day. Sweat contains approximately 0.4 mg iron/liter (Vellar, 1968). Since athletes may lose as much as 5-8 liters sweat/day during heavy training in hot environments, the amount of iron lost by the athlete could be considerably greater than that of the average person. Iron loss through the menses also varies considerably depending on the volume of flow (Beaton, Thein, Milne, & Veen, 1970; Hallberg, Hogdahl, Nilsson, & Rybo, 1966). The amount of iron stored by the body as ferritin and hemosiderin probably does not exceed 20 mg/kg (Finch, 1976). Low serum ferritin levels are an early indicator of low iron stores.

Research Findings of Increased Need

Several studies of the iron status of athletes have reported 22 to 25% of the female athletes to be low in iron (DeWijn, DeJongste, Mosterd, & Willebrand, 1971; Haymes, Harris, Beldon, Loomis, & Nicholas, 1972). While iron deficiency was found in only 10% of the male athletes (DeWijn et al., 1971), one recent study reported little iron stored in the bone marrow of distance runners (Ehn, Carlmark, & Hoglund, 1980). Ehn et al. calculated the iron loss to be 2 mg/day, but the runners were in iron balance due to their high iron intake.

Australian athletes who had low hemoglobin levels were reported to have performed less well in endurance events at the 1968 Olympic Games than those athletes with normal hemoglobin levels (Stewart, Steel, Toyne, & Stewart, 1972). Stewart et al. concluded the low hemoglobin levels were not due to low dietary iron intake. Low hemoglobin levels have been reported for both male and female athletes participating in endurance sports (Clement, Asmundson, & Medhurst, 1977); however, there has been speculation that this could be a hemodilution effect of plasma volume expansion. Dill and associates (Dill, Braithwaite, Adams, & Bernauer, 1974) believe the lower hemoglobin concentration may be beneficial in reducing resistance to blood flow. The studies that have examined blood volume in athletes are equivocal. Several studies have reported no significant difference between athletes and nonathletes in either blood volume or total hemoglobin (Cook, Gualtiere, & Galla, 1969; Glass, Edwards, DeGarreta, & Clark, 1969; Moore & Buskirk, 1974) whereas Brotherhood, Borzovic, and Pugh (1975) and Dill et al. (1974) reported athletes have 20 and 21% more blood volume, respectively, than nonathletes.

Significant reductions in the erythrocyte count have been observed during the early phase of training, which is usually followed by an increase back to normal levels (Puhl & Runyan, 1980; Yoshimura, 1970; Yoshimura et al., 1980). Kilbom (1971) found serum iron levels of sedentary females were significantly reduced following 6 weeks of training while the plasma volume remained relatively constant. Frederickson, Puhl, and Runyan (1980) found decreases in serum iron and percentage iron saturation in runners during 10 weeks of training. Ericsson (1970) reported an inverse relationship between improvement in physical work capacity and changes in the iron content of the bone marrow among subjects who were not receiving iron supplements. Because the myoglobin and cytochrome content of the muscle increase during training, the iron needed for their formation could be supplied by the destruction of erythrocytes, the plasma iron, or taken out of storage in the bone marrow (Yoshimura, 1966).

Iron deficiency anemia has been shown to lower maximal oxygen intake (Sproule, Mitchell, & Miller, 1960) and physical work capacity (Gardner, Edgerton, Senewiratne, Barnard, & Ohira, 1977), increase the heart rate at submaximal work loads (Davies, Chukweumeka, & Van Haaren, 1973; Gardner et al., 1977), increase the postexercise lactate levels (Gardner et al., 1977), and prolong the time needed for recovery from exercise (Anderson & Barkve, 1970). Experiments with iron-deficient rats whose hemoglobin levels had been restored by transfusion suggest that tissue iron deficiency reduces aerobic metabolism and endurance and results in elevated blood lactate levels (Finch, Gollnick, Hlastala, Miller, Dillmann, & Mackler, 1979). Iron supplementation increased performance to normal levels within 4 days in anemic rats (Edgerton, Bryant, Gillespie, & Gardner, 1972; Finch, Miller, Inamdar, Person, Seiler, & Mackler, 1976). Finch et al. (1976, 1979) suggested that restoration of alpha glycerolphosphate oxidase activity was responsible for the improvement in performance since myoglobin and cytochrome levels were still depressed. Anemic persons given iron supplements have lower heart rates at submaximal work loads compared to subjects given placebos (Gardner, Edgerton, Barnard, & Bernauer, 1975; Ohira, Edgerton, Gardner, Senewiratne, Barnard, & Simpson, 1979).

There is some evidence that iron supplements may be beneficial during training in subjects who are iron deficient but not anemic. Plowman and McSwegin (1980) reported a significant increase in hemoglobin and an almost significant increase in serum iron levels in female runners who received 234 mg of iron during training. The percentage of runners who were classified as iron deficient decreased from 37 to 9% in the iron supplement group. Serum ferritin and percentage iron saturation increased to normal when the diet of seven iron-deficient athletes was supplemented with 900 mg iron/day for 10-14 days (Nilson, Schoene, Robertson, Escourrou, & Smith, 1981). Maximal lactate levels were reduced following exercise, but no significant changes in maximal oxygen intake or performance time were observed following therapy.

Research Findings of Indefinite Effects

Although total hemoglobin has been found to be significantly related to maximal oxygen intake, both total hemoglobin and maximal oxygen intake increase with body size (Vellar & Hermansen, 1971). When subjects were subdivided into groups of similar body size and the same sex, Vellar and Hermansen found the relationship between hemoglobin and maximal oxygen intake was reduced. Runyan and Puhl (1980) also found no significant relationship between hemoglobin and distance running performance.

Little change in hemoglobin or serum iron levels was observed in a group of females undergoing a physical training program for 10 weeks (Wirth, Lohman, Avallone, Shire, & Boileau, 1978). Puhl and Runyan (1980b) found no significant change in serum iron and percentage iron saturation in female distance runners during a 10-week competitive season.

There is little evidence that supplementing the diet with iron when hemoglobin levels are normal improves performance. Vellar and Hermansen (1971) found little difference in maximal oxygen intake, hemoglobin concentration, or iron levels between groups receiving iron and a placebo. Several studies have reported no significant improvement in iron status or hemoglobin levels among athletes in training who received iron supplements compared to those receiving placebos (Cooter & Mowbray, 1978; Pate, Maguire, & Van Wyk, 1979; Weswig & Winkler, 1974).

Summary

Iron deficiency occurs more frequently among females than males, but the occurrence among athletes appears to be no more frequent than among the general population. There may be a redistribution of iron from erythrocytes to the tissues at the beginning of training with a restoration of hemoglobin occurring after several weeks of training. There is little doubt that iron deficiency anemia impairs aerobic endurance and that iron supplements are beneficial in restoring performance in anemic persons. However, iron supplements appear to have little effect, when hemoglobin levels are normal, on either hemoglobin levels or performance.

Reference Note

1. *Ten State Nutrition Survey 1968-1970: IV. Biochemical.* Department of Health, Education and Welfare Pubs. No. (HMS) 72-8132, 1972.

References

ANDERSEN, H.T., & Barkve, H. Iron deficiency and muscular work performance. *Scandinavian Journal of Clinical Laboratory Investigation,* 1970, **25**. (Supplement 114)

ARCHDEACON, J.W., & Murlin, J.R. The effect of thiamin depletion and restoration on muscular efficiency and endurance. *Journal of Nutrition,* 1944, **28**, 241-254.

BAILEY, D.A., Carron, A.V., Teece, R.G., & Wehner, H. Effect of vitamin C supplementation upon the physiological response to exercise in trained and untrained subjects. *International Journal of Vitamin Research,* 1970, **40**, 435-441.

BARBORKA, C.J., Foltz, E.E., & Ivy, A.C. Relationship between vitamin B complex intake and work output in trained subjects. *Journal of the American Medical Association,* 1943, **122**, 717-720.

BASS, D.E., Buskirk, E.R., Iampietro, P.F., & Mager, M. Comparison of blood volume during physical conditioning, heat acclimatization and sedentary living. *Journal of Applied Physiology,* 1958, **12**, 186-188.

BEATON, G.H., Thein, M., Milne, H., & Veen, M.J. Iron requirements of menstruating women. *American Journal of Clinical Nutrition,* 1970, **23**, 275-283.

BENTIVEGNA, A., Kelley, E.J., & Kalenak, A. Diet, fitness and athletic performance. *The Physician and Sportsmedicine,* 1979, **7**(10), 99-105.

BERGSTROM, J., Hultman, E., Jorfeldt, L., Pernow, B., & Wahren, J. Effect of nicotinic acid on physical working capacity and on metabolism of muscle. *Journal of Applied Physiology*, 1969, **26**, 170-176.

BERRYMAN, G.H., Henderson, C.R., Wheeler, N.C., Cogswell, R.C., & Spinella, J.R. Effects in young men consuming restricted quantities of B complex vitamins and proteins, and changes associated with supplementation. *American Journal of Physiology*, 1947, **148**, 618-647.

BIALECKI, M., & Nijakowski, F. Influence of physical effort on the level of thiamine in tissues and blood. *Acta Physiologica Polonica*, 1964, **15**, 192-197.

BIALECKI, M., & Nijakowski, F. Behavior of pantothenic acid in tissues and blood of white rats following short and prolonged physical strain. *Acta Physiologica Polonica*, 1967, **18**, 25-29.

BODDY, K., Hume, R., King, P.C., Weyers, E., & Rowan, T. Total body, plasma and erythrocyte potassium and leucocyte ascorbic acid in "ultra-fit" subjects. *Clinical Science and Molecular Medicine*, 1974, **46**, 449-456.

BROTHERHOOD, J., Brozovic, B., & Pugh, L.G.C. Haematological status of middle and long-distance runners. *Clinical Science and Molecular Medicine*, 1975, **48**, 139-145.

CARLSON, L.A., Havel, R.J., Ekelund, L.G., & Holmgren, A. Effect of nicotinic acid on the turnover rate and oxidation of the free fatty acids of plasma in man during exercise. *Metabolism Clinical and Experimental*, 1963, **12**, 837-845.

CELEJOWA, I., & Homa, M. Food intake, nitrogen and energy balance in Polish weight lifters during a training camp. *Nutrition and Metabolism*, 1970, **12**, 259-274.

CERNY, F. Protein metabolism during two hour ergometer exercise. In H. Howald & J.R. Poortmans (Eds.), *Metabolic adaptation to prolonged physical exercise*. Basel: Birkhauser Verlag, 1975.

CLEMENT, D.B., Asmundson, R.C., & Medhurst, C.W. Hemoglobin values: Comparative survey of the 1976 Canadian Olympic team. *Canadian Medical Association Journal*, 1977, **117**, 614-616.

CONSOLAZIO, C.F., Johnson, H.L., Nelson, R.A., Dramise, J.G., & Skala, J.H. Protein metabolism during intensive physical training in the young adult. *American Journal of Clinical Nutrition*, 1975, **28**, 29-35.

COOK, D.B., Gualtiere, W.S., & Galla, S.J. Body fluid volumes of college athletes and non-athletes. *Medicine and Science in Sports*, 1969, **1**, 217-220.

COOTER, G.R., & Mowbray, K. Effects of iron supplementation and activity on serum iron depletion and hemoglobin levels in female athletes. *Research Quarterly*, 1978, **49**, 114-118.

COTES, J.R., Dabbs, J.M., Elwood, P.C., Hall, A.M., McDonald, A., & Saunders, M.J. The response to submaximal exercise in adult females; Relation to hemoglobin concentration. *Journal of Physiology*, 1969, **203**, 79P.

CURETON, T.K. *The physiological effects of wheat germ oil on humans in exercise.* Springfield, IL: Charles C. Thomas, 1972.

CURETON, T.K., & Pohndorf, R.H. Influence of wheat germ oil as a dietary supplement in a program of conditioning exercises with middle-aged subjects. *Research Quarterly,* 1955, **26**, 391-407.

DARLING, R.C., Johnson, R.E., Pitts, G.C., Consolazio, C.F., & Robinson, P.F. Effects of variations in dietary protein on the physical well being of men doing manual work. *Journal of Nutrition,* 1944, **28**, 273-281.

DAVIES, C.T.M., Chukweumeka, A.C., & Van Haaren, J.P.M. Iron deficiency anemia: Its effect on maximum aerobic power and responses to exercise in African males aged 17-40 years. *Clinical Science,* 1973, **44**, 555-562.

DECOMBAZ, J., Reinhardt, P., Anantharaman, K., von Glutz, G., & Poortmans, J.R. Biochemical changes in a 100 km run: Free amino acids, urea, and creatinine. *European Journal of Applied Physiology,* 1979, **41**, 61-72.

DEWIJN, J.F., DeJongste, J.L., Mosterd, W., & Willebrand, D. Haemoglobin, packed cell volume, serum iron and iron binding capacity of selected athletes during training. *Journal of Sports Medicine,* 1971, **11**, 42-51.

DILL, D.B., Braithwaite, K., Adams, W.C., & Bernauer, E.M. Blood volume of middle-distance runners: Effect of 2300-m altitude and comparison with non-athletes. *Medicine and Science in Sports,* 1974, **6**, 1-7.

DILLARD, C.J., Litov, R.E., Savin, W.M., Dumelin, E.E., & Tappel, A.L. Effects of exercise, vitamin E, and ozone on pulmonary function and lipid peroxidation. *Journal of Applied Physiology: Respiratory, Environmental, Exercise Physiology,* 1978, **45**, 927-932.

DOHM, G.L., Puente, F.R., Smith, C.P., & Edge, A. Changes in tissue protein levels as a result of endurance exercise. *Life Sciences,* 1978, **23**, 845-850.

DURNIN, J.V.G.A. Protein requirements and physical activity. In J. Parizkova & V.A. Rogozkin (Eds.), *Nutrition, physical fitness, and health.* Baltimore: University Park Press, 1978.

EARLY, R.G., & Carlson, B.R. Water-soluble vitamin therapy in the delay of fatigue from physical activity in hot climatic conditions. *Internationale Zeitschrift für Angewandte Physiologie,* 1969, **27**, 43-50.

EDGERTON, V.R. Exercise and the growth and development of muscle tissue. In G.L. Rarick (Ed.), *Physical activity: Human growth and development.* New York: Academic Press, 1973.

EDGERTON, V.R., Bryant, S.L., Gillespie, C.A., & Gardner, G.W. Iron deficiency anemia and physical performance and activity of rats. *Journal of Nutrition,* 1972, **102**, 381-400.

EGANA, E., Johnson, R.E., Bloomfield, R., Brouha, L., Meiklejohn, A.P., Whittenberger, J., Darling, R.C., Heath, C., Graybiel, A., & Consolazio, F. The effects of a diet deficient in the vitamin B complex on sedentary man. *American Journal of Physiology,* 1942, **137**, 731-741.

EHN, L., Carlmark, B., & Hoglund, S. Iron status in athletes involved in intense physical activity. *Medicine and Science in Sports and Exercise*, 1980, **12**, 61-64.

ERICSSON, P. The effect of iron supplementation on the physical work capacity in the elderly. *Acta Medica Scandinavica*, 1970, **188**, 361-374.

FINCH, C.A. *Nutrition reviews' present knowledge in nutrition* (4th ed.). New York: The Nutrition Foundation, 1976.

FINCH, C.A., Gollnick, P.D., Hlastala, M.P., Miller, L.R., Dillmann, E., & Mackler, B. Lactic acidosis as a result of iron deficiency. *Journal of Clinical Investigation*, 1979, **64**, 129-137.

FINCH, C.A., Miller, L.R., Inamdar, A.R., Person, R., Seiler, K., & Mackler, B. Iron deficiency in the rat. *Journal of Clinical Investigation*, 1976, **58**, 447-453.

FREDERICKSON, C., Puhl, J., & Runyan, W. Iron status of high school women cross country runners. *Medicine and Science in Sports and Exercise*, 1980, **12**, 81.

FUGE, K.W., Crews, E.L., Pattengale, P.K., Holloszy, J.O., & Shank, R.E. Effects of protein deficiency on certain adaptive responses to exercise. *American Journal of Physiology*, 1968, **215**, 660-663.

GARDNER, G.W., Edgerton, V.R., Barnard, R.J., & Bernauer, E.M. Cardiorespiratory, hematological and physical performance responses of anemic subjects to iron treatment. *American Journal of Clinical Nutrition*, 1975, **28**, 982-988.

GARDNER, G.W., Edgerton, V.R., Senewiratne, B., Barnard, R.J., & Ohira, Y. Physical work capacity and metabolic stress in subjects with iron deficiency anemia. *American Journal of Clinical Nutrition*, 1977, **30**, 910-917.

GEY, G.O., Cooper, K.H., & Bottenberg, R.A. Effect of ascorbic acid on endurance performance and athletic injury. *Journal of the American Medical Association*, 1970, **211**, 105.

GLASS, H.J., Edwards, R.H.T., DeGarreta, A.C., & Clark, J.C. [11]CO red cell labeling for blood volume and total hemoglobin in athletes: Effect of training. *Journal of Applied Physiology*, 1969, **26**, 131-134.

GOLDBERG, A.L., Etlinger, J.D., Goldspink, D.F., & Jablecki, C. Mechanism of work-induced hypertrophy of skeletal muscle. *Medicine and Science in Sports*, 1975, **7**, 185-198.

GONTZEA, I., Sutzescu, R., & Dumitrache, S. The influence of muscular activity on nitrogen balance and on the need of man for proteins. *Nutrition Reports International*, 1974, **10**, 35-43.

GONTZEA, I., Sutzescu, R., & Dumitrache, S. The influence of adaptation to physical effort on nitrogen balance in man. *Nutrition Reports International*, 1975, **11**, 231-236.

GUTHRIE, H.A. *Introductory nutrition* (4th ed.). St. Louis: C.V. Mosby, 1979.

HALLBERG, L., Hogdahl, A.M., Nilsson, L., & Rybo, G. Menstrual blood loss and iron deficiency. *Acta Medica Scandinavica*, 1966, **180**, 639-650.

HAYMES, E.M., Harris, D.V., Beldon, M.D., Loomis, J.L., & Nicholas, W.C. *Abstracts of Research Papers 1972 AAHPER Convention*. Washington, DC: AAHPER, 1972.

HELGHEIM, I., Hetland, O., Nilsson, S., Ingjer, F., & Stromme, S.B. The effects of vitamin E on serum enzyme levels following heavy exercise. *European Journal of Applied Physiology*, 1979, **40**, 283-289.

HENSCHEL, A., Taylor, H.L., Brozek, J., Mickelsen, O., & Keys, A. Vitamin C and ability to work in hot environments. *American Journal of Tropical Medicine*, 1944, **24**, 259-265.

HILSENDAGER, D., & Karpovich, P.V. Ergogenic effect of glycine and niacin separately and in combination. *Research Quarterly*, 1964, **35**, 389-392.

HOOGERWERF, A., & Hoitink, A.W.J.H. The influence of vitamin C administration on the mechanical efficiency of the human organism. *Internationale Zeitschrift für Angewandte Physiologie*, 1963, **20**, 164-172.

HOWALD, H., Segesser, B., & Korner, W.F. Ascorbic acid and athletic performance. *Annals of the New York Academy of Sciences*, 1975, **258**, 458-463.

IYENGAR, A., & Narasinga Rao, B.S. Effect of varying energy and protein intake on nitrogen balance in adults engaged in heavy manual labour. *British Journal of Nutrition*, 1979, **41**, 19-25.

JOHNSON, R.E., Darling, R.C., Forbes, W.H., Brouha, L., Egana, E., & Graybiel, A. The effects of a diet deficient in part of the vitamin B complex upon men doing manual labor. *Journal of Nutrition*, 1942, **24**, 585-596.

KEREN, G., & Epstein, Y. The effect of high dosage vitamin C intake on aerobic and anaerobic capacity. *Journal of Sports Medicine*, 1980, **20**, 145-148.

KEYS, A., & Henschel, A.F. Vitamin supplementation of U.S. Army rations in relation to fatigue and the ability to do muscular work. *Journal of Nutrition*, 1942, **23**, 259-269.

KEYS, A., Henschel, A.F., Mickelsen, O., & Brozek, J.M. The performance of normal young men on controlled thiamine intakes. *Journal of Nutrition*, 1943, **26**, 399-415.

KEYS, A., Henschel, A.F., Mickelsen, O., Brozek, J., & Crawford, J.H. Physiological and biochemical function in normal young men on a diet restricted in riboflavin. *Journal of Nutrition*, 1944, **27**, 165-178.

KEYS, A., Henschel, A.F., Taylor, H.L., Mickelsen, O., & Brozek, J. Absence of rapid deterioration in men doing hard physical work on a restricted intake of vitamins of the B complex. *Journal of Nutrition*, 1944, **27**, 485-496.

KILBOM, A. Physical training with submaximal intensities in women. I. Reaction to exercise and orthostasis. *Scandinavian Journal of Clinical Laboratory Investigation*, 1971, **28**, 141-161.

KOBAYASHI, Y. *Effect of vitamin E on aerobic work performance in man during acute exposure to hypoxic hypoxia*. Unpublished doctoral dissertation, University of New Mexico, 1974.

LARITCHEVA, K.A., Yalovaya, N.I., Shubin, V.I., & Smirnov, P.V. Study of energy expenditure and protein needs of top weight lifters. In J. Parizkova & V.A. Rogozkin (Eds.), *Nutrition, Physical Fitness, and Health*. Baltimore: University Park Press, 1978.

LAWRENCE, J.D., Bower, R.C., Riehl, W.P., & Smith, J.L. Effects of α -tocopherol acetate on the swimming endurance of trained swimmers. *American Journal of Clinical Nutrition*, 1975, **28**, 205-208.

LAWRENCE, J.D., Smith J.L., Bower, R.C., & Riehl, W.P. The effect of α -tocopherol (vitamin E) and pyridoxine HC1 (vitamin B_6) on the swimming endurance of trained swimmers. *Journal of the American College Health Association*, 1975, **23**, 219-222.

LEMON, P.W.R., & Mullin, J.P. Effect of initial muscle glycogen levels on protein catabolism during exercise. *Journal of Applied Physiology: Respiratory, Environmental, Exercise Physiology*, 1980, **48**, 624-629.

LEMON, P.W.R., & Nagle, F.J. Effects of exercise on protein and amino acid metabolism. *Medicine and Science in Sports and Exercise*, 1981, **13**, 141-149.

LINDSAY, D.B. Amino acids as energy sources. *Proceedings of the Nutrition Society*, 1980, **39**, 53-59.

MARABLE, N.L., Hickson, J.F., Korslund, M.K., Herbert, W.G., Desjardins, R.F., & Thye, F.W. Urinary nitrogen excretion as influenced by a muscle-building exercise program and protein intake variation. *Nutrition Reports International*, 1979, **19**, 795-805.

MARGARIA, R., Aghemo, P., & Rovelli, E. The effect of some drugs on the maximal capacity of athletic performance in man. *Internationale Zeitschrift für Angewandte Physiologie*, 1964, **20**, 281-287.

MOLE, P., & Johnson, R. Disclosure by dietary modification of an exercise-induced protein catabolism in man. *Journal of Applied Physiology*, 1971, **31**, 185-190.

MONTOYE, H.J., Spata, P.J., Pickney, V., & Barron, L. Effects of vitamin B_{12} supplementation on physical fitness and growth of young boys. *Journal of Applied Physiology*, 1955, **7**, 589-592.

MOORE, R., & Buskirk, E.R. Exercise and body fluids. In W.R. Johnson & E.R. Buskirk (Eds.), *Science and medicine of exercise and sport* (2nd. ed.). New York: Harper & Row, 1974.

NIJAKOWSKI, F. Assays of some vitamins of the B complex group in human blood in relation to muscular effort. *Acta Physiologica Polonica*, 1966, **16**, 397-404.

NILSON, K., Schoene, R.B., Robertson, H.T., Escourrou, P., & Smith, N.J. The effect of iron repletion on exercise-induced lactate production in minimally iron-deficient subjects. *Medicine and Science in Sports and Exercise*, 1981, **13**, 92.

OHIRA, Y., Edgerton, V.R., Gardner, G.W., Senewiratne, B., Barnard, R.J., & Simpson, D.R. Work capacity, heart rate and blood lactate responses to iron treatment. *British Journal of Haematology*, 1979, **41**, 365-372.

OSCAI, L.B., Williams, B.T., & Hertig, B.A. Effects of exercise on blood volume. *Journal of Applied Physiology*, 1968, **24**, 622-624.

PATE, R.R., Maguire, M., & Van Wyk, J. Dietary iron supplementation in women athletes. *The Physician and Sportsmedicine*, 1979, **7**(9), 81-88.

PERNOW, B., & Saltin, B. Availability of substrates and capacity for prolonged heavy exercise in man. *Journal of Applied Physiology*, 1971, **31**, 416-422.

PITTS, G.C., Consolazio, F.C., & Johnson, R.E. Dietary protein and physical fitness in temperature and hot climates. *Journal of Nutrition*, 1944, **27**, 497-508.

PLOWMAN, S.A., & McSwegin, P.J. *Abstracts of Research Papers 1980 AAHPERD Convention*, Washington, DC: AAHPERD, 1980.

POORTMANS, J.R. Effects of long lasting physical exercise and training on protein metabolism. In H. Howald & J.R. Poortmans (Eds.), *Metabolic Adaptation to Prolonged Physical Exercise*. Basel: Birkhauser Verlag, 1975.

PUHL, J.L., & Runyan, W.S. Hematological variations during aerobic training of college women. *Research Quarterly for Exercise and Sport*. 1980, **51**, 533-541. (a)

PUHL, J.L., & Runyan, W.S. Hematology of women cross-country runners during training. *Medicine and Science in Sports and Exercise*, 1980, **12**, 108. (b)

RASCH, P.J., Hamby, J.W., & Burns, H.J. Protein dietary supplementation and physical performance. *Medicine and Science in Sports*, 1969, **1**, 195-199.

RASCH, P.J., & Pierson, W.R. Effect of a protein dietary supplement on muscular strength and hypertrophy. *American Journal of Clinical Nutrition*, 1962, **11**, 530-532.

REFSUM, H.E., Gjessing, L.R., & Stromme, S.B. Changes in plasma amino acid distribution and urine amino acids excretion during prolonged heavy exercise. *Scandianvian Journal of Clinical Laboratory Investigation*, 1979, **39**, 407-413.

REFSUM, H.E., & Stromme, S.B. Urea and creatinine production and excretion in urine during and after prolonged heavy exercise. *Scandinavian Journal of Clinical Laboratory Investigation*, 1974, **33**, 247-254.

RODAHL, K., Horvath, S.M., Birkhead, N.C., & Issekutz, B. Effects of dietary protein on physical work capacity during severe cold stress. *Journal of Applied Physiology*, 1962, **17**, 763-767.

RUNYAN, W.S., & Puhl, J. Relationships between selected blood indices and competitive performance in college women cross-country runners. *Journal of Sports Medicine*, 1980, **20**, 207-212.

SHARMAN, I.M., Down, M.G., & Sen, R.N. The effects of vitamin E and training on physiological function and athletic performance in adolescent swimmers. *British Journal of Nutrition*, 1971, **26**, 265-276.

SHEPHARD, R.J. Vitamin E and physical performance. In G.A. Stull (Ed.), *Encyclopedia of physical education, fitness, and sports. Training, environment, nutrition, and fitness*. Salt Lake City: Brighton, 1980.

SHEPHARD, R.J., Campbell, R., Pimm, P., Stuart, D., & Wright, G. Vitamin E, exercise and recovery from physical activity. *European Journal of Applied Physiology*, 1974, **33**, 119-126.

SHIRAKI, K., Yamada, T., & Yoshimura, H. Relation of protein nutrition to the reduction of red blood cells induced by physical training. *Japanese Journal of Physiology*, 1977, **27**, 413-421.

SPIOCH, F., Kobza, R., & Mazur, B. Influence of vitamin C upon certain functional changes and the coefficient of mechanical efficiency in humans during physical effort. *Acta Physiologica Polonica*, 1966, **17**, 204-215.

SPROULE, B.J., Mitchell, J.H., & Miller, W.F. Cardiopulmonary physiological responses to heavy exercise in patients with anemia. *Journal of Clinical Investigation*, 1960, **39**, 378-388.

STATON, W.M. The influence of ascorbic acid in minimizing post-exercise muscle soreness in young men. *Research Quarterly*, 1952, **23**, 356-360.

STEWART, G.A., Steel, J.E., Toyne, A.H., & Stewart, M.J. Observations on the haematology and the iron and protein intake of Australian Olympic athletes. *Medical Journal of Australia*, 1972, **2**, 1339-1343.

TORUN, B., Scrimshaw, N.S., & Young V.R. Effect of isometric exercises on body potassium and dietary protein requirements of young men. *American Journal of Clinical Nutrition*, 1977, **30**, 1983-1993.

UNITED States Senate. *Proper and improper use of drugs by athletes. Hearings before the subcommittee to investigate juvenile delinquency*, June 18 and July 12-13, 1973. Washington, US Government Printing Office, 1973.

VAN HUSS, W.D. What made the Russians run? *Nutrition Today*, 1966, **1**, 20-23.

VAN HUSS, W.D. Vitamin C. In G.A. Stull (Ed.), *Encyclopedia of physical education, fitness, and sports. Training, environment, nutrition, and fitness.* Salt Lake City: Brighton, 1980.

VELLAR, O.D. Studies on sweat losses of nutrients. I. Iron content of whole body sweat and its association with other sweat constituents, serum iron levels, hematological indices, body surface area, and sweat rate. *Scandinavian Journal of Clinical Laboratory Investigation*, 1968, **21**, 157-167.

VELLAR, O.D., & Hermansen, L. Physical performance and hematological parameters. *Acta Medica Scandinavica*, 1971. (Supplement 522)

VITALE, J.J. *Vitamins.* Kalamazoo: Upjohn, 1976.

WATT, T., Romet, T.T., McFarlane, I., McGuey, D., Allen, C., & Goode, R.C. Vitamin E and oxygen consumption. *Lancet*, 1974, **2**, 354-355.

WERBLOW, J.A., Fox, H.M., & Henneman, A. Nutritional knowledge, attitudes, and food patterns of women athletes. *Journal of the American Dietetic Association*, 1978, **73**, 242-245.

WESWIG, P.J., & Winkler, W. Iron supplementation and hematological data of competitive swimmers. *Journal of Sports Medicine*, 1974, **14**, 112-119.

WHITE, H.S. Iron nutriture of girls and women—a review. *Journal of the American Dietetic Association*, 1968, **53**, 563-569.

WIRTH, J.C., Lohman, T.G., Avallone, J.P., Shire, T., & Boileau, R.A. The effect of physical training on the serum iron levels of college-age women. *Medicine and Science in Sports*, 1978, **10**, 223-226.

YOSHIMURA, H. Adult protein requirements. *Federation Proceedings*, 1961, **20**, 103-110.

YOSHIMURA, H. Sports anemia. In K. Evang & K.L. Andersen (Eds.), *Physical activity in health and disease.* Baltimore: Williams & Wilkins, 1966.

YOSHIMURA, H. Anemia during physical training (sports anemia). *Nutrition Reviews*, 1970, **28**, 251-253.

YOSHIMURA, H., Inoue, T., Yamada, T., & Shiraki, K. Anemia during hard physical training (sports anemia) and its causal mechanism with special reference to protein nutrition. *World Review of Nutrition and Dietetics*, 1980, **35**, 1-86.

3

Water and Electrolytes

William G. Herbert

Consumption of water has long been regarded as important by industrial workers and soldiers who labor in warm environments. In such settings, water has been empirically effective in affording relief from thirst, allaying fatigue, and reducing the occurrence of heat exhaustion. Although less attention has been given to electrolyte replacement in these circumstances, salt tablets are generally provided near water supplies, and their use has been suggested when sweat losses are extensive. The opportunities for taking fluids and electrolytes during physical labor are very good in comparison to the conditions encountered in exercise and sports participation. In labor, the intensity of the effort is usually light to moderate, the activity is intermittent and often self-regulated, and the water and salt sources are close at hand.

In contrast, sports participation imposes constraints on drinking behavior. For example, in wrestling, boxing, and lightweight football, many athletes voluntarily deplete body water by rapid and extreme weight reductions over 2-4 days to qualify for competitive

William G. Herbert, Ph.D., F.A.C.S.M., is with the Human Performance Laboratory at Virginia Polytechnic Institute & State University in Blacksburg.

classifications in which they expect to gain a physical advantage over opponents who are thought to be smaller and weaker. These wrestlers may lose 4-7% of their body weight by such means as sweating in saunas, exercising in impermeable suits, withholding water and food, and taking diuretics and laxatives. Although weight reduction by artificial means is contrary to the spirit of the rules and has been criticized on the grounds that it may be potentially harmful to health (American Medical Association, 1967; Buskirk, 1978; National Research Council, Note 1), the practice is widespread and suggests a common belief that a normal (or even supernormal) performance can be expected despite a substantial depletion of body fluids. Under the current amateur rules, wrestlers are given 1-5 hours between the official weigh-in and competition in which they can drink and eat. With regard to these circumstances, what detrimental effects, if any, can be ascribed to the rapid loss of body fluids in such sports, and can water/electrolyte intake in the few hours that follow cause exercise functions and sports performance to be increased?

In endurance sports, such as distance road racing, competitive cycling, football, soccer, and basketball, profuse sweating during the activity can cause substantial losses of fluid that may lead to impaired function, premature fatigue, and reduced performance. These losses are particularly great when the environment is warm, but even on cool days it has been demonstrated that individuals who compete in marathon races may produce 3-5 liters of sweat during the event and show postrace weight deficits of more than -3% despite periodic drinking along the course (Cohen & Zimmerman, 1978; Pugh, Corbett, & Johnson, 1967). On hot, humid days, these losses have been associated with an increased risk of exertional hyperthermia (American College of Sports Medicine, 1975; England, Varsha, Tirinnanzi, Greenberg, Powell, & Slovis, 1980; Hanson, 1979). As indicated earlier, the circumstances of the contest often facilitate the development of these fluid deficits. Thus, distance races are conducted on warm, sunny days, which induce the greatest sweat losses, and the participant's desire to finish the course in the briefest time mitigates against adequate drinking at aid stations. Although controlled breaks and substitution allowances in sports like football and soccer perhaps provide reasonable opportunities for fluid replacement, a player's attention during a break is usually directed more to matters of the contest than to drinking. A number of questions may be posed about the efficacy of water and electrolytes which have implications for these sports. To what extent can water/electrolyte consumption before and during the contest influence exercise functions and performance? If benefits are scientifically verifiable, what should be the feeding schedule and composition of beverages taken in connection with these sports? Finally, for individuals who frequently incur large sweat losses as a result of training, are daily electrolyte losses sufficient to justify dietary supplementation so that exercise function and competitive performance can be optimized?

Through the 1970s there was a burgeoning participation in distance running and racing in the United States (Maron & Horvath, 1979). These fitness enthusiasts along with the competitive athletes in this country constitute a substantial and attractive economic market for manufacturers of equipment, clothing, and aids that are purported to enhance the activity experience or even increase performance, that is, ergogenic effects. In this arena, several commercially prepared glucose-electrolyte (GE) drinks are successfully marketed for sports and fitness activities with implicit or explicit promises of ergogenic effects. Each is advertised to give the consumer an ideal replacement formula for sweat losses, and the commercial brand names typically include word elements like "fit," "ade," or "erg," suggesting extraordinary benefits. This issue will be addressed within the limits of the questions posed in the foregoing paragraphs.

Prior to examining the research evidence, it is first necessary to develop a theoretical framework describing the importance of water and the principal electrolytes in the body known to be affected by sweating. This section includes a summary of the physiological effects of water and electrolytes under normal body fluid conditions. A review of the physiological and performance effects of water depletion (i.e., hypohydration) and sweat loss of electrolytes is also included in the section on theoretical considerations. The latter parts of this chapter contain a discussion of the research evidence on the efficacy of water and electrolyte administration under specific types of sports situations.

Theoretical Considerations

Physiological Importance of Water and Electrolytes

Water is the most plentiful substance in the constitution of the body, representing about 60% of weight in men and 50% in women (Pitts, 1968). Figure 1 shows the hypothetical composition; both solid and fluid components are illustrated. Solids compose about 25% of the body mass, and fat tissues represent a smaller fraction in nonobese individuals. About half the total body water is contained within the cells, providing form for the organelles and an essential reaction medium for a host of life-giving processes. Of the extracellular portion, the great majority is distributed in the interstitium. The remainder is contained in plasma ($\approx 4.6\%$ of body mass) and lymph (2%), and these volumes play vitally important roles in regulating body fluids at rest and in exercise, far beyond the small quantity they represent. The extracellular fluid provides the milieu for transport of respiratory gases, nutrients, byproducts of cellular metabolism, and metabolic heat. In addition, water serves several extracorporeal functions, including elimination of waste via urine, feces, and sweat and removal of excess heat in exercise through evaporation of sweat from skin surfaces. Above environmental temperatures of $17°$ C, vaporization of sweat is the principal avenue for heat dissipation in vigorous exercise (Mitchell, 1977).

Electrolytes are positively or negatively charged particles that are soluble in body fluids. The major cations are metallic monovalent or divalent species and include Na^+, K^+, Ca^{2+}, and Mg^{2+}, whereas the anions include both inorganic and organic particles, that is, Cl^-, HCO_3^-, HPO_4^{2-}, SO_4^{2-}, organic acids, and proteins. Table 1 presents these ions in summary. Within each body fluid compartment, a cation-anion balance exists to provide an electrically neutral environment. However, the various ion species are not equally distributed *within* or *between* the compartments. For instance, plasma and interstitial fluids have higher concentrations of Na^+, Cl^-, and HCO_3^-, whereas muscle water contains relatively higher concentrations of K^+, Mg^{2+}, HPO_4^{2-}, and protein anion. Although free Ca^{2+} is essentially absent in resting muscle, a small but functionally significant amount is available in a form bound to the sarcoplasmic reticulum (SR); this is released transiently on excitation of the muscle fiber, serving as the "trigger" mechanism that leads to actomyosin coupling and hence muscle contraction.

This ion distribution is most important for maintenance of fluid balance among the compartments. Because water can move freely across membranes, it distributes in a manner that tends to equalize the concentration of osmotically active particles in the compartments. The cell membrane exerts an important effect on the intra- and extracellular distribution of ions by virtue of the Na^+-K^+ pump (active transport) that accumulates K^+ intracellularly against a concentration gradient and extrudes Na^+. The ion, Mg^{2+}, seems necessary for normal function of this pump. Thus, the tendency for Na^+ to passively diffuse into cells and K^+ to diffuse out is opposed by the ion pump, and a resting transmembrane potential in excitable cells can be maintained at -88 mv (Cunningham, Carter,

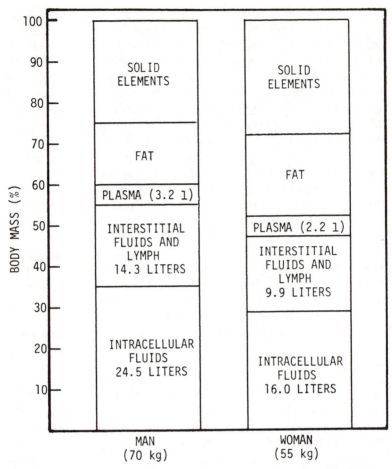

Figure 1—Hypothetical body composition and body water distribution. Modified with permission from Costill, D.L. In W.P. Morgan (Ed.), *Ergogenic Aids and Muscular Performance*. New York: Academic Press, 1972.

Rector, & Seldin, 1971). Normal bioelectric function in nerve and muscle depends on these Na^+-K^+ gradients, and factors that diminish the gradients or alter the exchangeable reserves for K^+, Na^+, or Mg^{2+} would apparently compromise ion pump function and disturb nerve transmission and muscle activation. It should also be mentioned that intracellular protein contributes uniquely to transcellular water distribution. With the relatively large molecular size of protein as contrasted to Na^+ and K^+, these particles cannot diffuse through the small pores of the cell membrane. According to the Gibbs-Donnan equilibrium concept, the presence of relatively more nondiffusible protein anions in muscle tends to cause some

Table 1
Electrolyte Composition and Total Osmolarity in Selected Body Fluid Compartments (mEq·liter^{-1})

	Plasma	Interstitial Fluid	Skeletal Muscle Cells[a]
Na$^+$	142	144	10
K$^+$	4	4	148
Ca^{2+}	2.5-5	2.5	0-2
Mg^{2+}	1.5-3	1.5	30-40
Cl$^-$	103	114	2
HCO$_3$$^-$	27	30	8
HPO$_4$$^{2-}$ H$_2$PO$_4$$^-$	2	2	140
SO$_4$$^{2-}$	1	1	0
Organic acid	5	5	0
Protein	16	0	55
Total osmolarity (mOsmol·liter^{-1})	304	304	302

[a]Sum of ionic contents of cells does not equal total cellular osmolarity because it is accepted that osmotic behavior for certain of these ions is reduced in the intracellular fluids (Pitts, 1968). From Pitts, R.F., *The Physiological Basis of Diuretic Therapy*. Springfield, IL: Charles C. Thomas, 1959. Reprinted with permission.

intracellular cation accumulation (and consequently diffusible anions); a slightly greater cellular influx of water follows. The conformation of the cells is apparently protected from this hydrostatic force by the important Na$^+$ extrusion function of the ion pump (Pitts, 1968). The biophysical factors that influence water and electrolyte distribution in body fluids are quite complex, but it should be appreciated that the resulting balances effected by these factors have implications for physiological processes essential to exercise performance. Interested readers are referred to Guyton (1968) and Pitts (1968) for detailed presentations.

Electrolytes are regulated in the fluid compartments within narrow limits. Stresses that induce moderate changes in the ionic contents can disturb functions. Marked derangements are life threatening. Because the major electrolytes under question in this chapter are the cations lost in sweat, discussion on effects of electrolyte disturbance will largely be limited to these species. The clinically normal range for the concentration of serum Na$^+$ is 136-145 mEq·liter^{-1} (Marcus, 1962). The level of Na$^+$ in serum may be considered as one component of the body's exchangeable sodium. About 70% of the body's total sodium is exchangeable, is distributed within the extracellular fluids, and is in equilibrium between body fluids and cancellous bone. The nonexchangeable amount is bound within long bones. Under normal circumstances, acute changes in serum [Na^+] (and consequent changes in osmolarity) stimulate renal effector mechanisms that exert precise feedback control of plasma volume and serum Na^+. It might be suspected that extensive sweat losses during prolonged exercise would reduce Na^+ in extracellular fluids (ECF), but the opposite, that is, a relative hypernatremia and hyperosmolarity accompanied by water depletion occurs because sweat is hypotonic to body fluids. The low ion concentrations for sweat are evident in Table 2. The rising extracellular Na^+ and osmolarity that occur with hypohydration stimulate an increased output of antidiuretic hormone (ADH) from the CNS and this leads to reduced urinary water excretion and sweat gland secretion. Thirst is stimulated in the ensuing period, but this sensation seems less than adequate to fully restore sweat losses and osmotic balance when individuals perform prolonged work in the heat. Thirst is more effective in restoring water balance, if adequate opportunity is given to take foods and fluids together in the hours following hypohydration (Adolph, 1947). If dietary sodium falls below or exceeds 2-10 g•day^{-1}, then aldosterone output is adjusted to effect renal conservation or dump Na^+ and normalize this ion in the ECF (Pitts, 1968). Some of the body's reservoir of exchangeable Na^+ can be mobilized to temporarily offset Na^+ deficits caused by sweat, urine, or fecal losses or reduced dietary intake. It should be recognized that Na^+ plays a key role in extracellular volume regulation through the ADH-aldosterone mediated renal mechanisms and through stimulation of drinking behavior. The mechanisms for regulating Na^+ seem most effective in preventing marked disturbances in body fluid levels of this ion.

Table 2
Losses of Electrolytes in Thermal Sweating by Man (mEq^2•liter^{-1})

Ion Losses			
Na^+	K^+	Cl^-	Mg^{2+}
40-45	3.9	39	3.3

From Costill, Cote, Miller, Miller, and Wynder (1975)

Nearly all the body K^+ stores are exchangeable and restricted intracellularly. The small extracellular quantity results in a normal plasma K^+ of $\simeq 4$ mEq·liter^{-1}. Plasma K^+ levels below 2-3 mEq· liter^{-1} are sometimes regarded as indirect evidence of cellular potassium depletion; in fact, if intracellular K^+ is depleted, then excitable tissues show depressed function, including cardiac rhythm abnormalities, muscular weakness, and impaired nerve conduction. However, the degree of K^+ depletion necessary to elicit these impairments is unlikely to occur except in disease states or as a result of excessive use of K^+-depleting agents. Moreover, hypokalemia alone cannot be accepted as evidence of a K^+ deficit because this ion is principally maintained intracellularly (Pitts, 1968). If plasma K^+ rises to 7-8 mEq·liter^{-1}, as in renal disease, abnormalities of cardiac electrical conduction and rhythm are often seen along with reduced chronotropic and inotropic responses (Guyton, 1968). Muscular weakness may also develop in hyperkalemia. As plasma K^+ rises above 8 mEq·liter^{-1}, resting membrane potentials apparently cannot be maintained by the ion pump, and ventricular fibrillation and cardiac arrest may occur (Pitts, 1968). Beyond its role in membrane excitation, K^+ is intimately involved in transport of glucose across cell membranes, storage of glycogen in muscle and liver, protein synthesis, and enzymatic regulation of many important cellular reactions (Lehninger, 1975). Also, the extracellular flux of K^+ from contracting muscle promotes local vasodilation, thereby helping to sustain blood flow in regions of increased metabolic demand. Small amounts of K^+ are routinely lost from the body via sweat and urine, but these losses are very low in relation to total body stores ($\simeq 3000$ mEq for a 70-kg man, [Pitts, 1968]). On the basis of the K^+ content for sweat shown in Table 2, it can be estimated that a 5-liter sweat loss during a marathon run would induce a K^+ loss of only $\simeq 20$ mEq, or $< 1.0\%$ of the total stores. Daily losses of K^+ through urine and feces normally does not exceed 100 mEq (Table 3). Episodes of diarrhea precipitate extensive and rapid K^+, Na^+, and water losses due to increased fluxes from the mucosa of the small intestine and a failure by the colon to reabsorb Na^+ and H_2O (Davenport, 1966). In vomiting, a substantial Cl^- loss occurs, and to counteract the resulting tendency for acidification of ECF, renal mechanisms are subsequently activated to reestablish pH by K^+ excretion. In the absence of such problems, the normal daily K^+ losses are offset by a modest dietary intake of 70-80 mEq (see Table 3). The estimated dietary requirement of $\cong 1$ g·day^{-1} seems easily satisfied by consumption of K^+-containing fruits and vegetables in the normal diet (Guyton, 1968). Thus, the body's K^+ stores are safeguarded by active transport mechanisms that concentrate this ion within cells. Substantial and sudden losses of K^+ in illness can compromise function, but the normal daily losses in the healthy individual seem small in relation to total body stores.

Ca^{2+} and Mg^{2+} have functional importance that belies the low content of these ions in body fluids. Their role in activation of muscle contraction is particularly important. Calcium is bound to the SR in resting muscle cells. On excitation, Ca^{2+} is released from the SR and rapidly flows to the troponin binding sites on actin filaments where, in the presence of adequate ATP, it activates the electromechanical bridges to initiate the muscle contraction. Conversely, the metabolically driven SR rebinding of Ca^{2+} initiates muscle relaxation (Lehninger, 1975). Mg^{2+} in resting muscle has a high affinity for ATP and thus forms $MgATP^{2-}$; this stabilizes the energy reservoirs by inhibiting ATP degradation by myosin. Upon Ca^{2+} release from the SR, this inhibition is released, and dissociation of Mg^{2+} from ATP allows splitting of the phosphate high energy bonds to fuel muscle contraction. Mg^{2+} also serves as a cofactor in many other intracellular enzyme reactions that involve ATP energy release (Lehninger, 1975). There is a Ca^{2+} reservoir in humans of about 1.2 kg. Probably 1% of this is exchangeable and the rest constitutes an unexchangeable matrix in bone (Guyton, 1968). The distribution and exchangeability of Mg^{2+} is similar to that for Ca^{2+}, but the total amount is much smaller (i.e., only ≈ 20 g [Guyton, 1968]) and the majority is located intracellularly (Pitts, 1968). In plasma, distortions in Ca^{2+} and Mg^{2+} found in disease states or induced in experimental animals cause abnormalities in excitable tissues. For example, low Ca^{2+} in extracellular fluids increases nerve membrane permeability and excitability. This can

Table 3
Typical Daily Exchanges of Sodium and
Potassium for Healthy Man in Caloric Balance

Ions	Intake ($mEq \cdot day^{-1}$)	Output ($mEq \cdot day^{-1}$) Urine	Feces
Na^+	100-120[a]	70-90[b]	5-10[a]
K^+	70-80[a]	30-70[b]	6-20[a]

[a]From Davenport (1966)
[b]From Guyton (1968)

lead to spontaneous activation of muscle and tetany. In contrast, hypercalcemia is characterized by weakened muscle contractions, accelerated electrical conductivity in the heart (shortened QT interval in the ECG complex) and vasoconstriction of vascular smooth muscle. An extracellular Mg^{2+} below the normal concentration of 2-3 in $Eq \cdot liter^{-1}$ is associated with increased nerve and muscle irritability, whereas high extracellular Mg^{2+} depresses nerve and muscle activity (Guyton, 1968).

Both Ca^{2+} and Mg^{2+} seem precisely regulated in the absence of disease states. Any tendency for plasma Ca^{2+} to decrease is opposed through actions of circulating parathyroid hormone. This hormone regulates Ca^{2+} and phosphate exchanges between plasma and bone as well as Ca^{2+} absorption and excretion rates in the intestine and kidney, respectively (Davenport, 1966). Regulation of extracellular Mg^{2+} is effected through adjustments in renal reabsorption similar to that for K^+ regulation (Guyton, 1968). Some Mg^{2+} is lost in sweat (see Table 2), but the amount is small compared to total body reserves (Costill, Cote, & Fink, 1976).

Any theoretical consideration of water and electrolytes in exercise must encompass a discussion of volume, osmolarity, and acid-base regulation of body fluids. These controls are complex and involve a number of neurohumoral mechanisms which mediate their effects mainly through renal clearance or conservation of water and electrolytes. Detailed presentations are available elsewhere (e.g., Guyton, 1968; Hultman & Sahlin, 1980; Pitts, 1968). With regard to regulation of water, a multifaceted process controls extracellular volume when changes in water or electrolyte content are imposed in the healthy individual. It has been postulated that this regulation depends on a highly sensitive glomerular filtration that is responsive to slight changes in arterial blood pressure brought about either by plasma volume contraction (hypohydration) or expansion (hyperhydration). Aldosterone and ADH circulate in the plasma and interact with this basic volume regulator to alter water exchange and reabsorption of certain ions at the kidney. Aldosterone increases renal tubule reabsorption of Na^+ and Cl^- and, as a result, also influences passive tubular reabsorption of water. ADH also acts at the renal tubule, specifically to increase water absorption. Low plasma Na^+, high plasma K^+, reduced cardiac output, and intense exercise all can stimulate increased aldosterone output from the adrenal cortex (Guyton, 1968). The process by which aldosterone secretion is regulated is complex and ultimately controlled by renin formation in the kidney; formation of renin is stimulated by reduced renal blood flow. In turn, the resulting elevated plasma renin leads to an increased angiotensin formation from a precursor in the blood. Elevated angiotensin then induces increased aldosterone secretion, giving rise to the aforementioned renal effects on water and ions. ADH output is believed to be mediated by increased osmolality of ECF, acting on osmoreceptors located at the base of the brain in the anterior hypothalamus. Stimulation of the osmoreceptors leads to increased ADH secretion by the neurohypophysis; a reduction in ECF osmolality has the opposite effect. The resultant change in circulating ADH will then alter tubular reabsorption of water to increase or decrease urinary output. Excretory and secretory mechanisms for water conservation and selective elimination of electrolytes represent only the output side of the regulatory process. Drinking of fluids (input) also represents an important but imprecise factor in these regulations. The drive to drink increases when the hypothalamic osmoreceptors are stimulated by a rising ECF osmolality. This stimulus, coupled with sensations of dryness in the mouth and absence of fullness in the stomach, seems to dictate the amount of drinking that is done to achieve satiation (Guyton, 1968).

Water and electrolytes play an integral part in acid-base regulation of body fluids. The extent to which these constituents can influence H^+ and buffering capacity has important implications for setting the limits of physical performance, because acidification of muscle in heavy exercise is believed to powerfully suppress Ca^{2+} activation of muscle contraction and the enzymatic reactions involved in energy metabolism (Hultman & Sahlin, 1980). There is also some evidence that accumulation of excess hydrogen ions in ECF may interfere with lactate elimination from exercising muscle, perhaps leading to premature feelings of fatigue and diminished performance (Hultman & Sahlin, 1980). How might alterations in body water or electrolyte balance affect acid-base status and buffering capacity in ways to impinge on physical performance?

First, it should be recognized that the H^+ in biological systems is so low under any metabolic circumstances that values are expressed as a negative log function, that is, pH. In healthy humans, the extracellular fluid is slightly more basic than water and regulated within narrow limits (pH = 7.35-7.45). Marked derangements in ECF beyond the limits of pH = 6.8-7.8 are inconsistent with survival (Marcus, 1962). Muscle cells maintain a slightly lower $pH \approx 7.0$ at rest and can become even more acidic in heavy exercise as a result of accumulating anaerobic metabolites. It has been reported that muscle pH may be as low as 6.4-6.6 immediately after exhaustive work (Hultman & Sahlin, 1980).

The mechanisms that regulate pH include a chemical acid-base buffer system, a respiratory compensation that controls pulmonary elimination of CO_2, and a renal compensation that involves excretion of either an acid or alkaline urine (Guyton, 1968). Each mechanism differs in its response time and buffering potency; the chemical system acts instantly but weakly and the renal mechanism acts much more slowly (24 hours) but potently (Guyton, 1968). The fundamental chemical buffer system in ECF comprises carbonic acid (H_2CO_3) and its salt, sodium bicarbonate ($NaHCO_3$). The bicarbonates of potassium, calcium, and magnesium also contribute to this chemical buffering system, as does the protein anion in extracellular fluid. Both red blood cells and muscle cells are intimately involved with this chemical buffer system in ECF and participate in ion shifts to protect the extracellular environment against changes in $[H^+]$. Guyton (1968) suggests that three-quarters of the body's chemical buffer capacity resides in the cellular contributions. In this regard, hemoglobin contained in red blood cells plays a key role in plasma buffering by temporarily binding H^+ and releasing HCO_3^- in association with transport of CO_2 from active tissues to the lung for elimination. Moreover, the sizable anion reserve in muscle (protein and phosphate) suggests a considerable potential for intracellular buffering of metabolically produced H^+. To simply illustrate buffering by the chemical system, consider that if H^+ increases as a result of accumulation of lactic acid in ECF, the tendency for acidification will be countered by a rightward shift in the reaction: $H^+ + lactate^- + Na^+ + HCO_3^- \longrightarrow Na \cdot lactate + H_2CO_3$. Because carbonic acid weakly dissociates, the increased amount formed from buffering lactic acid in the foregoing reaction will result in a minimal increase of H^+. If sufficient H^+ accumulate, pH is lowered despite the action of bicarbonate and the other chemical buffers. At this point, the H^+ increase stimulates increased respiration to promote further buffering via increased pulmonary elimination of CO_2. This compensation increases the ratio of HCO_3^- to CO_2 in ECF toward the normal value of 20:1 and, because H^+ varies inversely with this ratio (Henderson-Hasselbach equation), the pH will shift toward basic. The chemical-respiratory buffer systems only effect a temporary binding of hydrogen in some nonionizable form. When alteration in H^+ content of the body fluids must be achieved, renal mechanisms must be engaged. The kidney can make extensive corrections for acid-base disturbance by H^+ excretion and by adjusting urinary elimination of bicarbonate as needed. The kidney has the capacity to eliminate H^+ in association with phosphate buffers or via secretion with ammonia, but these avenues are not of principle concern here (Guyton, 1968; Pitts, 1968). It is important to note that the kidney can actively concentrate H^+ in urine to a level that is

$\simeq 1,000$-fold higher than levels in ECF; this capacity is evidenced by the high acidity of urine, that is, pH $\simeq 4.5$ (Guyton, 1968).

If water is removed (hypohydration) from a fluid system with a particular acid-base balance, a proportional increase in HCO_3^- occurs, but H^+ remains essentially unchanged because its concentration is infinitely small compared to HCO_3^-. Moreover, the H_2CO_3 and CO_2 in this fluid would not be affected by the water removal (Hultman & Sahlin, 1980) and therefore the HCO_3^-/CO_2 ratio would increase. This tendency toward anion excess would be buffered by removal of HCO_3^- via the reaction $HCO_3^- + H^+ \longrightarrow H_2CO_3$. The consequence would be binding of H^+ and a slight alkalinization of the fluid. Addition of water (hyperhydration) to the system would apparently have the opposite effect, that is, slight acidification. Unfortunately, it is difficult to speculate how the addition or removal of water may affect acid-base regulation of ECF, because the latter undergoes continuous ion exchange with the intracellular compartment.

The influence of altered concentration of various electrolytes on acid-base regulation is somewhat difficult to postulate. The most important of these may relate to the manner by which electrolyte balances across cell membranes influence fluxes of H^+, OH^-, or HCO_3^- (Hultman & Sahlin, 1980). For example, it is known that extrusion of H^+ from active muscle is linked to influx of Na^+ and exchanges of Cl^- and HCO_3^- (Aickin & Thomas, 1977). Moreover, the electronegativity of the internal cell environment attributable to the transmembrane potential actually favors retention of H^+ internally and release of HCO_3^- to ECF (Hultman & Sahlin, 1980). These exchanges appear to serve a buffer role that protects the ECF against further acidification. There may be some basis for speculating that the transcellular concentration and distribution of at least Na^+ or K^+ can influence pH regulation in exercise by altering the transmembrane potential and thereby the velocity of and metabolic cost for H^+ and HCO_3^- transport. To extend this example, any changes in intracellular-extracellular balances for Na^+ or K^+ that decreased the membrane potential might increase H^+ elimination and decrease HCO_3^- release, thus leading to more rapid acidification of ECF. In addition, alterations in Mg^{2+} and Ca^{2+} in either fluid compartment might alter acid-base regulation by affecting cell membrane permeability to Na^+ and K^+; such effects would change ion pump function and perhaps lead to altered membrane transport of H^+ and HCO_3^-, consequently changing the buffering capacity of ECF. Unfortunately, there is little direct evidence to elucidate the effects of altered electrolyte status on acid-base regulations under exercise conditions. Many of the important questions await future technological advances that will permit *in vivo* measurements in the active muscle.

Effects of Water and Electrolyte Losses on Physical Performance

A sweat loss equal to as little as 2% of weight causes noticeable impairments in circulatory and thermoregulatory functions that can compromise endurance performance (Adolph, Brown, Goddard, Gosselin, Kelly, Molnar, Rahn, Rothstein, Towbin, Wills, & Wold, 1947; Astrand & Saltin, 1964; Saltin, 1964b; Saltin & Stenberg, 1964). Uncertainty exists concerning the exact mechanism(s) responsible for this impairment, and the experimental evidence suggests at least three possibilities: (a) a reduced hemodynamic capacity to achieve maximal cardiac output and/or peripheral circulation (Claremont, Costill, Fink, & Van Handel, 1976); (b) an altered autonomic nervous control of sweat gland function and/or peripheral circulation (Ekblom, Greenleaf, & Hermansen, 1970; Harrison, Edwards, & Fennessy, 1978; Senay, 1979); and (c) an impairment in skeletal muscle fibers leading to a suppressed capacity for anaerobic exercise (Astrand & Saltin, 1964; Saltin, 1964a).

Regardless of which factor may predominate, reductions in circulating blood volume and cell water are fundamental to the problem. Investigations published prior to the mid-1970s yielded conflicting evidence regarding the quantitative reductions in plasma volume that occur with thermal- vs. exercise-induced sweat losses. Some early reports indicated that thermal sweating reduces plasma volume roughly 3-6% for each percentage reduction in body weight (Adolph et al., 1947; Kozlowski & Saltin, 1964; Saltin, 1964a). Other evidence from that period indicated that sweat losses in exercise were almost completely covered by the intracellular compartment (Astrand & Saltin, 1964; Saltin, 1964b; Saltin & Stenberg, 1964). Using improved hematological techniques, Costill and his colleagues (Costill, Branam, Eddy, & Fink, 1974; Costill & Fink, 1974; Costill & Saltin, 1974a; Dill & Costill, 1974) later resolved this conflict by demonstrating that both exercise and thermal hypohydration result in nearly equivalent fractional reductions in plasma volume (PV) that are approximately twice the percentage reduction in body weight. The same group (Claremont et al., 1976) also demonstrated that only one depletion method, that is, diuretic hypohydration, causes a greater fractional reduction. They showed that use of a diuretic will cause a sudden contraction of PV that is threefold greater than the percentage reduction in weight. This diuretic hypohydration also induced substantial losses of Na^+, K^+, and Cl^-, and, although plasma concentrations of these ions were not significantly lowered, the exchangeable reserves for these ions were definitely diminished. Costill et al. (1976) measured blood, urine, and muscle biopsy parameters after three different levels of hypohydration in an attempt to clarify the effects on body water and electrolytes. The heat-exercise hypohydration reduced plasma and muscle water by about -2.4% and -1.2%, respectively, for each percentage decline in body weight. However, since more than half the total body water is distributed in the cells, calculation was done to show that this small fractional cellular contribution actually represented 30-50% of the total water loss at each level of hypohydration. Concerning electrolyte changes in the Costill et al. study (1976), the concentrations of extracellular and intracellular Na^+, K^+, and Cl^- increased progressively in proportion to the level of hypohydration, but when corrections were calculated for water loss it was determined that neither ECF nor cellular contents for these ions were affected. In contrast, Mg^{2+} content of muscle declined by -12%. Computed values for resting membrane potential suggested that muscle tissue excitability was unaffected by hypohydration to -5.8% of body weight. Although the moderate reduction in cellular Mg^{2+} apparently had no functional importance, further investigation to clarify the mechanisms of its loss seems warranted. The investigators noted that K^+ was well maintained in both plasma and cells despite some K^+ losses in sweat. This led to speculation that interstitial fluid may give up some K^+ to plasma and cells in hypohydration to safeguard the latter two compartments against losses. Another attractive possibility is that during glycolysis release of K^+ and water sequestered with muscle glycogen (2-3 liters) may provide reserves to offset losses caused by sweating (Olsson & Saltin, 1971). Unfortunately, experimental evidence to indicate how release of this metabolic water affects body fluids is lacking (Ryan, Costill, Gisolfi, Murphy, & Westerman, 1975).

The effects of hypohydration on exercise and sports performance have been evaluated under a variety of circumstances. Water deficits to -5% of body weight caused by sweating seem to have little detrimental effect upon oxygen transport either at submaximal or maximal loads (Bock, Fox, & Bowers, 1967; Craig & Cummings, 1966; Greenleaf, Matter, Bosco, Douglas, & Averkin, 1966; Saltin, 1964a; Saltin & Stenberg, 1964) or the ability to attain maximal cardiac output or heart rate (Saltin, 1964a, 1964b; Saltin & Stenberg, 1964). However, after imposing a diuretic hypohydration to -3% of weight, Costill (Note 2) observed that $\dot{V}O_2$ max in treadmill running was reduced by $\approx 6\%$. Apparently, the fully upright posture of running coupled with the exaggerated hypovolemia of diuretic hypohydration compromised central blood volume, cardiac filling pressure, and stroke volume to a greater extent than for subjects who have been tested for $\dot{V}O_2$ max in cycling exercise following comparable water losses by sweating (Saltin, 1964a). Other investigations (Saltin, 1964a, 1964b) have consistently shown that sweat losses beyond -2 or -3% of weight are associated with sharp reductions in performance time and peak blood lactic acid levels at standardized heavy loads; these effects are most pronounced after exercise hypohydration.

Under environmental heat stress, impairments in endurance performance after hypohydration are more pronounced. This increased deterioration is largely related to the added thermoregulatory demands imposed on the circulation during exercise in the heat. Skin and active muscle compete for peripheral blood flow to serve both heat transfer and metabolic needs under circumstances in which the central blood volume is contracted by a high rate of sweating. The demands for increased muscle blood flow then take priority over any further increased skin flow needs for cooling. Thereafter, body heat storage rises (Johnson, 1977). As sweat losses increase, plasma Na^+ and osmolarity rise and sweat gland output declines due to effects mediated by the hypothalamus (Claremont et al., 1976; Greenleaf, Note 3). Despite a preferential blood flow to the active muscle, perfusion still becomes inadequate due to the hypohydration. Consequently, anaerobic metabolites accumulate at a faster rate than normal and premature exhaustion occurs (Saltin, Gagge, Bergh, & Stolwijk, 1972). Impaired circulation and thermoregulation become apparent during exercise in the heat when sweat losses exceed -2% of weight. Beyond this deficit, impairments progressively increase in proportion to sweat losses, and the resultant elevation in exercise core temperature toward maximum tolerable levels of 40-41° C is a precursor of early heat fatigue in an endurance sports event (Saltin et al., 1972). Episodes of hyperthermic injury or death, although infrequent, have occurred in football and distance running in individuals who evidence extreme hypohydration (Mathews, Fox, & Tanzi, 1969; Murphy, 1963; Ryan et al., 1975).

The effects of hypohydration relative to other parameters of physical and motor fitness have also been examined. A majority of studies (Ahlman & Karvonen, 1961; Greenleaf et al., 1966; Saltin, 1964a; Singer & Weiss, 1968; Tuttle, 1943) have indicated that static strength and reaction time are not affected by water deficits to -5% of weight. Torranin, Smith, and Byrd (1979) reported significant declines of $\approx 30\%$ in static and dynamic muscular endurance after a -4% weight loss with tasks involving the arms and legs. A number of investigations dealing specifically with the effects of rapid weight reduction in wrestlers have indicated that between 6 and 9% of body weight may be shed through several days of hypohydration-semistarvation without detrimentally affecting strength, coordination, or reaction time (Doscher, 1944; Singer & Weiss, 1968; Elfenbaum, 1966; Jennings, 1951). Houston, Marrin, Green, and Thomson (1981) recently reported that an -8% rapid weight reduction in collegiate wrestlers incurred over 4 days was associated with significant impairments in peak torque attainable in a slow isokinetic knee extension exercise. However, the significant reductions found in muscle glycogen (biopsy) underscore the contribution of caloric factors to rapid weight reduction in wrestlers. Since weight deficits in many of these studies with wrestlers involved variable contributions from caloric restriction, interpreting the specific effects of hypohydration in the subjects is difficult.

Since psychological factors can exert important influences on physical performance, it would be advantageous to consider effects of hypohydration in this domain. Unfortunately, there is a paucity of research on this issue. Morgan (1969) has conducted a relevant study investigating the effects of a -5% rapid weight reduction incurred over 5 days by wrestlers. Morgan found no evidence of any ergogenic or detrimental effects on state anxiety levels as a result of this weight reduction. Another study by Skinner, Hutsler, Bergsteinova, and Buskirk (1973) may have some pertinence to individuals who are exposed to higher-than-normal core temperatures during exercise as a result of sweat losses. Skinner et al. (1973) observed that subjects who performed progressive aerobic exercise in a hot environment rated their effort at a higher level than at the same loads under cool conditions. Although core temperatures were not measured by these investigators, an increased deep body temperature would be expected. Thus, there is some support for speculating that one consequence of an elevated deep body temperature in hypohydration might be a reduced ability to perceive accurately the effort level. There is a clear need for research in this area, particularly to determine whether salient measures of psychological state and perceptual competence are altered by hypohydration in ways that might influence physical performance.

There is a limited research literature dealing with the effects of electrolyte deficits on muscular performance in healthy subjects. As indicated at an earlier point in this discussion, sweat is hypotonic to body fluids so that even a substantial sweat loss will reduce exchangeable stores for Na^+, K^+, Cl^-, and Mg^{2+} by such slight amounts that detrimental effects on neuromuscular function would seem unlikely. Moreover, the function of these electrolytes is dependent upon their concentration in plasma and cells, and sweating has the immediate effect of elevating rather than reducing these concentrations. Knochel (1977) cautioned that extended periods of daily physical activity can deplete K^+ through combined losses via sweat, urine, and feces even when K^+ intake is normal. He further postulated that K^+ deficiencies arising under such conditions might induce syncope, impair regulation of regional blood flow in active muscle, suppress insulin release in response to a rising blood glucose, reduce muscle membrane potential, and impair glycogen synthesis in muscle. He further hypothesized that K^+ depletion is a principal precipitating cause of exertional heat stroke. Despite these potential detrimental effects, Lowensohn, Patterson, and Olsson (1978) were unable to induce any detrimental effects in exercise hemodynamic response or performance in dogs after 4 weeks of feeding K^+-free diets that reduced skeletal muscle K^+ by 25%.

Findings of Increased Performance

It might be expected that replenishing fluids lost in exercise or preloading fluids before exercise would be beneficial to performance. An important assumption that underpins this expectation is that drinking will be associated with rapid assimilation. Actually, the uptake of various beverages is dependent on several factors, including the solute and thermal properties of the drink, the volume and frequency of feeding, and the intensity of any ongoing exercise performed while drinking. The timing of intake before initiating exercise is also important if water or hypotonic beverages are drunk, because the tendency for dilution of plasma volume caused by water influx from intestinal absorption is known to trigger a large diuresis within 40-80 minutes (Pitts, 1968). Neophyte distance runners who have tried preloading with dilute fluids too far in advance of the race quickly learn the problems with such a strategy! Concerning these matters, Fordtran and Saltin (1967) investigated gastric emptying and intestinal absorption of fluids in subjects who performed 1 hour of aerobic exercise at 70% of $\dot{V}O_2$ max. In two different trials, either tap water or a GE solution (glucose, $13.3 \text{ g} \cdot \text{dl}^{-1}$) was drunk in 150-ml portions at 10-minute intervals during exercise until the total intake reached 750 ml. Identical trials were also performed at rest. At the end of each trial, aspiration of gut residue via a Levine tube allowed indirect determination of the fluid volume and solutes that were absorbed. The results in both the exercise and resting conditions showed that about 600 ml of water (75% of intake) were absorbed in contrast to only 250 ml of the GE drink. Comparative measurements of absorptive rates for solutes showed that glucose content was responsible for the marked delay in GE fluid uptake, and the electrolytes Na^+, K^+, Cl^- and HCO_3^- exerted no retarding effect. It was also concluded that exercise at intensities up to 70% $\dot{V}O_2$ max does not compromise absorption of water or any of the solutes tested, but Fordtran and Saltin (1967) apparently conducted this study in a normothermic environment, so their findings may not be applicable to heavy exercise in the heat, where increased peripheral circulatory demands might limit fluid absorption. Costill and Saltin (1974) extended the aforementioned research design in an effort to determine optimal circumstances for fluid replenishment during prolonged exercise. Again, postexercise gastric emptying gave indirect measures of uptake in several different trials; various fluid-exercise combinations were tested in each case. In each trial, the subjects drank a particular volume of test fluid, then ran for 15 minutes at a predetermined intensity before the gastric emptying procedure was performed. The findings of this study indicated that uptake was highest (60%) with ingestion of cool fluids in larger volumes (up to 600 ml) that contained only trace amounts of glucose (≤ 150 mM•liter^{-1}) and were taken at exercise intensities lower than 70% of $\dot{V}O_2$ max. More recently, Coyle, Costill, Fink, and Hoopes (1978) evaluated gastric emptying rates in 12 resting subjects for water and three different commercial GE beverages. Each test beverage was drunk cold (6° C) and rapidly in 400-ml volumes, and gastric residues were collected at 15 minutes postingestion. It was found that absorption of the GE beverage with a glucose content of 4.6 g•dl^{-1} was significantly retarded in comparison to the other beverages (glucose ≤ 2.5 g•dl^{-1}) and water, that is, only 39% absorbed as opposed to 55% for the other fluids. Differences in Na^+ (10-23 mEq•liter^{-1}), K^+ (2-10 mEq•liter^{-1}), and Cl^- (8-15 mEq•liter^{-1}) content of the fluids had no apparent effect on uptake.

These investigations collectively demonstrate that body fluid losses can be partially offset in exercise by frequent consumption of cold, lightly salted (0.1-0.2 g•dl^{-1}) fluids which contain little or no glucose. In distance runners producing sweat at rates up to 1.8 liters•hour^{-1}, assimilation of these fluids could cover almost half the losses. As to the utility of preloading with fluids before distance running (hyperhydration), body fluids might be expanded by ≈ 400 ml if a total of 800 ml were taken in two feedings spaced at 15-minute intervals; increasing the pre-exercise drinking period would surely be counterproductive due to the diuretic effect.

Replacement of Sweat Losses Prior to Physical Activity

The efficacy of rapid fluid intake following various combinations of
acute hypohydrative and metabolic weight loss have special relevance to wrestling, boxing, and lightweight football. A majority of
studies in this area have employed rehydration intervals of 1-5
hours, which correspond to the time constraints imposed on
wrestlers between the official weigh-in and their competitive
match. In this regard, Herbert and Ribisl (1972) investigated the effects of *ad libitum* food and fluid intake in collegiate wrestlers who
had undergone a -4.8% rapid weight reduction in the previous 2
days. Then, in the 5 hours between weight certification and the
varsity meet, these athletes replenished all but -2.2% of their
deficits. These weight changes are illustrated in Figure 2 along with
the associated changes in exercise performance. Physical working
capacity after rehydration showed significant restoration as compared to the weigh-in condition, but a significant impairment persisted relative to the normal condition. In a study of similar design,
Allen, Smith, and Miller (1977) provided high school wrestlers
with *ad lib* quantities of a commercial GE beverage (glucose, 4.6
mg•dl^{-1}) after they had reduced by -4.6% over 48 hours. Voluntary drinking within 1 hour of the weigh-in resulted in a partial
rehydration, but average body weight and estimated plasma
volume remained -2.6% and -1.6% below normal. Submaximal bicycle exercise tests (65% $\dot{V}O_2$ max) were administered before and
after weight reduction and after the rehydration period. Partial
rehydration was fully effective in relieving the observed impairments in exercise hemodynamic responses that were evident
after weight reduction.

The potential benefit to performance of fully replacing weight
deficits with fluids has also been evaluated. In different studies,
Palmer (1968), Ribisl and Herbert (1970), and Herbert and Ribisl
(1972) investigated the physiological and performance effects of
forced fluid intake after subjects had undergone rapid weight reduction. Palmer (1968) fed glucose-sweetened water and a salt supplement to physically trained men following a -5% weight loss induced by several hours of sweating in the sauna. During rehydration, fluid intake was distributed over 5 hours to exactly match
sweat losses. Examination of exercise data from a standard
10-minute treadmill run given during each body weight condition
showed that complete rehydration fully relieved exercise tachycardia and the reduction in oxygen pulse that had been observed in
hypohydration. The studies by Ribisl and Herbert (1970) and
Herbert and Ribisl (1972) involved forced weight reduction to

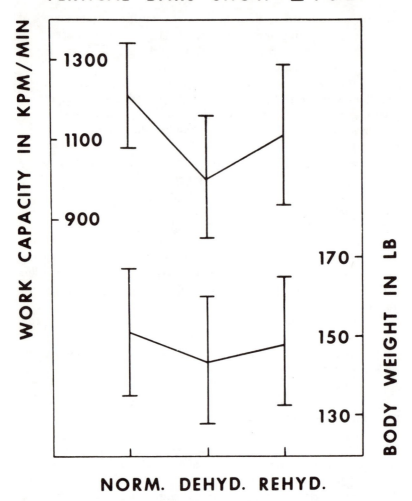

Figure 2—Changes in physical working capacity and body weight after rapid weight reduction (DEHYD) and rehydration in a group of college wrestlers.

specified deficits over 2-3 days in wrestlers by methods individually selected to reproduce the practices usually followed by these athletes under competitive conditions. After reduction, a cold commercial GE solution (glucose, 4.6 mg·dl⁻¹) was taken in volumes to completely replace the deficits within 5 hours. Moderate-intensity fixed-load exercise tests were performed in both of these studies at normal, reduced, and rehydrated body weight conditions. The significant impairment in cardiovascular endurance observed with weight deficits to -7% were completely relieved by fluid replacement. When these deficits exceeded -4%, however, subjects had great difficulty in consuming the required volumes and diuresis began well before drinking was completed. In another study, Costill and Sparks (1973) compared the rehydrative value of water and a cold GE solution (glucose, 10.6 $g \cdot dl^{-1}$) following a thermal hypohydration to -4% of weight. In different trials, fluids were taken in volumes to replace the deficits over 3 hours. By the third hour of rehydration with both water and the GE drink, heart rates during a submaximal treadmill test decreased to control levels. Despite this normalization of cardiovascular response, neither water nor the GE drink reduced serum osmolarity or restored plasma volume to normal, and a large diuresis resulted in retention of only 62% of the ingested fluid.

Replacement of Sweat Losses During Exercise

There has been considerable interest in assessing various strategies for fluid replacement during prolonged exercise. It has been well documented that frequent drinking to offset sweat losses under these exercise conditions will reduce thermoregulatory strain and prevent premature fatigue. In this regard, Strydom, Wyndham, van Graan, Holdsworth, and Morrison (1966) found that *ad lib* consumption of water by men performing a prolonged march with backpacks was associated with lower heart rates, lower rectal temperatures, and fewer dropouts than when only 1 liter was taken by a comparable group under the same march conditions. Despite the advantages observed in the *ad lib* drinkers, their thirst was apparently inadequate to prevent hypohydration because they incurred end-march deficits equal to -2.9% of weight. Wyndham and Strydom (1969) observed that runners who drank sufficiently during a marathon to keep their weight deficits below -3% had end-race rectal temperatures no higher than 38.9° C (102° F). Costill, Kammer, and Fisher (1970) evaluated the benefits of fluid replacement in elite marathoners during 2 hours of treadmill running at 70% $\dot{V}O_2$ max. In different trials, subjects were fed 2,000 ml of either cold water or a cold GE solution (glucose, 4.5 $g \cdot dl^{-1}$) in 120 ml-quantities every 5 minutes over the first 1.5 hours of running. A third run trial with no fluid was also performed. Exercise was accomplished in both fluid trials with lower rectal temperatures, but the heart rates and the pulmonary and metabolic responses were similar in the fluid and no-fluid trials. After 2 hours of running, serum Na^+ and Cl^- were slightly lower in the GE trial and thus nearer to normal values than in the water and no-fluid trials. Since sweat rates were similar in all three trials, the lower core temperatures observed in the fluid trials may have been partly due to conductive effects of the cold drinks rather than an enhanced capacity for heat dissipation.

The results of a recent unpublished case study in our laboratory (Herbert & Smith, Note 4) provide a reasonable illustration of the performance-enhancing effects of fluid replacement during distance racing in the heat. A physically active middle-aged male, $\dot{V}O_2$ max = 52 ml$\cdot$kg^{-1}min^{-1}, performed treadmill simulations of 10-mile (16-km) races on two separate days in a heated chamber. In the first trial, running velocity was frequently adjusted by the subject in an attempt to complete the distance in the briefest possible time; he varied the pace through speed adjustments that represented 65-95% of $\dot{V}O_2$ max. A cold, dilute GE beverage (glucose, 2.0 g$\cdot$dl^{-1}) was force-fed in 400-ml volumes at 20-minute intervals before and throughout the run. Drinking was accomplished without interrupting exercise by having the subject use a squeeze bottle with a tapered delivery tube. In the second trial, the exercise protocol was repeated exactly as before, but no fluids were given. The data for this experiment, shown in Figures 3 and 4, indicate that beyond 4 miles the benefits of fluid intake were manifested by substantially lower heart rate and core temperature responses as well as a lower skin temperature. As in the Costill et al. (1970) study, some of the physiological benefits during the fluid run trial may be attributable to conductive effects of the cold drink rather than rehydrative effects *per se*. In the no-fluid trial, the sweat rate was about 15% higher and premature exhaustion occurred at 6.8 miles coincident with exertional hyperthermia (T_c = 40.5° C) and a cumulative weight deficit of -2.8%. These results suggest that inexperienced distance runners who compete in the heat and drink adequately at aid stations may be able to maintain a somewhat faster race pace without increased risk of hyperthermic injury that would arise if no fluids were taken.

The value of complete rehydration in prolonged exercise as contrasted with *ad lib* drinking was clearly demonstrated by Pitts, Johnson, and Consolazio (1944). In their study, subjects who drank exactly enough water to replace sweat losses every 15 minutes during heat-walk trials had rectal temperatures well below that for trials in which they received water *ad lib* or no water. Dill, Yousef, and Nelson (1973) fed cold, lightly salted water (NaCl, 0.1 g$\cdot$dl^{-1}) at 7-minute intervals in exact volumes to replace sweat losses in subjects who performed prolonged desert walks. This strategy was effective in preventing hypohydrative impairments in circulation

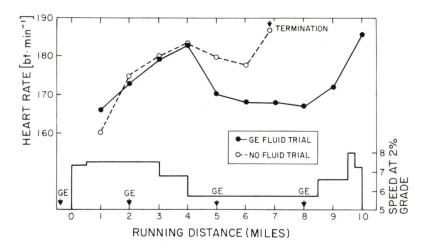

Figure 3—Heart rate responses for one male subject running a 10-mile race simulation in the heat (DBT = 35°C, RH = 50%) during trials with and without forced drinking. (Treadmill speed is shown in miles·hr^{-1}.)

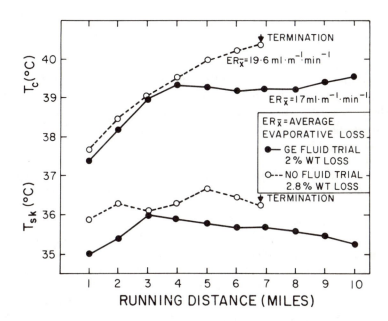

Figure 4—Rectal and skin temperature responses for male subject under conditions described in Figure 3. Weight deficits and estimated sweat losses (ER) are indicated for each trial.

and thermoregulation, and the findings led the investigators to suggest that inclusion of salt in the drink facilitated water balance better than would be expected with water alone. Their reasoning was that a slight elevation of plasma Na^+ would result with absorption of the salt water and this would trigger increased renal conservation of water via the ADH mechanism. A recent investigation by Bar-Or, Dotan, Inbar, Rotshtein, and Zonder (1980) involved a comparison of voluntary vs. forced cold water consumption in pre-adolescent boys during prolonged intermittent leg cycling in the heat (45% $\dot{V}O_2$ max). Forced drinking at frequent intervals was effective in replacing nearly all sweat losses and in keeping exercise heart rates and core temperatures at lower levels than in the water *ad lib* trials. In the *ad lib* condition, these boys voluntarily replaced only 72% of the volume taken in the forced drinking trial and this resulted in final weight deficits of 1-2%. Although the subjects did not perceive exercise in the *ad lib* condition to be more difficult, they evidenced elevations in heart rate and core temperature that suggested a poorer tolerance to heat-exercise hypohydration than indicated in the literature for mature lean males.

Hyperhydration Before Exercise

A number of investigations have been conducted to evaluate the efficacy of hyperhydration prior to prolonged exercise in anticipation of forestalling body fluid depletion from sweat losses. Blyth and Burt (1961) investigated the effects of a preliminary feeding of 1 liter of dilute saline followed by 1 liter of water in three normally hydrated subjects before they performed an exhaustive aerobic treadmill run in the heat (49° C). Running time to exhaustion was slightly greater in the hyperhydrated condition (17.5 vs. 16.9 minutes). Moroff and Bass (1965) also investigated the effects of hyperhydration preliminary to endurance exercise. Each of their subjects took 2 liters of tepid water in distributed feedings during the 50 minutes before a 90-minute treadmill walk in the heat. To prevent exercise hypohydration from confounding the interpretation of results, water was also given in 300-ml portions every 20 minutes during walking. In a second trial, the same subjects walked in the heat with sweat replacement but without preliminary hyperhydration. Exercise in the hyperhydrated condition was associated with significantly lower heart rates and core temperatures and significantly higher sweat rates. Greenleaf and Castle (1971) also assessed the effects of preliminary hyperhydration on temperature regulation during 70 minutes of cycling exercise at 50% $\dot{V}O_2$ max. On three different days, their subjects performed in

either euhydrated, hypohydrated (-5% of weight) or hyperhydrated conditions. Hyperhydration was achieved by drinking 2.7
liters of warm tap water within the hour before work. During work
in each body fluid condition, subjects were required to drink warm
saline (NaCl, 0.9 g•dl^{-1}) or, in the hyperhydrated condition, to
drink water at 10-minute intervals to offset sweat losses. The findings showed nonsignificant but systematic variations in core temperatures and sweat rates that suggested favorable effects of hyperhydration. Specifically, rectal temperatures were lowest and
sweat rates highest in hyperhydration. The use of saline rather
than water for offsetting sweat losses in two of the experimental
conditions (euhydration and hypohydration) could have resulted
in slight hypernatremia leading to ADH-mediated suppression of
sweat rate. Whether this possibility biased thermoregulatory
responses in favor of hyperhydration cannot be stated because
blood electrolytes were not reported.

What are the mechanisms whereby hemodynamic and thermoregulatory functions in prolonged exercise are improved with ingestion of various rehydrative drinks? This question is complex
and the pertinent published research is limited. Myhre and Robinson (1977) demonstrated that unacclimatized men exposed to hot,
dry conditions at rest were able to effectively attenuate reductions
in plasma volume by replacing sweat losses with dilute saline
(NaCl, 0.1 g•dl^{-1}). Their data indicated that plasma volumes were
reduced by only -2.9% with the saline drinking, as compared to a
passive thermal sweating condition in which PV was reduced by
-7.8% after a weight loss of -2.6%. Fortney, Nadel, Wenger, and
Bove (1981) induced a 7.9% hypervolemia by infusing isotonic
serum albumin into the vascular systems of physically fit men and
observed 1 hour later that the subjects were able to maintain a
higher circulating blood volume during moderate exercise in the
heat. Although this hypervolemia was not associated with either a
lowering of the thermal threshold of sweating onset or an increase
in sweating rate per unit rise in core temperature, the subjects' internal temperatures were consistently lower after the 20th minute
of exercise than in a comparable trial administered under normovolemic conditions.

Electrolyte Intake and Exercise Performance

In the sports community, ergogenic effects have been ascribed to
electrolytes when these are taken as constituents of athletic
beverages or as supplements. The sites of potential physiological
effect are manifold, and the intracellular measurements necessary

to directly study the impact of these substances on the critical cellular processes are not available. There is some supportive indirect evidence, however. Cade, Spooner, Schlein, Pickering, and Dean (1972) compared the effects of a GE solution (glucose, 3 $g \cdot dl^{-1}$), dilute saline (0.1 $g \cdot dl^{-1}$), or water during two different types of endurance exercise trials. Unfortunately, their report does not directly address some critical aspects of the research design; it is uncertain whether intake volumes were equated for the different drinks tested or whether subject participation in the trials was randomized. It is clear that the drinks were treated with lemon juice and citric acid in an effort to mask the composition from the subjects. When subjects received the GE beverage, they ran the equivalent of a 7-mile distance under normothermic conditions on the treadmill in 78.4 minutes. For two comparable trials in which either water or no fluids was administered, the 7-mile runs were performed significantly slower (83.2 and 82.1 minutes). With a second type of endurance exercise evaluated in the Cade et al. (1972) study, subjects walked at a fixed rate to exhaustion in a hot, dry condition, consuming the citrus-flavored GE beverage in one trial and either the citrus-flavored saline or no fluid in the other two trials. Subjects walked substantially farther (7 miles) with the GE beverage than in the saline or no-fluid trials (5.5 vs. 4.7 miles). Exercise with the GE beverage (Na^+ = 17 $mEq \cdot liter^{-1}$) resulted in the lowest elevations in core temperatures and serum Na^+ and the lowest sweat rates of all trials performed. The saline and water trials were of intermediate effectiveness as compared to the no-fluid trial. Unfortunately, the aforementioned research design uncertainties, the metabolic effects of the glucose in the GE beverage, and the failure to include a water trial in the heat-walk experiment confounds any interpretation regarding the specific effects of the electrolytes contained in the beverage.

Nielsen (1974) compared the effects of taking 1-liter solutions of either hypertonic (2 $g \cdot dl^{-1}$) NaCl or $CaCl_2$ several hours before a 1-hour cycling exercise at 40% $\dot{V}O_2$ max in a warm environment. Exercise in the $CaCl_2$ trial was associated with an earlier sweating onset, a higher sweat rate, and a lower core temperature. The NaCl solution had the opposite effect, that is, a delayed sweating onset, a lower sweat rate, and a higher core temperature. It was postulated that alteration in the thermoregulatory "set-point" occurred as a result of introducing these cations into the extracellular fluids; Ca^{2+} mediated a lowering effect on the set-point (lower T_c for sweat onset) and Na^+ caused an elevating effect. Greenleaf and Brock (1980) also compared the use of solutions containing Na^+ vs. Ca^{2+} on exercise responses. In several different experiments, their subjects hyperhydrated over 1 hour with 1-1.5 liters of either isotonic NaCl (0.9 $g \cdot dl^{-1}$), hypertonic NaCl (1.5 $g \cdot dl^{-1}$), or hypertonic saccharin-sweetened calcium glutonate (Ca-glutonate, 1.5 $g \cdot dl^{-1}$) prior to 1 hour of supine moderate-intensity cycling in either hot or cool conditions. The findings of this investigation indicated that the iso- or hypertonic NaCl drinks were effective in counteracting the transient plasma volume reductions that normally occur with exercise onset in both cool and hot environments. However, consumption of the hypertonic Ca^{2+} drink did not expand the pre-exercise plasma volume, and exercise was associated with a markedly lower circulating blood volume, particularly in the heat.

Harrison et al. (1978) reported that replacement of sweat losses *after a preliminary hypohydration* with isotonic saline vs. water or no fluid resulted in maintenance of plasma volume during moderate-intensity cycling in hot conditions. In the saline trials, reductions in PV never exceeded -3%, as compared to -9% and -13% with the water and no-fluid exercise-heat trials. Although vascular volume during exercise was well maintained by saline drinking in the Harrison et al. study (1978), higher core temperature, plasma osmolarity, and plasma K^+ levels were observed in this condition than in the water drinking trial. These latter findings are suggestive of impaired exercise thermoregulation associated with the saline. In another series of trials, these same investigators (Harrison et al., 1978) showed that exercise hemodynamics are benefited by sweat replacement with saline as long as the environment remains cool. In this regard, they reported that heart rates during moderate-to-heavy work in cool conditions were significantly lower after replacement of sweat losses with saline than with water. Francis and MacGregor (1978), concerned about the health implications of high urinary K^+ levels associated with prolonged work in the heat, replaced sweat losses during exercise with either water or a K^+-rich GE solution (glucose, 2.3 $g \cdot dl^{-1}$; K^+ and Na^+, 20 mEq $\cdot$ liter^{-1} each). The GE solution caused slight elevation of serum K^+ and significantly lowered both plasma renin activity and aldosterone. Urinary volumes were also significantly reduced during exercise and at 1 hour afterward with the K^+-rich drink. This beverage appeared to suppress aldosterone-mediated Na^+ and K^+ excretion and thereby conserved these ions. Thus, 42% of the Na^+ and 100% of the K^+ lost through sweat and urine during exercise were effectively replaced with the K^+-rich drink.

A number of investigators have attempted to determine possible ergogenic effects of such salt preparations as potassium-magnesium-aspartate, $NaHCO_3$, and NH_4Cl (e.g., Ahlborg,

Ekelund, & Nilsson, 1968). It has been hypothesized that such substances may exert physiological effects to somehow alter acid-base status and delay fatigue during exercise. In an excellent analysis of the factors affecting acid-base balance in exercise, Hultman and Sahlin (1980) have considered the conflicting state of this research literature and the adequacy of available experimental evidence that might indicate a biological basis for ergogenic effects by these substances. They have suggested that verification of bene-fit should be achieved through reconciling performance effects with *in vivo* evidence of a reduced intracellular accumulation of fatigue-producing substances (e.g., H^+), an enhanced physico-chemical state of substrates (e.g., glycogen sparing), or improve-ments in metabolic control (e.g., improved enzyme function). It seems that even well designed double-blind experimental trials showing increased performance are not a sufficient basis for con-firming ergogenic properties. A detailed discussion of these sup-plements is beyond the scope of this chapter.

Findings of Indefinite or Detrimental Effects

The evidence on uncertain or deleterious effects with water and electrolyte use will be considered within the same sports-specific framework just utilized for the review of studies showing benefi-cial effects.

Replacement of Sweat Losses Prior to Physical Performance

Bock et al. (1967) evaluated the effect of rehydration in wrestlers who had previously incurred rapid weight reductions (-3.8%) over a 40-hour period. During rehydration, one subgroup of wrestlers ate and drank as they normally would before a meet. A 5-minute near-maximal bicycle ergometer test administered before and after weight reduction and after rehydration provided a basis for assess-ing the performance effects of rehydration. Although $\dot{V}O_2$ max was unaffected in the final 2 minutes of the postrehydration test, core temperatures were significantly higher and sweat rates signifi-cantly lower than in the control condition. These results imply that thermoregulatory capacity was reduced by rehydration, but it was stated that this effect was probably related to specific dynamic ef-fects of digesting the food eaten during the rehydration period. Results of a study by Costill and Sparks (1973) indicate that com-plete restoration of normal cardiovascular endurance after a brief rehydration period is unlikely if the foregoing hypohydration has been extreme. Their subjects attempted to completely replace a -4% thermally induced weight loss by drinking either water or a GE beverage (glucose, 10.6 $g \cdot dl^{-1}$) at 15-minute intervals over 3 hours. Beyond the third hour of rehydration, a large diuresis occurred with ingestion of either fluid. At this point plasma volumes still remained -5 to -10% below normal. Diuresis was most pronounced with the water ingestion trial (380 $ml \cdot hr^{-1}$). Analysis of group data showed that restoration of the cardiovascular response to a submaximal treadmill run was achieved by the 2nd hour of rehydration with the GE drink and by the 3rd hour with water. However, many individuals still showed weight deficits greater than -1.5% after this 3rd hour of rehydration and showed elevations in exercise heart rates and core temperatures that would be predictive of an impaired endurance capacity. Torranin et al. (1979) imposed rapid rehydration on wrestlers after a thermal hypohydration to -4% of weight to determine the effects on isometric and isotonic muscular endurance. Despite restoration of body weight with a GE drink (glucose, 5 $g \cdot dl^{-1}$), estimated plasma volume remained -5% below normal, and both isometric and isotonic endurance were still depressed (as in hypohydration) by -13% and -21%, respectively. It was speculated that the relatively greater endurance impairment in the isotonic mode might have been related to reduced perfusion of active tissues attributable to the hypovolemia that persisted after rehydration. Houston et al. (1981) also evaluated the effects of rehydration in wrestlers. After reducing weight by -8% over 4 days in a carefully prescribed regimen of food and fluid restriction, their subjects ate and drank *ad lib* within 3 hours before postrehydration performance and muscle biopsy procedures were administered. A weight deficit of -3.4% was observed after rehydration, but the magnitude of the body water deficit at that point is uncertain because fluid intakes and indicators of water balance (e.g., hematocrit [Hct] and hemoglobin [Hb]) were not reported. Peak torque in an isokinetic knee extension task performed at a slow velocity was significantly lower than normal. There was also a trend for reductions in leg torque at high velocities, but these differences were not significant in relation to values for the pre-reduction test. These impairments correlated with muscle glycogen levels in vastus lateralis that were 50% below normal, but muscle phosphagen content was not reduced. No measures of intracellular or extracellular water or electrolyte status were made in this study. It is attractive to speculate that possible fluid or electrolyte imbalances still present after rehydration may have somehow impaired cellular function and contributed to the reduced isokinetic performance.

Replacement of Sweat Losses During Exercise

A search of the literature did not reveal any investigations that indicated equivocal or detrimental effects of taking water and electrolytes concomitantly with exercise. This is not surprising since any performance of sufficient intensity and duration to induce hypohydration from sweat losses will also depend heavily on the equanimity of thermoregulatory and circulatory functions. The benefits of frequent water or dilute saline consumption in such exercise and sports situations has been unequivocally demonstrated. Complaints are sometimes heard from highly competitive runners that drinking at aid stations during a race would slow their overall pace sufficiently that the physiological benefits of drinking would not be offsetting in all but the longest event (≥ 15 miles). No controlled studies that directly address this empirical criticism could be found.

Hyperhydration Before Exercise

The efficacy of hyperhydration in exercise and sport seems dependent upon the extent of sweat loss that occurs in the activity and whether thermoregulatory and circulatory factors may be limiting. Thus, for activities in which performance is limited primarily by anaerobic capacity, sweat losses and thermoregulatory involvement would be insignificant and hyperhydration would not be expected to augment performance. The findings of Blank (1959) offer some support for this expectation. Blank had trackmen sprint 220 yards in three different conditions in which water consumption was manipulated prior to the trials as follows: no water within 60 minutes; water *ad lib* (80-530 ml); and 500 ml of water taken in a single feeding 5 minutes before the sprint. Participation in the trials was randomized and subjects were not told the results of their performances until completion of the study. No systematic differences were found in sprint times between the euhydrated and hyperhydrated conditions. Blank expressed uncertainty about the subjects' adherence to the drinking restriction procedure in the no-water trial (unsupervised) and about their consistency in performing at maximal effort in each trial. This study illustrates the experimental difficulties which can confound the determination of ergogenic effects in human subjects. A study by Gisolfi and Copping (1974) also has pertinence to the issue of hyperhydration and performance. These investigators gave numerous trials of prolonged running (2 hours) in the heat at 75% $\dot{V}O_2$ max to six physically trained males. The potential of various techniques for minimizing thermal strain was examined, including the value of preliminary hyperhydration with warm or cold water. When the subjects drank 1 liter of water 30 minutes before exercise, the progressive rise in core temperature during the first 60 minutes of running was not suppressed nearly as well as when equal quantities of warm or cold water were fed in 200-ml volumes at 20-minute intervals during running. Even when hyperhydration was combined with drinking during the run, no supplemental thermoregulatory benefit was evidenced in core temperature changes during the final 60 minutes. Furthermore, sweat rates were well maintained in the subjects when water was fed during the run and sweating was not further increased when hyperhydration was combined with this rehydration procedure. Consequently, preliminary drinking prior to distance running in the heat may not forestall hyperthermic fatigue at maximal performance levels as well as if water is drunk during the race.

Electrolyte Intake and Exercise Performance

Electrolytes in rehydrative drinks such as Na^+, K^+, Ca^{2+}, Cl^-, and HPO_4^{2-} are readily absorbed through the intestine and do not retard gastric emptying of water as long as the concentrations are low, the beverage is not hyperosmolar to body fluids and the glucose content is minimal (Fordtran & Saltin, 1967; Hunt & Pathak, 1960). What evidence can be cited to show that electrolyte supplementation with rehydrative drinks or other sources may be ineffective or detrimental to performance?

Pitts et al. (1944) studied the response of heat-acclimatized men to prolonged periods of intermittent brisk treadmill walking in the heat. When subjects replaced their sweat losses with dilute saline (NaCl, 0.2 $g \cdot dl^{-1}$), heart rates, core temperatures, sweat rates, serum chloride levels, and performances were essentially the same as when equivalent amounts of water were drunk. On outdoor marches of 10 miles in summer heat, these investigators gave subjects three enteric coated salt tablets (9 g) within a 3-hour period before the trial began. In an alternative trial, no tablets were given to the same subjects before they marched. Water was taken periodically in both trials. No advantages were observed with salt administration relative to exercise core temperatures, pulse rates, or the subjects' reported feelings of exertional discomfort. Some subjects did complain of gastrointestinal discomfort in the salt trial, thus supporting the observation that intake of salt tablets or concentrated salt solutions (NaCl, ≥ 10 $g \cdot dl^{-1}$) may cause gastrointestinal distress (Pitts et al., 1944). Although the report of Taylor, Henschel, Mickelsen, and Keys (1944) gives evidence that men who do heavy daily work in the heat need a salt intake of $\simeq 15$ g•day^{-1}, it also indicates that cardiovascular function or work tolerance in the heat will not be further improved by raising the salt intake to 30 g•day^{-1}. Moreover, a daily salt intake above the 15-g level seemed to promote an increase in urinary water and electrolyte loss in the Taylor et al. study (1944).

Knochel (1977) has expressed concern over the possibility of runners developing K$^+$ deficiency during physical training in the heat. The occurrence of K$^+$ deficiency has been linked to increased susceptibility for heat stroke and rhabdomyolosis (muscle necrosis). Knochel (1977) hypothesized that the K$^+$ content of the normal diet ($\simeq 100$ mEq•day^{-1}) is inadequate to protect K$^+$ reserves against sweat and urinary K$^+$ losses during repeated days of work in the heat. However, in testing this hypothesis experimentally, he found that subjects showed only a slight K$^+$ deficit during the first 3 weeks of work in the heat and that total exchangeable K$^+$ was subsequently reestablished by the 25th day of the experiment. The measured daily K$^+$ losses in sweat and urine never seemed sufficient to account for the negative K$^+$ balance noticed early in the experiment. Knochel ascribed the restoration of exchangeable K$^+$ to a diminished K$^+$ loss in sweat and perhaps a reduced total sweating response attendant to cooler weather that prevailed toward the end of the experiment. Thus, the need to supplement the normal diet with K$^+$ preparations during heavy exercise in warm climates to assure normal body K$^+$ levels can be questioned. Knochel and Vertel (1967) and Knochel (1977) have cautioned against the use of chemical K$^+$ and Na$^+$ salts. They suggest that intake of K$^+$ salts might conceivably lead to sharp elevations in serum K$^+$ that might provoke myocardial toxicity. They further suggest that consumption of NaCl supplements by individuals in the transition of heat-exercise acclimatization might lead to increased urinary wasting of K$^+$ because increased aldosterone production during acclimatization is associated with greater renal absorption of Na$^+$ and loss of K$^+$. No published evidence could be found to confirm or dispute these possible effects for healthy subjects undergoing controlled feeding and exercise training in the heat.

A final study by Costill, Cote, Miller, Miller, and Wynder (1975), has relevance to the question of K$^+$-supplement value in physically active individuals. These investigators conducted a controlled metabolic study to determine the effects of consuming water vs. a GE beverage (glucose, 13 g•dl^{-1}; Na$^+$, 23 mEq•liter^{-1}; K$^+$, 9.3 mEq•liter^{-1}) in trained acclimatized men performing prolonged work in the heat on consecutive days. The duration of the exercise each day was sufficient to induce a sweat loss equivalent to -3% of weight. In the first 5-day test series, the GE drink was consumed with food *ad lib*, whereas in the second series an equivalent volume of water was given. In both series, water, electrolyte, and caloric intakes, as well as water and electrolyte losses in sweat and urine, were carefully measured. The dietary patterns resulted in total daily K^+ and Na^+ intakes of about 70 and 260 mEq in the water trial and 100 and 330 mEq in the GE trial. Plasma volumes were also measured on selected days. The treatments in both series were associated with reduced daily urinary volumes and reduced urinary losses of Na^+ and Cl^-. In the water feeding series, there was also a substantial renal conservation of Na^+. Weight, exercise sweat rate, plasma ions (Na^+, K^+, Cl^-), and plasma osmolality were all maintained at normal levels throughout both series. By the fifth day, plasma volume had expanded by 12% and 8%, respectively, in the water and GE series; this effect was attributed to elevated aldosterone activity stimulated by the daily exercise-heat hypohydration. Within 3 days after cessation of the daily heat-exercise bouts, PV returned to pretreatment levels in both series. The investigators concluded that unless sweat losses during periods of daily exercise exceed -3% of weight, supplementation of the normal diet with K^+ and Na^+ is not necessary to protect against electrolyte depletion. Furthermore, consumption of the additional electrolytes (GE trial) did not result in elevations of serum Na^+ or K^+. Neither did these added electrolytes result in an increased sweating response during exercise or in an enhanced plasma volume expansion arising from the daily heat-exercise stimulus.

Summary and Conclusions

As the most abundant constituent in the body, water is intimately involved in many physiological processes. Among their many functions, electrolytes play a crucial role in regulation of body water distribution between various fluid compartments. Sodium in particular has a major influence on fluid regulation, and changes in its extracellular concentration will stimulate adjustments in thermoregulation, water and ion excretion, and drinking behavior. In addition, electrolytes are essential to muscle and nerve excitation, electromechanical coupling in muscle contraction, and enzymatic control of cellular reactions. There are exquisite neurohumoral mechanisms that regulate the balances for water and ions in the body, and only in certain disease states is it likely that marked disturbances that might impair function or threaten life can occur. It should also be recognized that sudden water and electrolyte disturbances can exert subtle effects on acid-base regulation, but current research does not clearly indicate how these disturbances may influence the biochemical processes in the exercising muscle. It is certain, however, that sudden losses of water induced by extensive sweating or losses of water and ions associated with laxative or diuretic administration must be compensated for by the body's chemical, respiratory, and renal acid-base buffer mechanisms if pH is to remain in normal limits. In view of the precise controls for water, electrolyte, and acid-base balances in healthy individuals, some skepticism seems justified regarding the expectation that water and/or electrolyte supplementation can actually potentiate a normal exercise performance. In contrast, it seems likely that functional integrity in exercise could be compromised if normal water and ion balance are not maintained.

The evidence is unequivocal that depletion of body water beyond -2% of weight will cause significant impairments in thermal and circulatory regulations during exercise. These effects can lead to decrements in endurance performance that are proportional to the degree of hypohydration and are especially pronounced when sweat losses have been induced by exercise and the activity environment is hot. The capacity to sustain exercise at near-maximal loads is sharply reduced when sweat losses exceed -5% of weight; blood lactic acid accumulation is substantially reduced under these conditions, suggesting a decrement in anaerobic functions. Although maximal oxygen uptake and cardiac output can still be attained after a -5% weight loss caused by sweating, even these functions are impaired if the loss is diuretically induced. Muscular endurance and some muscular power measures deteriorate after a -5% hypohydration, but strength and reaction time are not impaired. To date, there is no published evidence to indicate whether hypohydration interferes with effort perception in ways that might degrade performance. The mechanisms of functional and performance deterioration in hypohydration have not been fully elucidated, but contraction of the vascular volume and consequent impairments in central hemodynamic and peripheral perfusion are basic to the problem. Since the content of electrolytes in sweat is very low in comparison to body fluids, sweating results in an increased concentration of electrolytes in extracellular fluids, and it is actually a hypernatremia (and hyperosmolarity) that increasingly impairs exercise thermoregulation as hypohydration progresses. How electrolyte losses in sweat affect cellular electrolytes and biochemistry *in vivo* remains largely unknown.

The efficacy of water and electrolyte intake is dependent upon a host of factors, including the characteristics of the rehydrative fluid, the feeding schedule, the performer's state of hydration, the type of exercise to be performed, and the extent of thermal stress imposed by the environment. The present research evidence related to beverage consumption indicates that optimal uptake is achieved if either water or hypotonic saline is drunk in volumes of ~400 ml every 15-20 minutes during exercise. If individuals drink while exercising under normothermic conditions, fluid uptake is not retarded until intensities exceed 70% $\dot{V}O_2$ max; whether performing heavy exercise in the heat retards this uptake is uncertain. Up to 60% of the volume ingested by these feedings may be absorbed, resulting in replenishment of almost half the sweat losses incurred in an ongoing exercise. If hypotonic fluids are taken earlier than 20 minutes before the exercise is begun, a significant diuresis will occur coincident with the start of the event.

When individuals try to rehydrate within a few hours to relieve pre-existing body water deficits greater than -2 to -3% of weight, full restoration cannot be achieved. Attempts at replacing deficits beyond this level will be associated with a substantial diuresis and even after 3 hours of drinking, the plasma volume may still be significantly lower than normal. Furthermore, if forced drinking is not done to fully replace even relatively small deficits (i.e., -2%), there is likely to be some persistence of thermoregulatory and hemodynamic impairments in exercise. Unfortunately, the research literature related to performance effects of fluid administration after preliminary hypohydration is so varied with regard to weight reduction regimes and the composition of the rehydrative beverages that it is most difficult to make comprehensive interpretations.

The literature relating to fluid replacement during exercise is somewhat more uniform with regard to methodology. There is good agreement that fluid replacement is most effective when individuals attempt to fully replace their sweat losses. Without forced drinking, deficits greater than -3% are likely to develop and lead to reductions in maximal endurance capacity and an increased risk of heat injury. Hyperhydration prior to prolonged exercise appears to offer only limited advantage; this procedure does not offset losses, promote sweating, or reduce body heat storage as well as an equivalent rehydration during exercise.

Ergogenic outcomes that may be attributed specifically to administration of electrolytes are most difficult to verify physiologically, since correlated evidence of enhanced muscle cell biochemistry cannot be experimentally demonstrated with currently available research techniques. Until such evidence can be obtained, the effect of electrolyte supplementation must be tentatively interpreted from research in which experimentally observed changes in performance are systematically associated with alterations in electrolyte or acid-base balance of extracellular fluids. In this regard, it has been demonstrated that hypotonic NaCl drinks maintain plasma volume and hemodynamic function in exercise more effectively than water alone. In contrast, hypertonic saline has been shown to be associated with some impairment in thermoregulatory function. In addition, ingestion of hypertonic saline or more than 2-3 salt tablets with water (NaCl, ≥ 10 g$\cdot$dl^{-1}) may cause gastric distress. Furthermore, high daily intake of salt during extended periods of heavy training in the heat may promote sufficient urinary K^+ losses to jeopardize the stores of this important ion. Interestingly, a few recent studies have demonstrated that inclusion of Ca^{2+} in rehydrative drinks results in effects that are nearly opposite to those of Na^+, that is, a relative hypovolemia and lower core temperature in exercise. With regard to K^+, there is currently no substantial evidence to support the use of supplements or K^+-rich beverages, even for individuals who perform prolonged exercise in the heat on repeated days. Under such conditions, daily K^+ losses remain low and should easily be offset by slightly increasing the natural K^+-containing foods in the diet. Moreover, ingestion of K^+ in chemical forms has been discouraged, because these might possibly cause sharp elevations in plasma K^+ and a risk of cardiac toxicity.

Reference Notes

1. National Research Council Committee on Nutritional Misinformation, National Academy of Sciences. *Water deprivation and performance of athletes.* A statement of the Food and Nutrition Board, Division of Biological Sciences, Assembly of Life Sciences, National Research Council, 1972.
2. Costill, D.L. *Electrolytes and water.* Unpublished manuscript presented in Symposium on Regulatory Mechanisms in Metabolism During Exercise. Third International Symposium on Biochemistry of Exercise, Quebec City, Quebec, Canada, 1976.
3. Greenleaf, J.E. *Blood electrolytes and exercise in relation to temperature regulation.* Unpublished manuscript presented in Symposium on the Pharmacology of Thermoregulation, San Francisco, 1972.
4. Herbert, W.G., & Smith, L.C. *A fluid replacement schedule to avoid hyperthermia in novice distance runners: Report of a laboratory case study.* Poster presented at the Research Section, Annual Meeting of the Virginia Association of Health, Physical Education and Recreation, Norfolk, 1979.

References

ADOLPH, E.R., Brown, A.H., Goddard, D.R., Gosselin, R.C., Kelly, J.J., Molnar, G.W., Rahn, H., Rothstein, A., Towbin, E.J., Wills, J.H., & Wold, A.V. *Physiology of man in the desert.* New York: Interscience, 1947.

AHLBORG, B., Ekelund, L.G., & Nilsson, C.G. Effect of potassium-magnesium-aspartate on the capacity for prolonged exercise in man. *Acta Physiologica Scandinavica,* 1968, **74**, 238-245.

AHLMAN, K., & Karvonen, M.J. Weight reduction by sweating in wrestlers and its effect on physical fitness. *Journal of Sports Medicine,* 1961, **1**, 58-62.

AICKIN, C.C., & Thomas, R.C. Micro-electrode measurement of the intracellular pH and buffering power of the mouse soleus muscle fibers. *Journal of Physiology (London),* 1977, **267**, 791-810.

ALLEN, T.E., Smith, D.P., & Miller, D.K. Hemodynamic response to submaximal exercise after dehydration and rehydration in high school wrestlers. *Medicine and Science in Sports,* 1977, **9**, 159-163.

AMERICAN College of Sports Medicine. Position statement: Prevention of heat injuries during distance running. *Medicine and Science in Sports,* 1975, **1**, vii-viii.

AMERICAN Medical Association Committee on Medical Aspects of Sports. Wrestling and weight control. *Journal of the American Medical Association,* 1967, **201**, 541-543.

ÅSTRAND, P.O., & Saltin, B. Plasma and red cell volume after prolonged severe exercise. *Journal of Applied Physiology,* 1964, **19**, 829-832.

BAR-OR, O., Dotan, R., Inbar, O., Rotshtein, A., & Zonder, H. Voluntary hypohydration in 10- to 12-year-old boys. *Journal of Applied Physiology: Respiratory, Environmental and Exercise Physiology,* 1980, **48**, 104-108.

BLANK, L.B. An experimental study of the effect of water ingestion upon athletic performance. *The Research Quarterly,* 1959, **30**, 131-135.

BLYTH, C.S., & Burt, J.J. Effect of water balance on ability to perform in high ambient temperatures. *The Research Quarterly,* 1961, **32**, 301-307.

BOCK, W., Fox, E.L., & Bowers, R. The effects of acute dehydration upon cardiorespiratory endurance. *Journal of Sports Medicine,* 1967, **7**, 67-72.

BUSKIRK, E.R. Weight loss in wrestlers. *American Journal of Diseases of Children,* 1978, **132**, 355-356.

CADE, R., Spooner, G., Schlein, E., Pickering, M., & Dean, R. Effect of fluid, electrolyte, and glucose replacement during exercise on performance, body temperature, rate of sweat loss, and compositional changes of extracellular fluid. *Journal of Sports Medicine and Physical Fitness,* 1972, **12**, 150-156.

CLAREMONT, A.D., Costill, D.L., Fink, W., & Van Handel, P. Heat tolerance following diuretic induced dehydration. *Medicine and Science in Sports*, 1976, **8**, 239-243.

COHEN, I., & Zimmerman, A.L. Changes in serum electrolyte levels during marathon running. *South African Medical Journal*, 1978, **53**, 449-453.

COSTILL, D.L., Branam, L., Eddy, D., & Fink, W. Alterations in red cell volume following exercise and dehydration. *Journal of Applied Physiology*, 1974, **37**, 912-916.

COSTILL, D.L., Cote, R., & Fink, W. Muscle water and electrolytes following varied levels of dehydration in man. *Journal of Applied Physiology*, 1976, **40**, 6-11.

COSTILL, D.L., Cote, R., Miller, E., Miller, T., & Wynder, S. Water and electrolyte replacement during repeated days of work in the heat. *Aviation and Space Environmental Medicine*, 1975, **46**, 795-800.

COSTILL, D.L., & Fink, W.J. Plasma volume changes following exercise and thermal dehydration. *Journal of Applied Physiology*, 1974, **37**, 521-525.

COSTILL, D.L., Kammer, W.F., & Fisher, A. Fluid ingestion during distance running. *Archives of Environmental Health*, 1970, **21**, 520-525.

COSTILL, D.L., & Saltin, B. Changes in the ratio of venous to body hematocrit following dehydration. *Journal of Applied Physiology*, 1974, **36**, 608-610. (a)

COSTILL, D.L., & Saltin, B. Factors limiting gastric emptying during rest and exercise. *Journal of Applied Physiology*, 1974, **37**, 679-683. (b)

COSTILL, D.L., & Sparks, K.E. Rapid fluid replacement following thermal dehydration. *Journal of Applied Physiology*, 1973, **34**, 299-303.

COYLE, E.F., Costill, D.L., Fink, W.J., & Hoopes, D.G. Gastric emptying rates for selected athletic drinks. *The Research Quarterly*, 1978, **49**, 119-124.

CRAIG, F.N., & Cummings, E.G. Dehydration and muscular work. *Journal of Applied Physiology*, 1966, **21**, 670-674.

CUNNINGHAM, J.N., Carter, N.W., Rector, F.C., & Seldin, D.W. Resting transmembrane potential difference of skeletal muscle in normal subjects and severely ill patients. *The Journal of Clinical Investigation*, 1971, **50**, 49-59.

DAVENPORT, H.W. *Physiology of the digestive tract* (2nd ed.). Chicago: Yearbook Medical Publishers, 1966.

DILL, D.B., & Costill, D.L. Calculation of percentage changes in volumes of blood plasma, and red cells in dehydration. *Journal of Applied Physiology*, 1974, **37**, 247-248.

DILL, D.B., Yousef, M.K., & Nelson, J.D. Responses of men and women to two-hour walks in desert heat. *Journal of Applied Physiology*, 1973, **35**, 231-235.

DOSCHER, N. The effects of rapid weight loss upon the performance of wrestlers and boxers, and upon the physical proficiency of college students. *Research Quarterly*, 1944, **15**, 317-324.

EKBLOM, B., Greenleaf, C.J., Greenleaf, J.E., & Hermansen, L. Temperature regulation during exercise dehydration in man. *Acta Physiologica Scandinavica*, 1970, **79**, 475-483.

ELFENBAUM, L. *The physiological effects of rapid weight loss among wrestlers.* Unpublished doctoral dissertation, Ohio State University, 1966.

ENGLAND, A.C., Varsha, R.A., Tirinnanzi, R., Greenberg, D.J., Powell, K.E., & Slovis, C.M. Epidemiology of severe heat injury occurring among participants of the 1979 Peachtree Road Race. *Medicine and Science in Sports and Exercise*, 1980, **12**, 102. (Abstract)

FORDTRAN, J.S., & Saltin, B. Gastric emptying and intestinal absorption during prolonged severe exercise. *Journal of Applied Physiology*, 1967, **23**, 331-335.

FORTNEY, S.M., Nadel, E.R., Wenger, C.B., & Bove, J.R. Effect of blood volume on sweating rate and body fluids in exercising humans. *Journal of Applied Physiology: Respiratory, Environmental and Exercise Physiology*, 1981, **51**, 1594-1600.

FRANCIS, K.T., & MacGregor, R. Effect of exercise in the heat on plasma renin and aldosterone with either water or a potassium-rich electrolyte solution. *Aviation and Space Environmental Medicine*, 1978, **19**, 461-465.

GISOLFI, C.V., & Copping, J.R. Thermal effects of prolonged treadmill exercise in the heat. *Medicine and Science in Sports*, 1974, **6**, 108-113.

GREENLEAF, J.E., & Brock, P.J. Na^+ and Ca^{2+} ingestion: Plasma volume-electrolyte distribution at rest and exercise. *Journal of Applied Physiology: Respiratory, Environmental and Exercise Physiology*, 1980, **48**, 838-847.

GREENLEAF, J.E., & Castle, B.L. Exercise temperature regulation in man during hypohydration and hyperhydration. *Journal of Applied Physiology*, 1971, **30**, 847-853.

GREENLEAF, J.E., Matter, M., Bosco, J.S., Douglas, L.G., & Averkin, E.G. Effects of hypohydration on work performance and tolerance to $+G_z$ acceleration in man. *Aerospace Medicine*, 1966, **37**, 34-39.

GUYTON, A.C. *Textbook of medical physiology* (3rd ed.). Philadelphia: W.B. Saunders, 1968.

HANSON, P.G. Heat injury in runners. *The Physician and Sportsmedicine*, 1979, **7**, 91-96.

HARRISON, M.H., Edwards, R.J., & Fennessy, P.A. Intravascular volume and tonicity as factors in the regulation of body temperature. *Journal of Applied Physiology: Respiratory, Environmental and Exercise Physiology*, 1978, **44**, 69-75.

HERBERT, W.G., & Ribisl, P.M. Effects of dehydration upon physical working capacity of wrestlers under competitive conditions. *Research Quarterly*, 1972, **43**, 416-422.

HOUSTON, M.E., Marrin, D.A., Green, H.J., & Thompson, J.A. The effect of rapid weight loss on physiological functions in wrestlers. *The Physician and Sportsmedicine*, 1981, **9**, 73-78.

HULTMAN, E., & Sahlin, K. Acid-base balance during exercise. In R.W. Hutton & D.I. Miller (Eds.), *Exercise and sport sciences reviews*. Philadelphia: The Franklin Institute, 1980.

HUNT, J.N., & Pathak, J.D. The osmotic effects of some simple molecules and ions on gastric emptying. *Journal of Physiology*, 1960, **154**, 254-269.

JENNINGS, B.E. *A study of the effect of semi-starvation on strength and endurance with reference to college wrestling*. Unpublished master's thesis, University of North Carolina, 1951.

JOHNSON, J.M. Regulation of skin circulation during prolonged exercise. *Annals of the New York Academy of Sciences*, 1977, **301**, 195-212.

KNOCHEL, J.P. Potassium deficiency during training in the heat. *Annuals of the New York Academy of Sciences*, 1977, **301**, 175-189.

KNOCHEL, J.P., & Vertel, R.M. Salt loading as a possible factor in the production of potassium depletion, rhabdomyolysis, and heat injury. *The Lancet*, 1967, **9**, 659-661.

KOZLOWSKI, S., & Saltin, B. Effect of sweat loss on body fluids. *Journal of Applied Physiology*, 1964, **19**, 1119-1124.

LEHNINGER, A.L. *Biochemistry* (2nd ed.). New York: Worth, 1975.

LOWENSOHN, H.S., Patterson, R.E., & Olsson, R.A. Exercise performance and hemodynamics during dietary potassium depletion in dogs. *Journal of Applied Physiology: Respiratory, Environmental and Exercise Physiology*, 1978, **45**, 728-732.

MARCUS, E. Problems in fluid and electrolyte imbalance and their management. *The Surgical Clinics of North America*, 1962, **42**, 35-54.

MARON, M.B., & Horvath, S.M. The marathon: A history and review of the literature. *Medicine and Science in Sports*, 1979, **11**, 137-150.

MATHEWS, D.K., Fox, E.L., & Tanzi, D. Physiological responses during exercise and recovery in a football uniform. *Journal of Applied Physiology*, 1969, **26**, 611-615.

MITCHELL, J.W. Energy exchanges during exercise. In E.R. Nadel (Ed.), *Problems with temperature regulation during exercise*. New York: Academic Press, 1977.

MORGAN, W.P. Psychological effect of weight reduction in the college wrestler. *Medicine and Science in Sports*, 1969, **2**, 24-27.

MOROFF, S.V., & Bass, D.E. Effects of overhydration on man's physiological responses to work in the heat. *Journal of Applied Physiology*, 1965, **20**, 267-270.

MURPHY, R.J. The problems of environmental heat in athletics. *Ohio State Medical Journal*, 1963, **59**, 799-803.

MYHRE, L.G., & Robinson, S. Fluid shifts during thermal stress with and without fluid replacement. *Journal of Applied Physiology*, 1977, **42**, 252-256.

NIELSEN, B. Effect of changes in plasma Na^+ and Ca^{++} ion concentration on body temperature during exercise. *Acta Physiologica Scandinavica*, 1974, **91**, 123-129.

OLSSON, K.E., & Saltin, B. Diet and fluids in training and competition. *Scandinavian Journal of Rehabilitation Medicine*, 1971, **3**, 31-38.

PALMER, W.K. Selected physiological responses of normal young men following dehydration and rehydration. *The Research Quarterly*, 1968, **39**, 1054-1059.

PITTS, G.L., Johnson, R.E., & Consolazio, F.C. Work in the heat as affected by intake of water, salt and glucose. *American Journal of Physiology*, 1944, **142**, 253-259.

PITTS, R.F. *Physiology of the kidney and body fluids* (2nd ed.). Chicago: Yearbook Medical Publishers, 1968.

PUGH, L.G.C.E., Corbett, J.L., & Johnson, R.H. Rectal temperatures, weight losses and sweat rates in marathon running. *Journal of Applied Physiology*, 1967, **23**, 347-352.

RIBISL, P.M., & Herbert, W.G. Effects of rapid weight reduction and subsequent rehydration upon the physical working capacity of wrestlers. *Research Quarterly*, 1970, **41**, 536-541.

RYAN, A.J., Costill, D.L., Gisolfi, C., Murphy, R.J., & Westerman, R.L. Balancing heat stress, fluids, and electrolytes. *The Physician and Sportsmedicine*, 1975, **3**, 43-52.

SALTIN, B. Aerobic and anaerobic work capacity after dehydration. *Journal of Applied Physiology*, 1964, **19**, 1114-1118. (a)

SALTIN, B. Circulatory response to submaximal and maximal exercise after thermal dehydration. *Journal of Applied Physiology*, 1964, **19**, 1125-1132. (b)

SALTIN, B., Gagge, A.P., Bergh, V., & Stolwijk, J.A.J. Body temperatures and sweating during exhaustive exercise. *Journal of Applied Physiology*, 1972, **32**, 635-643.

SALTIN, B., & Stenberg, J. Circulatory response to prolonged severe exercise. *Journal of Applied Physiology*, 1964, **19**, 833-838.

SENAY, L.C. Temperature regulation and hypohydration: A singular view. *Journal of Applied Physiology: Respiratory, Environmental and Exercise Physiology*, 1979, **47**, 1-7.

SINGER, R.N., & Weiss, S.A. Effects of weight reduction on selected anthropometric, physical, and performance measures of wrestlers. *The Research Quarterly*, 1968, **39**, 361-369.

SKINNER, J.S., Hutsler, R., Bergsteinova, V., & Buskirk, E.R. Perception of effort during different types of exercise and under different environmental conditions. *Medicine and Science in Sports*, 1973, **5**, 110-115.

STRYDOM, N.B., Wyndham, C.H., van Graan, C.H., Holdsworth, L.D., & Morrison, J.F. The influence of water restriction on the performance of men during a prolonged march. *South African Medical Journal*, 1966, **40**, 539-544.

TAYLOR, H.L., Henschel, A., Mickelsen, O., & Keys, A. The effect of the sodium chloride intake on the work performance of man during exposure to dry heat and experimental heat exhaustion. *American Journal of Physiology*, 1944, **140**, 439-451.

TORRANIN, C., Smith, D.P., & Byrd, R.J. The effect of acute thermal dehydration on isometric and isotonic endurance. *The Journal of Sports Medicine and Physical Fitness*, 1979, **19**, 1-7.

TUTTLE, W.W. The effect of weight loss by dehydration and the withholding of food on the physiologic responses of wrestlers. *Research Quarterly*, 1943, **14**, 158-166.

WYNDHAM, C.H., & Strydom, N.B. The danger of an inadequate water intake during marathon running. *South African Medical Journal*, 1969, **43**, 893-896.

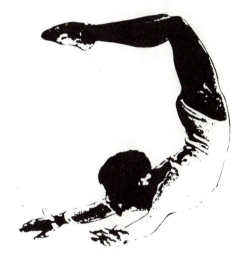

Part 2
Pharmacological Ergogenic Aids

4

Amphetamines

John L. Ivy

Stimulants have been used for many years with the idea that they could increase physical performance. The first stimulants were of plant origin. For example, the leaves of the coca plant and of the African plant *Catha edulis* contain the psychomotor stimulant drugs cocaine and norpseudoephedrine, respectively. Both are believed, by the people in the regions where these plants grow, to increase strength and to delay the onset of fatigue (Van Rossum, 1970).

Very similar in structure to the naturally occurring stimulants ephedrine and norpseudoephedrine is 2-phenyl-isopropylamine, better known as amphetamine. This white, odorless, crystalline powder was first synthesized in 1887, and its N-methylated derivative, methamphetamine, was produced in 1919 (Hart & Wallace, 1975). During World War II, amphetamine and methamphetamine were used extensively by army troops to combat fatigue and to improve endurance (Ivy & Krasno, 1941; Van Rossum, 1970). Amphetamine abuse in sports became prominent following World

John L. Ivy, Ph.D., F.A.C.S.M., is with the Exercise Physiology Laboratory, School of Health and Physical Education, at the University of Texas, Austin.

War II when veterans carried the drug from the battlefields to the athletic fields (Mandell, 1979).

An American College of Sports Medicine survey (Note 1) revealed that 35% of the respondents, including professional and amateur coaches, trainers, and physicians, expressed knowledge of situations in which athletes had used drugs. The drugs they mentioned most frequently were amphetamine derivatives, and the stated purpose of their use was to improve performance.

More recent surveys (Gilbert, 1969a, 1969b, 1969c; Johnson, 1972) would lead one to believe that the abuse of amphetamines in sports is on the rise, despite condemnation by many athletic and medical associations involved in the conduct of athletics. This increased drug abuse is also documented in such contemporary writings as *Ball Four* (Bouton, 1970) and *The Nightmare Season* (Mandell, 1976). Both picture the openness and routinely indiscriminate use of the drug in the locker room. Probably Mandell's calculations best reflect the use and abuse of amphetamines in sports today. On the basis of the drug purchase record of several professional football teams, Mandell (1979) found that the average consumption for each game in 1969 was 70.0 mg/person.

Athletes resort to amphetamines for many reasons, but the ones they cite most often are to ward off fatigue (Golding, 1972), to get "psyched up," and to improve performance (American College of Sports Medicine, Note 1; Gilbert, 1969a). Whether amphetamines actually enhance performance, however, is still under debate within the scientific community. After reviewing the literature, Weiss and Laties (1962) in 1962 and again in 1967 (Laties & Weiss, 1967) concluded that amphetamines can enhance athletic performance. This also was the conclusion drawn by Pfeiffer and Symthies (1970). On the other hand, Golding (1972) and Williams (1974) felt that the results of contemporary laboratory research did not indicate that amphetamines have a beneficial effect on athletic performance.

This review will not resolve the debate of whether or not amphetamines are capable of increasing physical and athletic performance; it will, however, provide a new interpretation of the available data. The final decision on the effectiveness of amphetamines as an ergogenic aid has to rest with the reader. Other excellent reviews that should be consulted are those by Golding (1972), Pfeiffer and Smythies (1970), Van Rossum (1970), Weiss and Laties (1962), and Williams (1974).

Theoretical Benefits

To understand how amphetamine could possibly improve physical

performance, a knowledge of its modes of action and the physiological responses to those actions is essential. Amphetamine is an
optically active molecule, existing as dextrorotatory (or d-) amphetamine and levorotatory (or l-) amphetamine. The dextrorotatary
isomer is three to four times more potent than the levorotatory
isomer (Van Rossum, 1970). Amphetamines are usually administered orally as hydrochlorides or as other salts. They are readily absorbed from mucous membranes of the small intestines and reach a
peak in the blood 2 hours after ingestion (Quinn, Cohn, Reid,
Greengard, & Weiner, 1967). Campbell (1969) found that human
subjects given 10.0-15.0 mg of d-amphetamine sulfate had maximum blood levels of 0.04-0.05 mg/liter after 1½-2 hours. The peak
subjective and behavioral effects are seen 2-3 hours after ingestion
(Ray, 1972). Intraperitoneal injection produces maximum blood
levels within 30 minutes (Maickel, Cox, Segal, & Miller, 1966).

Animal studies have demonstrated that amphetamines pass
rapidly from blood to brain and that they are eliminated from the
system partly by renal excretion and partly by biotransformation
(Pfeiffer & Smythies, 1970). The biological half-life of amphetamines is about 12 hours (Van Rossum, 1970).

Central Effects

Amphetamines are both sympathomimetic and central nervous
system stimulants. Their mode of action on the central nervous
system is complex and not completely understood. One theory is
that amphetamines produce their effects by mimicking the neurotransmitters (Ray, 1972). Another theory assumes that amphetamines inhibit monoamine oxidase, thereby reducing the rate of
catecholamine destruction and allowing catecholamine accumulation (Van Rossum, 1970). Still others believe that these drugs affect
the disposition of catecholamines by altering their binding sites at
the nerve endings (Axelrod, Whitby, & Hertting, 1961) or cause
synthesis and release of norepinephrine from presynaptic sites
(Burger, 1968; Stone, 1970).

The most marked and consistent central effect of amphetamines
is their production of a state of arousal or wakefulness, probably
through a direct action upon the reticular activating system
(Bradley & Elkes, 1957; Kalant, 1973). This central stimulating effect is usually perceived subjectively as a sense of increased
energy, self-confidence, and faster and more efficient thought and
decision making. An associated feeling of well-being and euphoria
appears to be caused by stimulation of the forebrain bundle (Ray,
1972). The use of amphetamines to produce a state of arousal or

wakefulness and to reduce or to relieve the sense of fatigue is one of the predominant reasons for their use in athletics.

Amphetamines also increase cerebral activity and affect the hypothalamus directly (Van Rossum, 1970). It is conceivable that stimulation of the cerebral cortex could alter perception, attention, motivation, motor coordination, strength, and other faculties beneficial to athletic performance. The hypothalamus is associated with the reticular activating system of the midbrain, and such behavioral functions as excitability, pleasure, pain, and rage are under its control. The "psyched up" effect produced by amphetamines may be a result of their action on this area of the brain. In addition, the hypothalamus is the seat of the autonomic nervous system and is associated with the endocrine system via the pituitary gland. Therefore, stimulation of this area can have widespread results throughout the systems of the body.

Peripheral Effects

As sympathomimetic drugs, the amphetamines are capable of increasing systolic and diastolic blood pressure, heart rate, peripheral vascular tone, respiratory stimulation, bronchial tube dilation, pupillary dilation, and relaxation of the smooth muscles of the gastrointestinal tract (Kalant, 1973; Ray, 1972; Van Rossum, 1970). Further, amphetamines promote vasoconstriction of cutaneous blood vessels, vasodilation in the skeletal muscles, and a redistribution of blood from the skin and portions of the splanchnic bed to the skeletal muscles and brain (Beckman, 1958). This usually results in a rise in body temperature (Griffith, Canaugh, Held, & Oates, 1972).

Theoretically, an increased heart rate and myocardial contractility, in conjunction with a more efficient venous return due to an increased vascular tone, could increase cardiac output and oxygen delivery to the skeletal muscles during exercise. However, vasoconstriction of cutaneous tissue during exercise could result in hyperthermia.

Burger (1968) has argued that, in the periphery, amphetamines have the greatest effect on the effector cells by causing the release of catecholamines from functional storage pools located in the peripheral sympathetic nerve endings. Others have suggested a more direct action of amphetamines on the effector cells (Fuller & Hines, 1967). Such a direct action on muscle cells could possibly place these cells in a state of hyperirritability, thus enhancing their recruitment and rendering muscle groups more capable of executing speed and power movements.

Tissue respiration is also increased by amphetamines. Dembert and Harclerode (1974) found that homogenates of mouse brain and muscle prepared 2½ hours after administration of dl-amphetamine had significantly elevated oxygen consumption (state III respiration). Behavioral changes at the time of sacrifice included irritability and increased motor activity. Others have demonstrated an increased motor activity in animals following amphetamine administration (Grinker, Drewnoski, Enns, & Kissileff, 1980; Mantegazza, Müller, Naimzada, & Riva, 1970). Stimulated liver and muscle glycolysis (Beckman, 1958; Estler, Fickl, & Fröhlich, 1970), a rise in blood glucose, and mobilization of free fatty acids (Estler et al., 1970; Optiz, 1970; Pinter & Pattee, 1968) are also associated with this increased activity.

Studies using humans (Costill, Coyle, Dalsky, Evans, Fink, & Hoopes, 1977; Ivy, Costill, Van Handel, Essig, & Lower, 1981) and rats (Rennie, Winder, & Holloszy, 1976) have demonstrated that when free fatty acids are raised prior to submaximal exercise, there is an increased reliance on lipid oxidation, a sparing of carbohydrates, and an increased endurance capacity (Hickson, Rennie, Conlee, Winder, & Holloszy, 1977). Thus, amphetamines could possibly enhance endurance performance by increasing lipid oxidation and decreasing the rate of glycogen depletion.

Research Findings of Increased Performance

Aerobic Endurance

Studies on humans and animals, using such modes of exercise as cycling, running, swimming, and marching, have demonstrated that amphetamines can decrease the rate of fatigue and thus enhance endurance performance. One of the earlier studies investigating the effect of amphetamine on endurance performance was by Lehmann, Straub, and Szakall (1939). Making repeated studies on three subjects who rode a bicycle ergometer to exhaustion, they found that 5.0, 10.0, and 15.0 mg of methamphetamine effectively reduced the rate of fatigue and enhanced performance.

Studies of a similar nature were reported by other investigators in the next decade. Testing amphetamine and methamphetamine, Knoefel (1943) reported that both drugs effectively increased the work output of subjects riding to exhaustion on a bicycle ergometer. Using both hand and cycle ergometers, Cuthbertson and Knox (1947) found that 10.0 mg of methamphetamine or 15.0 mg of d-amphetamine, administered during work, restored performance to (and in some instances above) initial levels and increased the amount of work that could be performed over a 6-hour period. The effect took between ½-1½ hours to be seen and lasted for ¾-3 hours. Based on the participant dropout rate and questionnaire data, Cuthbertson and Knox (1947) also reported that 15.0 mg of methamphetamine diminished the fatigue and discomfort of an 18-mile march. In another study designed to investigate the effects of amphetamine on recovery, three groups of 50 subjects underwent a military exercise lasting 56 hours (Sommerville, 1946). During the last 22 hours, two groups took between 30.0 and 35.0 mg of amphetamine and one group received a placebo. At the end of the exercise, the subjects were required to negotiate an obstacle course as rapidly as possible. It was reported that the time to complete the course was significantly shorter for the groups receiving amphetamine (Sommerville, 1946).

In more recent years, use of swimming animals has proven to be a popular model for evaluating the effects of various experimental treatments on endurance capacity. Using a unique approach, Kay and Birren (1958) studied the effect of amphetamine on the swimming endurance of mice. Amphetamine (4.0 mg•kg^{-1} body wt) was administered intraperitoneally 30 minutes before the swim. The animals were placed in the water at one end of a trough. At the other end was an escape ramp. Upon reaching the escape ramp, the mice were returned to the starting point and this sequence repeated 30 times. The time to swim each length of the trough, called a trial, was recorded. The increase in swim time for each trial, with increasing number of trials completed, was presumed to be due to fatigue. The results indicated that amphetamine practically abolished the increase in swim time normally seen with an increase in completed trials and thus delayed the onset of fatigue.

Using a swimming protocol similar to that of Kay and Birren (1958), Bättig (1963), Kiplinger (1967), Kleinrok and Swiezynska (1966), and Molinengo and Orsetti (1976) also reported an increased endurance capacity for animals that had received amphetamine. Kleinrok and Swiezynska (1966) used a 3-meter-long trough and 25 consecutive swimming trials and found that only 92% of the control rats could complete the task, whereas 100% of the rats receiving amphetamine were able to complete it. When the animals were forced to swim pulling a weight equivalent to 5% of their body weight, the percentage of successful animals decreased to 79 and 96%, respectively. Amphetamine also successfully attenuated the increase in swim time with increasing trials.

It is interesting to note that neither Bättig (1963) nor Kiplinger (1967) could find an increase in performance with low dosages of amphetamine (1.0-2.0 mg·kg^{-1} body wt). However, Bättig (1963) reported that 4.0 mg·kg^{-1} body wt improved swimming endurance, and Kiplinger (1967) found that 4.0 and 8.0 mg·kg^{-1} body wt were effective dosages for delaying the onset of fatigue. Kiplinger (1967) also observed that 16.0 mg·kg^{-1} body wt appeared to cause confusion in the animals and to reduce their ability to swim the length of the trough.

Using the more traditional approach of determining endurance by swim time to exhaustion, Bhagat and Wheeler (1973a, 1973b) reported that 10.0 and 20.0 mg·kg^{-1} body wt of the d and ℓ isomers of amphetamine and 20.0 mg·kg^{-1} body wt of dl-amphetamine increased the swimming time of trained rats. Dosages of the d and l isomers below 5.0 mg·kg^{-1} body wt were ineffective.

A biphasic effect of amphetamine on running endurance has also been demonstrated (Gerald, 1978). Rats running at 18.8 m·min^{-1} were reported to have improved their treadmill endurance by 24-64% with low dosages of amphetamine (0.31-5.0 mg·kg^{-1} body wt) and reduced it by 18-47% with high dosages (7.5-10.0 mg·kg^{-1} body wt). At belt speeds ranging from 10.7 to 26.8 m·min^{-1}, a low dosage of amphetamine (2.5 mg·kg^{-1} body wt) increased running times by 33-101%, whereas a high dosage (10.0 mg·kg^{-1} body wt) reduced endurance by 17-43%. Amphetamine also effectively enhanced the endurance performance of fatigued rats.

Local Muscle Endurance

Foltz, Ivy, and Barborka (1943) had trained subjects ride a bicycle ergometer to exhaustion with the work rate held constant at 1,235 kgm·min^{-1}. Amphetamine (10.0-15.0 mg) or methamphetamine (5.0 mg) was injected intravenously 30 seconds to 30 minutes before the work period. Methamphetamine was found to increase ride time to exhaustion, whereas amphetamine had no effect on performance. Only two subjects, however, were tested with amphetamine, and the actual times of its administration were not given.

More recent studies have also demonstrated that subjects working at an intensive effort could increase work time after taking amphetamine. Using 10 maximum work (cycling) periods of 45 seconds duration with a 15-second pause between periods, Borg, Edström, Linderholm, and Marklund (1972) found that the final performances were significantly improved under the amphetamine (10.0 mg) condition as compared to a placebo condition. Improvements in work time to exhaustion were also reported for two

trained cyclists after they had ingested 10.0 mg of methamphetamine. Work rates were set above maximal oxygen consumption. Postexercise blood analysis indicated that blood lactates were
higher following the amphetamine rides than the control rides.
However, lactate levels were determined for only one of the two
subjects (Wyndham, Rogers, Benade, & Strydom, 1971). In a well
controlled study, Chandler and Blair (1980) found results similar to
that of Wyndham et al. (1971). Using a double-blind, placebo-
control design, they determined that d-amphetamine (15.0 mg•70
kg^{-1} body wt) increased run time to exhaustion and significantly
elevated postexercise blood lactates. No increase in submaximum
or maximum oxygen consumption could be attributed to the amphetamine.

Employing a Mosso-type finger ergograph to test muscle endurance, Hollister and Gillespie (1970) determined that fatigue
could be attenuated by 20.0 mg of d-amphetamine. Alles and
Feigen (1942) also used a finger ergometer and reported that dl-
amphetamine inhibited voluntary muscle fatigue. The experimental protocol used by Alles and Feigen, however, makes critical
evaluation of their results extremely difficult.

Using a repeated measures design, Wenzel and Rutledge (1962)
studied the effects of 2.5, 5.0, and 10.0 mg of d-amphetamine on
speed of tapping. The rate of decline in tapping speed was their
criterion for fatigue. It was noted that amphetamine reduced the
decline in tapping rate over a 60-second period, and that this effect
was dose related. Thornton, Holck, and Smith (1939) also noticed a
significant improvement in tapping tests of 2- and 5-minutes duration following amphetamine ingestion.

In tests of static muscular endurance, Thornton, Holck, and
Smith (1939), Bujas and Petz (1955), Costello (1963), Graham and
Bos (Note 2), and Ikai and Steinhaus (1961) reported a beneficial effect for amphetamine. Thornton and colleagues (1939) measured
the effect of 20.0 mg of d-amphetamine, administered 85 minutes
before testing, on the ability of three subjects to maintain two-
thirds of their maximum grip strength. Compared to a placebo condition, amphetamine improved performance by approximately
63%. Using a similar test of muscle endurance, Costello (1963)
reported that 10.0 mg of d-amphetamine increased the time that a
predetermined percentage of maximum handgrip strength could
be maintained. He conducted two tests, however. In the first test
he found a significant drug effect, but his *post hoc* analysis revealed
that only the control and amphetamine treatments were
significantly different. For the second test, he reported that amphetamine increased muscle endurance beyond that attained dur-

ing either the control or placebo treatments. Graham and Bos (Note 2) used a double-blind placebo protocol to test the effects of 15.0 mg of d-amphetamine on the isometric and isotonic endurance of the triceps brachii. Simultaneously, they monitored muscle action potentials by electromyography. They reported that amphetamine slowed the rate of fatigue and reduced the integrated action potential of the triceps during isometric contractions. Amphetamine, they found, had no effect on isotonic work. Ikai and Steinhaus (1961), using 10 trained subjects, observed the influence of dl-amphetamine on static contractions of the right forearm flexors over a 30-minute period. The results indicated that 10.0 mg of amphetamine, taken 25 minutes prior to testing, could significantly reduce the rate of musce fatigue. However, their subjects always knew when they were receiving the drug, and thus a confounding psychological variable was introduced into the experimental design.

Strength

A number of studies have demonstrated that maximum isometric strength can be improved by amphetamine. In an early study, Thornton et al. (1939) found that 20.0 mg of d-amphetamine improved grip strength by 2, 8, and 9% in three subjects. Ikai and Steinhaus (1961) tested several factors that could affect strength and reported that three 10.0-mg tablets of dl-amphetamine, ingested 25 minutes before testing, enhanced grip strength by 13.5%. However, as previously indicated, the subjects always knew when they were receiving the drug. To determine whether or not the increase in strength attributed to amphetamine was mediated by suggestion, Hurst, Radlow, and Bagley (1968) conducted a similar study to that of Ikai and Steinhaus (1961) but added a placebo group. In addition, prior to giving their maximum effort, the subjects were required to estimate their strength on the basis of perceived effort required to reach an assigned submaximal value. The results indicated that strength was significantly higher under d-amphetamine than under both the placebo and control conditions. Since the treatments did not differ significantly with respect to estimated strength, Hurst et al. (1968) concluded that the increase in strength was not psychologically motivated. An improvement in maximal isometric strength by ingestion of d-amphetamine was also demonstrated by Lovingood, Blyth, Peacock, and Lindsay (1967), Graham and Bos (Note 2), and Chandler and Blair (1980). However, Chandler and Blair found that only knee extension strength, but not elbow flexion strength, was improved. They postulated that the effect of amphetamine on muscular strength is directly proportional to the number of motor units recruited; that is, the greater the number of motor units involved in any particular strength performance, the greater the amphetamine effect.

Fowler, Filerich, and Leberer (1977) investigated the influence of d-amphetamine on the isometric force of rats. By water reinforcement, the rats were taught to paw-press a silent isometric force-sensing device. Dosages of 0.8, 1.6, and 3.2 mg·kg^{-1} body wt of d-amphetamine were administered. Amphetamine produced an interesting biphasic response, as has been found in many endurance studies. The lowest dose of amphetamine had no effect on peak force, the moderate dose increased peak force significantly, and the high dose decreased peak force but lengthened the duration of the response.

Only a few studies with regard to the effect of amphetamines upon isotonic, or dynamic, strength exist. Smith and Beecher (1959) reported the only study that demonstrated amphetamine significantly improved isotonic strength. Their criterion for isotonic strength was how far a 35-pound weight or 16-pound shot could be put. They found that the ingestion of 14.0 mg·70 kg^{-1} body wt of dl-amphetamine 2-3 hours before testing significantly improved the isotonic strength of 85% of their subjects. The average improvement ranged between 3 and 4%. This study, however, has come under strong criticism because of the inaccurate measuring technique used by these investigators to determine the distances the weights were thrown (Pierson, 1961).

Reaction Time

Only a few studies demonstrated that amphetamines decrease the reaction time of alert, nonfatigued subjects. Lehmann and Csank (1957) reported a significant reduction in simple reaction time after dosages of 12.5 and 15.0 mg of d-amphetamine. Testing subjects at a simulated altitude of 18,000 feet, Adler, Burkardt, Ivy, and Atkinson (1950) reported a decrease in discriminative reaction time following administration of 10.0 mg of d-amphetamine. More recently, Evans and Jewett (1962) demonstrated a significant decrease in discriminative reaction time after 15.0 mg of d-amphetamine. However, Laties and Weiss (1967) argued that the long intertrial intervals used by these investigators transformed their reaction time experiment into a vigilance experiment.

Several studies have been designed to assess how amphetamine improves reaction time after sleep deprivation. Kornetsky, Mirsky, Kessler, and Dorff (1959) reported that 10.0 mg of d-amphetamine, taken by subjects deprived of sleep for 44 hours, or 15.0 mg of d-amphetamine, taken after 68 hours of sleep deprivation, restored their reaction time to within normal limits. Seashore and Ivy (1953), using subjects deprived of sleep for 24 hours, found a significant decrease in discriminative reaction time following the administration of 10.0 mg of d-amphetamine or 5.0 mg of methamphetamine. Tyler (1947) also reported that the deterioration in reaction time that occurred after sleep deprivation or fatigue was counteracted by this drug.

Uyeda and Fuster (1962) examined the effect of amphetamine on the reaction time of the rhesus monkey (*Macaca rhesus*). They reported that an intramuscular injection of 1.5 mg of dl-amphetamine significantly decreased reaction time, compared to a placebo injection. Since similar effects had previously been produced in the monkey by stimulation of the mesencephalic reticular formation (Fuster, 1958), the authors suggested that amphetamine's action was the result of its stimulating effect on this brain system.

Speed

Rate of tapping is a popular means of measuring the speed of fine movement as well as of fine motor coordination. The usual procedure is to tap as fast as possible with a finger or stylus for a period of between 5 and 30 seconds. When tapping is performed for periods greater than 1 minute, however, an element of fatigue is introduced into the test. Only two studies show a positive effect of amphetamine on tapping rate for tests lasting less than 1 minute. Thornton et al. (1939) found that 20.0 mg of dl-amphetamine improved tapping rate by 10% when the test was conducted for 30 seconds. Lehmann and Csank (1957) also noted a rise in tapping rate with 12.5 and 15.0 mg of d-amphetamine.

The swimming of animals has also been utilized to study the effect of amphetamine on gross body speed. Kleinrok and Swiezynska (1966) tested the effects of 5.0 $mg \cdot kg^{-1}$ body wt of dl-amphetamine on the swimming speed of weighted and unweighted rats 1, 2, 3, 4, 6, and 24 hours after its administration. They found that amphetamine increased the swimming speed of unweighted rats, but not that of weighted rats, 3 hours after administration of the drug. The increase in speed persisted for 24 hours, at which time the weighted rats also demonstrated a significant improvement. Kay and Birren (1958) determined the speed at which rats could swim the length of a trough. They reported that during the initial swimming trials, following the injection of 4.0 $mg \cdot kg^{-1}$ body wt of amphetamine, the rats appeared uncoordinated and could not swim a straight line. During trials 5 through 8, however, the animals regained a smooth swimming style and surpassed their previous best times. Variant dosages of d-amphetamine were found to have a biphasic effect on the swimming speed of rats (Latz, Kornetsky, Bain, & Goldman, 1966). Compared to the placebo, dosages of 1.0 and 2.0 mg•kg^{-1} body wt had no significant effect on swimming speed, a dosage of 4.0 mg•kg^{-1} body wt enhanced swimming speed, and a dosage of 8.0 mg•kg^{-1} body wt impaired swimming speed. However, all dosages of amphetamine were found to impair swimming speed when compared with the pretreatment swim times, thus making interpretation of the results difficult.

Using highly trained runners and swimmers, Smith and Beecher (1959) conducted an extensive study on the effects of amphetamine on athletic performance. Many of the swimming and running events they tested were of such distance that the effect of amphetamine on speed was confounded by a possible endurance factor. However, their results are noteworthy. In general, swimming times for the 100-yard freestyle and butterfly and the 200-yard freestyle, breaststroke, and backstroke were improved by an average of 0.59-1.16%. All six runners who participated in races of 600 and 1,000 yards on an indoor track improved their times following ingestion of amphetamine. The average improvement was approximately 1.0%. In a follow-up study, Smith, Weitzner, and Beecher (1963) examined the effect of amphetamine on the swimming speed of expert and nonexpert swimmers. They found that 24 of the 32 experts had significantly better times with amphetamine than with placebo. Only 3 of 32 nonexperts showed significant improvement. They suggested that the performances by the nonexperts were so inconsistent that whatever effect amphetamine might have had was impossible to measure.

Research Findings of Detrimental or Indefinite Effects

Aerobic Endurance

Only two studies have found no improvement in aerobic endurance after acute administration of amphetamine. Sommerville (1946) subjected two groups of 50 subjects to a 17-hour march. One hour before the end of the march, one group received 15.0 mg of amphetamine and the other group a placebo. At the end of the march, the subjects' state of fatigue was evaluated by how fast they could negotiate an obstacle course. He observed no differences in performance between the groups. However, when amphetamine was given more time to take effect and its dosage increased, Sommerville (1946) found a significantly better performance by the amphetamine group. Thus, the failure of Sommerville to demonstrate a significant effect on the first experiment is probably attributable to an inadequate dose of amphetamine, administered at an inappropriate time.

Using a repeated measures design, Cooter and Stull (1974) reported that 4.0, 8.0, 12.0, and 16.0 mg•kg^{-1} body wt of dl-amphetamine, administered by stomach tube at 30, 60, 90, and 120 minutes prior to testing, had no effect on the swimming endurance of rats. Two points should be made about this study. First, the swim time to exhaustion for each amphetamine treatment was greater than that of the control. Second, Bhagat and Wheeler (1973b) have reported that, with repeated swims to exhaustion, rats learn that each submersion of sufficient duration is rewarded by rescue from the water, and therefore they are less motivated to swim to complete exhaustion. That the rats repeatedly refused to swim to exhaustion in Cooter and Stull's study is supported by the large standard deviations in swim time. In fact, the standard deviations indicate that some of the rats were thought to be exhausted after approximately 1 minute of swimming. Even though the rats were weighted (5.5% of body wt), this is highly unlikely and not supported by other studies (Bhagat and Wheeler, 1973a, 1973b).

Only one study has investigated the impact of chronic administration of amphetamine on endurance performance. Rats were treated with 10.0 mg•kg^{-1} body wt of methamphetamine/day for 6 weeks. The amphetamine was added to their drinking water. Following the 6 weeks' treatment, the average swim time for the rats receiving amphetamine was 18% greater than the swim time of the controls. This difference, however, was not statistically significant (Estler & Gabrys, 1979).

Local Muscle Endurance

Studies by Foltz, Schiffrin, and Ivy (1943), Karpovich (1959), and Golding and Barnard (1963) showed no beneficial effect of amphetamine during the performance of rapidly exhausting work. Foltz, Schiffrin, and Ivy (1943) did find that bench-stepping performance consistently improved with each additional trial. They suggested the use of trained subjects to stabilize performance so that a drug effect might be detectable. In addition to this confounding training effect, the amphetamine administration procedure used by Foltz and colleagues is also of concern. The oral administration of amphetamine 1 hour prior to testing is probably inadequate time for the drug to have its full effect on performance. This latency period between administration and testing also needs to be considered in evaluating the Karpovich (1959) study. In his study, amphetamine was ingested either 30 or 60 minutes before a run to exhaustion on the treadmill. Although Golding and Barnard (1963) waited an adequate amount of time for the amphetamine to take effect, one has to question whether or not their performance test could detect a drug effect. This test consisted of running to exhaustion on a treadmill at a speed of 10.0 miles/hour on an 8.5% grade. The average run time was less than 2 minutes. Chandler and Blair (1980) found that amphetamine significantly increased time to exhaustion by 19.44 seconds for an endurance test lasting slightly more than 7 minutes. Based on this data, the estimated difference in performance between an amphetamine treatment and control treatment, lasting only 2 minutes, would be approximately 5 seconds. It is interesting to note that in Golding and Barnard's study, the average run time to exhaustion for the amphetamine trial was 6 seconds longer than the placebo trial.

Hueting and Poulus (1970) and Williams and Thompson (1973) provided two of the better designed studies examining the effect of amphetamine on work of high intensity. Hueting and Poulus (1970) used dosages of 10.0, 20.0, and 30.0 mg of methamphetamine. They administered the drug intramuscularly 30 minutes before testing. Williams and Thompson (1973) used 5.0, 10.0, and 15.0 mg•70 kg^{-1} body wt of d-amphetamine. They administered the drug orally 2-3 hours before testing. Both studies employed a bicycle ergometer and a progressively increased work load each minute until the subjects could no longer maintain a predetermined cycle cadence, and both studies concluded that amphetamine had no effect on endurance performance.

Adamson and Finlay (1965) also found amphetamine had no effect on muscle endurance of an isotonic nature. The criterion used for muscle endurance was the maximum number of pull-ups that could be executed. Using a double-blind placebo protocol, Graham and Bos (Note 2) studied the effect of 15.0 mg of d-amphetamine on isotonic endurance of the triceps brachii. They recorded muscle action potentials concurrently by electromyography. In agreement with the findings of Adamson and Finlay (1965), Graham and Bos (Note 2) found that amphetamine had no significant effect on the isotonic muscle contractions.

Jacob and Michaud (1961) studied the effect of d-amphetamine on the endurance of mice during a rapidly exhausting swim test. To produce rapid exhaustion, the water temperature was maintained at 20° C. The average swim time was found to be 5.6 minutes. Amphetamine had no effect on muscle endurance. The investigators, however, point out that swimming mice in 20° C water introduces new and complex factors that make interpretation of the effects of the drug difficult.

Singh (1962) investigated the effect of 7.5 mg of d-amphetamine on the ability to maintain two-thirds maximal handgrip strength on a hand dynamometer. A similar study was conducted by Costello (1963) using 10.0 mg of d-amphetamine. Both Singh (1962) and Costello (1963) reported no significant difference between placebo and amphetamine on static muscular endurance. Costello, however, detected a significant improvement when amphetamine and control (no placebo) conditions were compared; and using only women as subjects, as opposed to men and women combined, Costello (1963) successfully demonstrated that amphetamine, in comparision to placebo, significantly enhanced static muscular endurance.

Strength

After examining the effects of d-amphetamine and methamphetamine on a battery of isometric strength tests, Cuthbertson and Knox (1947) concluded that these drugs had little effect on muscular strength. They provided little information about their experimental protocol; thus, a critical evaluation of the data is impossible. Blyth, Allen, and Lovingood (1960) studied the effects of 5.0 mg of d-amphetamine on strength before, during, and after exposure to a high ambient temperature. They measured strength by standard hand, back, and leg dynamometer tests and computed total strength by summation of the scores. Their results indicated that amphetamine had no effect on total strength under any of the conditions tested. However, the dosage of amphetamine they administered was small. As discussed previously, this same laboratory found a significant improvement in strength following the administration of 15.0 mg of d-amphetamine (Lovingood et al., 1967). Adamson and Finlay (1965) were also unable to demonstrate that amphetamine significantly enhanced isometric strength.

Graham and Bos (Note 2) investigated the effect of amphetamine on isotonic strength by monitoring the electrical activity of the triceps brachii during contraction. They observed similar electromyographic recordings for the amphetamine and placebo treatments and concluded that amphetamine did not affect isotonic strength. Chandler and Blair (1980) used a bicycle ergometer to test the effect of amphetamine on muscular power of the legs. After a

30-second warm-up at a light work rate, the resistance was increased to 4 kg and the subject was signaled to commence pedaling as fast as possible. The total time required to execute five cycling revolutions was determined and a power rating calculated. The results indicated that amphetamine had no effect on muscle power.

Reaction Time

Thornton et al. (1939) found no beneficial effect of 20.0 mg d-amphetamine on visual or auditory reaction time. However, their experiment involved only three subjects. Blyth et al. (1960) investigated the effects of 5.0 mg of d-amphetamine on simple reaction time and a number of other psychomotor parameters under normal and stress conditions. Their results indicated that amphetamine had neither a beneficial nor deleterious effect on any of the psychomotor measures used, including reaction time. In a follow-up study, they employed a similar experimental design but increased the dosage of d-amphetamine to 15.0 mg. Again the drug treatment did not significantly decrease reaction time, although a trend in this direction was noted ($p < .07$) (Lovingood et al., 1967). Kornetsky (1958) studied the effect of 5.0 and 15.0 mg of d-amphetamine, and Wenzel and Rutledge (1962) the effect of 2.5, 5.0, and 10.0 mg of d-amphetamine on simple and choice reaction time. Statistical analysis of the data revealed that amphetamine failed to enhance either type of reaction time. Goldstein, Searle, and Schimke (1960) studied the effect of amphetamine on simple and contingent reaction time. Their data did not indicate that amphetamine produced a beneficial effect. Pierson, Rasch, and Brubaker (1961) measured the reaction time and movement time of 26 subjects after each had ingested 20.0 mg of amphetamine or placebo. Each subject was tested under both conditions. They observed no drug effect. Studying decision reaction time and movement time, DiMascio and Buie (1964) concluded that 10.0 or 15.0 mg of d-amphetamine had no effect on either parameter. The only study that did not demonstrate a positive effect of amphetamine on the reaction time of fatigued subjects was by Cuthbertson and Knox (1947). However, because of the use of a novel task, a significant learning effect was found. Thus, Cuthbertson and Knox concluded that their reaction time test was invalid.

Speed

Goldstein et al. (1960) found no improvement in tapping rate following the ingestion of 10.0 mg of d-amphetamine. Similar results were reported by Blum, Stern, and Melville (1964) for 10.0 mg of dl-amphetamine. Blyth and others (1960) studied the effects of 5.0 mg of d-amphetamine under normal conditions and environmental stress. No significant effect was reported. In addition, Adler et al. (1950) found that 10.0 mg d-amphetamine did not restore tapping rate that had decreased in a simulated altitude of 18,000 feet.

Bättig (1963) investigated the effect of 1.5 and 4.0 mg•kg^{-1} body wt of dl-amphetamine on the swimming speed of rats. He reported that the 1.5 mg•kg^{-1} body wt dosage did not affect speed but that the 4.0 mg•kg^{-1} body wt dosage impaired swimming speed. Uyeno (1968) also found that a high dose of d-amphetamine (46.6 μmoles•kg^{-1} body wt, approximately 6 mg•kg^{-1} body wt) impaired the swimming speed of rats. Lower dosages, however (11.7 and 23.3 μmoles•kg^{-1} body wt), had no effect.

Using human subjects, Haldi and Wynn (1946) investigated the effects of 5.0 mg of dl-amphetamine on the time to swim 100 yards. Under the influence of the dl-amphetamine, time to swim the 100 yards was 0.6 seconds faster than after taking the placebo; however, this difference was not statistically significant. At any rate, 5.0 mg is a light dose and should not be expected to have too great an effect on performance. Karpovich (1959) examined the effect of 10.0-20.0 mg of dl-amphetamine on swimming and running speed. Using criterion swim tests of 100, 220, and 440 yards, he reported that amphetamine had no significant effect on performance. Karpovich also reported no significant effect upon the competitive running performance of 11 track men in events ranging from 100-yards to 2-mile runs. Obviously, an endurance component is inherent in some of these tests, but even in the shorter events amphetamine produced little alteration in performance. Chandler and Blair (1980) conducted probably the best study of the effects of amphetamine on speed. Their test was designed to measure peak running speed and acceleration. They reported that 15.0 mg•70 kg^{-1} body wt of d-amphetamine had no effect on peak running speed, although it significantly improved acceleration.

Summary and Conclusions

The evidence overwhelmingly suggests that amphetamines extend aerobic endurance and hasten recovery from fatigue. The mechanism by which amphetamines yield such effects has not been established. Lehmann and others (1939) could find no improved cardiovascular adjustments after amphetamine ingestion, although work time to exhaustion was increased. Other investigators have demonstrated that amphetamines have no effect on submaximum (Chandler & Blair, 1980; Pirnay, Petit, Dujardin, Deroanne, Juchmes, & Bottin, 1960; Venerando, Gesmundo, & Dal Monte, 1966) or maximum oxygen consumption (Chandler & Blair, 1980; Margaria, Aghemo, & Rovelli, 1964). Lehmann et al. (1939) concluded that amphetamines in no way improved physiological mechanisms. Instead they suggested that this drug increased motivation via central nervous system stimulation and extended the limits of performance of the subjects so that they could use up more of the reserves that normally protect the individual from excessive exhaustion. Although central nervous system stimulation is a feasible explanation, more recent studies suggest that metabolic alterations, particularly related to substrate availability, may contribute significantly to the improved endurance capacity seen following amphetamine administration.

It has been demonstrated that amphetamines cause a rise in blood free fatty acids (Estler et al., 1970; Opitz, 1970; Pinter & Pattee, 1968). Normally, the rate of free fatty acid uptake by the muscle cell is roughly proportional to the concentration of fatty acids to which it is exposed (Paul, 1970). Several investigators have shown that when free fatty acid levels are raised during muscle activity there is an increased reliance on fatty acid oxidation and a subsequent decrease in carbohydrate usage (Costill et al., 1977; Rennie et al., 1976). Moreover, this carbohydrate sparing mechanism has been shown to result in an increased endurance capacity (Hickson et al., 1977). There is some circumstantial evidence suggesting that the enhanced aerobic endurance produced by amphetamines is due to a similar process. First, propranolol, a beta adrenergic receptor blocker, inhibits the release of free fatty acids and attenuates the spontaneous motor activity caused by amphetamines (Estler et al., 1970; Mantegazza et al., 1970). Second, amphetamines lower the respiratory exchange ratio of resting animals (Estler et al., 1970), indicating an increased lipid oxidation. Third, Chatterjee, Jacob, Srivastava, Pabral, and Ghose (1970) found a decrease in blood lactate during a standardized submaximal exercise test following the administration of 1.0 to 2.0 mg kg^{-1} body wt of amphetamine. An increase in lipid oxidation during exercise produces the same effect (Hickson et al., 1977; Ivy et al., 1981).

Reduced endurance capacity has also been observed when high concentrations of amphetamines are administered. The reason for this reduced capacity has not been ascertained. However, Gerald and Hsu (1975) discovered that high concentrations produce neuromuscular blockade by a curare-like mechanism. High concentrations of amphetamines also cause disorientation and confusion (Griffith et al., 1972; Kay & Birren, 1958). The neuromuscular blockade could reduce endurance capacity by inhibiting motor unit recruitment. Disorientation and confusion could result in loss of motor control and a decreased metabolic efficiency. In addition, high concentrations of amphetamines have been shown to cause an abnormally high rise in blood lactate during exercise. Although it has been suggested that lactate *per se* may not cause impairment of muscle performance (Fitts & Holloszy, 1976), it has been demonstrated by Fuch, Reddy, and Briggs (1970) and Nakamura and Schwartz (1972) that the dissociated hydrogen ion from lactate can interfere with excitation-contraction coupling.

From the available information it would appear that aerobic endurance can be improved by an appropriate dosage of amphetamine. The literature is divided as to whether or not amphetamines are beneficial during intense endurance work. Assuming they are capable of increasing local muscle endurance, it is clear that this is not a result of improved cardiorespiratory function. It is also highly improbable that amphetamines directly improve anaerobic capacity. More likely, amphetamines delay the sensations of fatigue allowing the subjects to work longer and to accumulate more lactate. Blocking these sensations, however, could be potentially hazardous, especially under extreme environmental conditions.

The majority of studies tends to support the position that amphetamines can increase static muscular strength. As discussed by Graham and Bos (Note 2) and later by Williams (1974) the principal type of work during athletics is isotonic in nature. Thus, it is doubtful that increased static muscular strength would be of significant benefit to performance.

There is very little information concerning the effects of amphetamines on isotonic strength and power, and the data that are available are inconsistent. For example, Chandler (Note 3) reported an improvement in muscular power following the administration of amphetamine but reported just the opposite results in a later study (Chandler & Blair, 1980). Prudence, therefore, dictates that a decision concerning the effect of amphetamine on isotonic strength and power be withheld until more definitive information is available.

On the basis of recent literature, it is suggested that amphetamines are incapable of improving the reaction time of alert, motivated, not-fatigued subjects. On the other hand, amphetamines appear to be capable of restoring reaction time retarded by physiological or environmental stress. Davis (1947), Hauty and Payne (1957), and Kornetsky et al. (1959) all concluded that amphetamines improve performance on psychomotor tasks by increasing alertness and motivation. In this regard, the most documented effect of amphetamines is their ability to produce a state of arousal or wakefulness (Bradley & Elkes, 1957).

There appears to be no general trend related to the effect of amphetamines on speed. The contradictory results appear to be due to differences in experimental designs and the criteria for assessing speed.

Although amphetamines appear to improve several physiological components thought to be related to athletic success, it cannot be concluded with certainty that they can enhance athletic performance. This is particularly true for more complex sports activities such as baseball, basketball, and tennis. In addition, the use of amphetamines to improve performance is not without risk. Amphetamines reduce blood flow to the cutaneous tissue (Griffith et al., 1972), and thus could cause hyperthermia during physical activity, especially in a hot and humid environment. High concentrations of amphetamines can result in neuromuscular blockade (Gerald & Hsu, 1975); disorientation and confusion (Griffith et al., 1972; Kay & Birren, 1958); and hallucinations and increased anxiety (Kalant, 1973), all of which can be detrimental to performance. Chronic abuse of amphetamines can lead to addiction and damage to the heart and other organs of the body. Also, with repeated use, an increased tolerance to these drugs develops (Kalant, 1973). It therefore seems reasonable to suggest that the risks involved in the use of amphetamines to improve athletic performance far exceed their potential benefits.

Reference Notes

1. American College of Sports Medicine. Report of the committee to study the use of drugs in athletics, 1958.
2. Graham, G., & Bos, R. *The effect of dextro-amphetamine sulfate on integrated action potentials and local muscular fatigue.* Paper presented at AAHPER National Convention, Houston, Texas, 1972.
3. Chandler, J.V. *Effects of amphetamines on athletic performances.* Unpublished independent study, University of South Carolina, 1970.

References

ADAMSON, G., & Finley, S. The effects of two psycho-stimulant drugs on muscular performance in male athletes. *Ergonomics*, 1965, **8**, 237-241.

ADLER, H.F., Burkardt, W.L., Ivy, A.C., & Atkinson, A.J. Effects of various drugs on psychomotor performance at ground level and simulated altitudes of 18,000 feet in a low pressure chamber. *Journal of Aviation Medicine*, 1950, **21**, 221-236.

ALLES, G.A., & Feigen, G.A. The influence of benzedrine on work-decrement and patellar reflex. *American Journal of Physiology*, 1942, **136**, 392-400.

AXELROD, J., Whitby, L.G., & Hertting, G. Effect of psychotropic drugs on the uptake of H^3 - norepinephrine by tissue. *Science*, 1961, **133**, 383-384.

BÄTTIG, K. The effect of training and amphetamine on the endurance and velocity of swimming performance of rats. *Psychopharmacologia*, 1963, **4**, 15-27.

BECKMAN, H. *Drugs—Their nature, action, and use*. Philadelphia: W.B. Saunders, 1958.

BHAGAT, B., & Wheeler, N. Effect of amphetamine on the swimming endurance of rats. *Neuropharmacology*, 1973, **12**, 711-713. (a)

BHAGAT, B., & Wheeler, N. Effect of nicotine on the swimming endurance of rats. *Neuropharmacology*, 1973, **12**, 1161-1165. (b)

BLUM, B., Stern, M.J., & Melville, K.I. A comparative evaluation of the action of depressant and stimulant drugs on human performance. *Psychopharmacologia*, 1964, **6**, 173-177.

BLYTH, C.S., Allen, M., & Lovingood, B.W. Effect of amphetamine (Dexedrine) and caffeine on subjects exposed to heat and exercise stress. *Research Quarterly*, 1960, **31**, 553-559.

BORG, G., Edström, C.G., Linderholm, H., & Marklund, G. Changes in physical performance induced by amphetamines and amobarbital. *Psychopharmacologia*, 1972, **26**, 10-18.

BOUTON, J. *Ball four*. New York: World Publishing, 1970.

BRADLEY, P.B., & Elkes, J. The effects of some drugs on the electrical activity of the brain. *Brain*, 1957, **80**, 77-117.

BUJAS, Z., & Petz, B. Utjecaj fenamina na ekonomicnost staticnog rada. *Arhiz za Higijenu Rada*, 1955, **6**, 205-208.

BURGER, A. (Ed.). *Drugs affecting the central nervous system* (Vol. 2). New York: Marcel Dekker, 1968.

CAMPBELL, D.B. A method for the measurement of therapeutic levels of (+)-amphetamine in human plasma. *Journal of Pharmacy and Pharmacology*, 1969, **21**, 129-130.

CHANDLER, J.V., & Blair, S.N. The effect of amphetamines on selected physiological components related to athletic success. *Medicine and Science in Sports and Exercise*, 1980, **12**, 65-69.

CHATTERJEE, A.K., Jacob, S.A., Srivastava, R.K., Pabrai, P.R., & Ghose, A. Influence of methylamphetamine on blood lactic acid following exercise. *Japanese Journal of Pharmacology*, 1970, **20**, 170-172.

COOTER, G.R., & Stull, G.A. The effect of amphetamine on endurance in rats. *Journal of Sports Medicine*, 1974, **14**, 120-126.

COSTELLO, C. The effect of stimulant and depressant drugs on physical persistence. *American Journal of Psychology*, 1963, **76**, 698-700.

COSTILL, D.L., Coyle, E., Dalsky, G., Evans, W., Fink, W., & Hoopes, D. Effects of elevated plasma FFA and insulin in muscle glycogen usage during exercise. *Journal of Applied Physiology*, 1977, **43**, 695-699.

CUTHBERTSON, D.P., & Knox, J.A. The effects of analeptics on the fatigued subject. *Journal of Physiology*, 1947, **106**, 42-58.

DAVIS, D.R. Psychomotor effects of analeptics and their relation to fatigue phenomena in air crew. *British Medical Journal*, 1947, **5**, 43-45.

DEMBERT, M.L., & Harclerode, J. Effects of $1-\Delta^9$ - tetrahydrocannabinol, dl-amphetamine and pentobarbital on oxygen consumption by mouse brain and heart homogenates. *Biochemical Pharmacology*, 1974, **23**, 947-956.

DIMASCIO, A., & Buie, D.H. Psychopharmacology of chlorphentermine and d-amphetamine—A comparative study of their effects in normal males. *Clinical Pharmacology and Therapeutics*, 1964, **5**, 174-184.

ESTLER, C.J., Fickl, H.P.T., & Fröhlich, H.N. Substrate supply and energy metabolism of skeletal muscle of mice treated with methamphetamine and propranolol. *Biochemical Pharmacology*, 1970, **19**, 2957-2962.

ESTLER, C.J., & Gabrys, M.C. Swimming capacity of mice after prolonged treatment with psychostimulants. II. Effect of methamphetamine on swimming performance and availability of metabolic substances. *Psychopharmacologia*, 1979, **60**, 173-176.

EVANS, W.O., & Jewett, A. The effect of some centrally acting drugs on disjunctive reaction time. *Psychoparmacologia*, 1962, **3**, 124-128.

FITTS, R.H., & Holloszy, J.O. Lactate and contractile force in frog muscle during development of fatigue and recovery. *American Journal of Physiology*, 1976, **231**, 430-435.

FOLTZ, E.E., Ivy, A.C., & Barborka, C.J. The influence of amphetamine (Benzedrine) sulfate and desoxyephedrine hydrochloride (pervitin) and caffeine upon work output and recovery when rapidly exhausting work is done by trained subjects. *Journal of Laboratory and Clinical Medicine*, 1943, **28**, 603-606.

FOLTZ, E.E., Schriffin, J.M., & Ivy, A.C. The influence of amphetamine (Benzedrine) sulfate and caffeine on the performance of rapidly exhausting work by untrained subjects. *Journal of Laboratory and Clinical Medicine*, 1943, **28**, 601-603.

FOWLER, S.C., Filewich, R.J., & Leberer, M.R. Drug effects upon force and duration of response during fixed-ratio performance in rats. *Pharmacology Biochemistry and Behavior*, 1977, **6**, 421-426.

FUCH, F., Reddy, V., & Briggs, F.N. The interaction of cations with the calcium-binding site of troponin. *Biochemistry Biophysica Acta (Amsterdam)*, 1970, **221**, 407-409.

FULLER, R.W., & Hines, C.W. d-Amphetamine levels in brain and other tissues of isolated and aggregated mice. *Biochemical Pharmacology*, 1967, **16**, 11-16.

FUSTER, J.M. Effects of stimulation on brain stem on tachistoscopic perception. *Science*, 1958, **127**, 150-153.

GERALD, M.C. Effects of (+)-amphetamine on the treadmill endurance performance of rats. *Neuropharmacology*, 1978, **17**, 703-704.

GERALD, M.C., & Hse, S.Y. The effects of amphetamine isomers on neuromuscular transmission. *Neuropharmacology*, 1975, **14**, 115-123.

GILBERT, B. Drugs in sport. *Sports Illustrated*, June 23, 1969, **30**, 64-72, (a).

GILBERT, B. Something extra on the ball. *Sports Illustrated*, June 30, 1969, **30**, 30-42, (b).

GILBERT, B. High time to make some rules. *Sports Illustrated*, July 7, 1969, **31**, 30-35, (c).

GOLDING, L. Drugs and hormones. In W. Morgan (Ed.), *Ergogenic aids and muscular performance*. New York: Academic Press, 1972.

GOLDING, L.A., & Barnard, J.R. The effect of d-amphetamine sulfate on physical performance. *Journal of Sports Medicine and Physical Fitness*, 1963, **3**, 221-224.

GOLDSTEIN, A., Searle, B.W., & Schimke, R.T. Effects of secobarbital and d-amphetamine on psychomotor performance of normal subjects. *Journal pf Pharmacological Experimental Therapy*, 1960, **130**, 55-58.

GRIFFITH, J.D., Canaugh. J., Held. J., & Oates, J.A. Dextroamphetamine: Evaluation of psychomimetic properties in man, *Archives of General Psychiatry*, 1972, **26**, 97-100.

GRINKER, J.A., Drewnowski, A., Enns, M., & Kissileff, H. Effects of d-amphetamine and fenfluramine on feeding patterns and activity of obese and lean Zucker rats. *Pharmacology Biochemistry and Behavior*, 1980, **12**, 265-275.

HALDI, J., & Wynn, W. Action of drugs on efficiency of swimmers. *Research Quarterly*, 1946, **17**, 96-101.

HART. J.B., & Wallace, J. The adverse effects of amphetamines. *Clinical Toxicology*, 1975, **8**, 179-180.

HAUTY, G.T., & Payne, R.B. Effects of dextro-amphetamine upon judgment. *Journal of Pharmacology and Experimental Therapeutics*, 1957, **120**, 33-37.

HICKSON, R.C., Rennie, M.J., Conlee, R.K., Winder, W.W., & Holloszy, J.O. Effects of increased plasma fatty acids on glycogen utilization and endurance. *Journal of Applied Physiology*, 1977, **43**, 829-833.

HOLLISTER, L.E., & Gillispie, H.K. A new stimulant, prolintane hydrochloride, compared with dextroamphetamine in fatigued volunteers. *Journal of Clinical Pharmacology*, 1970, **10**, 103-109.

HUETING, J., & Poulus, A. Amphetamine, performance, effort and fatigue. *Pflügers Archives*, 1970, **318**, 260.

HURST, P.M., Radlow, R., & Bagley, S.K. The effects of d-amphetamine and chlordiazepoxide upon strength and estimated strength. *Ergonomics*, 1968, **11**, 47-52.

IKAI, M., & Steinhaus, A.H. Some factors modifying the expression of human strength. *Journal of Applied Physiology*, 1961, **16**, 157-163.

IVY, A.C., & Krasno, L.R. Amphetamine (Benzedrine) sulfate: A review of its pharmacology. *War Medicine*, 1941, **1**, 15-42.

IVY, J.L., Costill, D.L., Van Handel, P.J., Essig, D.A., & Lower, R.W. Alteration in the lactate threshold with changes in substrate availability. *International Journal of Sports Medicine*, 1981, **2**, 139-142.

JACOB, J., & Michaud. G. Actions of various pharmacologic agents on the exhaustion time and behavior of mice swimming at 20°C. I. Description of the technic actions of amphetamine, cocaine, caffeine, hexobarbital and meprobamate. *Archives Internationales de Pharmacodymamie et de Therapie*, 1961, **133**, 101-105.

JOHNSON, L.A. *Amphetamine use in professional football.* Unpublished doctoral dissertation, United States International University, 1972.

KALANT, O.J. *The amphetamines: Toxicity and addiction* (2nd ed.). Toronto: University of Toronto Press, 1973.

KARPOVICH, P.V. Effect of amphetamine sulfate on athletic performance. *Journal of American Medical Association*, 1959, **170**, 558-561.

KAY, H., & Birren, J.E. Swimming speed of the albino rat. II. Fatigue, practice, and drug effects on age and sex differences. *Journal of Gerontology*, 1958, **13**, 378-285.

KIPLINGER, G.F. The effects of drugs on the rate of development of fatigue in mice. *Texas Reports on Biological Medicine*, 1967, **25**, 531-540.

KLEINROK, Z., & Swiezynska, M. The effect on nialamid, pargylin, methylphenidan, amphetamine, carboethoxyphthalazinehydrazine, benzquinamide, and reserpine on the swimming speed of normal and weighted rats. *Acta Physiological Polonica*, 1966, **17**, 549-556.

KNOEFEL, P.K. The influence of phenisopropyl amine and phenisopropyl methyl amine on work output. *Federation Proceedings*, 1943, **2**, 83.

KORNETSKY, C. Effects of meprobomate, phenobarbial and dextro-amphetamine on reaction time and learning in man. *Journal of Pharmacology and Experimental Therapeutics*, 1958, **123**, 216-219.

KORNETSKY, C., Mirsky, A.F., Kessler, E.K., & Dorff, J.E. The effects of dextro-amphetamine on behavioral deficits produced by sleep-loss in humans. *Journal of Pharmacology and Experimental Therapeutics*, 1959, **127**, 46-50.

LATIES, V.G., & Weiss, B. Performance enhancement by the amphetamines: A new appraisal. In H. Brill, J.O. Cole, P. Deniker, H. Hippins, & P.B. Bradley (Eds.), *Proceedings Vth International Congress of the Collegium Internationnale Neuropsychopharmacologium, 1966*, 1967, 800-808.

LATZ, A., Kornetsky, C., Bain, G., & Goldman, M. Swimming performance of mice as affected by antidepressant drugs and baseline levels. *Psychopharmacologia*, 1966, **10**, 67-88.

LEHMANN, G., Straub, H., & Szakáll, A. Pervitan als Leistungssteigernds Mittel. *Arbeitsphysiologie*, 1939, **10**, 680-691.

LEHMANN, H.E., & Csank, J. Differential screening of phrentropic agents in man. *Journal of Clinical Psychopathology*, 1957, **18**, 222-235.

LOVINGOOD, B.W., Blyth, C.S., Peacock, W.J., & Lindsay, R.B. Effects of d-amphetamine sulfate, caffeine, and high temperature on human performance. *Research Quarterly*, 1967, **38**, 65-71.

MAICKEL, R.P., Cox, R.H., Segal, D.S., & Miller, F.P. Studies on psychoactive drugs. I. Physiological disposition and time course of behavioral effects of d-amphetamine in rats. *Federation Proceedings*, 1966, **25**, 385.

MANDELL, A.J. *The nightmare season.* New York: Random House, 1976.

MANDELL, J.A. The Sunday syndrome: A unique pattern of amphetamine abuse indigenous to American professional football. *Clinical Toxicology*, 1979, **15**, 225-232.

MANTEGAZZA, P., Müller, E.E., Naimzada, M.K., & Riva, M. Studies on the lack of correlation between hyperthermia, hyperactivity and anorexia induced by amphetamine. In E. Costa & S. Garattini (Eds.), *International Symposium on Amphetamines and Related Compounds.* New York: Raven Press, 1970.

MARGARIA, R., Aghemo, R., & Rovelli, E. The effect of some drugs on the maximal capacity of athletic performance in man. *Internationale Zeitschrift für Angewandte Physiologie Einschliesslich Arbeitsphysiologie*, 1964, **20**, 281-287.

MOLINENGO, L., & Orsetti, M. Drug action on the "grasping" reflex and on swimming endurance; an attempt to characterize experimentally anti-pressant drugs. *Neuropharmacology*, 1976, **15**, 257-260.

NAKAMURA, Y., & Schwartz, S. The influence of hydrogen ion concentration on calcium binding and release by skeletal muscle sarcoplasmic reticulum. *Journal of General Physiology*, 1972, **59**, 22-32.

OPITZ, K. Adipokinetic action of amphetamine—A study in the beagle dog. In E. Costa & S. Garattini (Eds.), *International Symposium on Amphetamines and Related Compounds*. New York: Raven Press, 1970.

PAUL, P. FFA metabolism of normal dogs during steady-state exercise at different workloads. *Journal of Applied Physiology*, 1970, **28**, 127-132.

PFEIFFER, C.C., & Symthies, J.R. *Neurobiology* (Vol. 12). New York: Academic Press, 1970.

PIERSON, W.R. Amphetamine sulfate and performance. A critique. *Journal of the American Medical Association*, 1961, **177**, 345-347.

PIERSON, W.R., Rasch, P.J., & Brubaker, M.L. Some psychological effects of the administration of amphetamine sulfate and meprobamate on speed of movement and reaction time. *Medicina Dello Sports*, 1961, **1**, 61-66.

PINTER, E.J., & Pattee, C.J. Fat-mobilizing action of amphetamine. *Journal of Clinical Investigation*, 1968, **47**, 394-402.

PIRNAY, F., Petit, J.M., Dujardin, J., Deroanne, R., Juchmes, J., & Bottin, R. Influence de l-amphetamine sur quelques exercises musculaires effectues par l' individu normal. *Internationale Zeitschrift für Angewandte Physiologie Einschliesslich Arbeitsphysiologie*, 1960, **18**, 280-284.

QUINN, G.P., Cohn, M.M., Reid, M.B., Greengard, P., & Weiner, M. The effect of formulation on phenmetrazine plasma levels in man studied by a sensitive analytic method. *Clinical Pharmacology and Therapeutics*, 1967, **8**, 369-373.

RAY, O.S. *Drugs, society, and human behavior*. St. Louis: C.V. Mosby, 1972.

RENNIE, M.J., Winder, W.W., & Holloszy, J.O. A sparing effect of increased plasma fatty acids on muscle and liver glycogen content in the exercising rat. *Biochemistry Journal*, 1976, **156**, 647-655.

SEASHORE, R.H., & Ivy, A.C. Effects of analeptic drugs in relieving fatigue. *Psychological Monographs*, 1953, **67**, 1-16.

SINGH, S.D. Effects of stimulant and depressant drugs on physical performance. *Perceptual and Motor Skills*, 1962, **14**, 270.

SMITH, G.M., & Beecher, H.K. Amphetamine sulfate and athletic performance. I. Objective effects. *Journal of the American Medical Association*, 1959, **170**, 542-557.

SMITH, G.M., Weitzner, M., & Beecher, H.K. Increased sensitivity of measurement of drug effects in expert swimmers. *Journal of Pharmacology and Experimental Therapeutics*, 1963, **139**, 114-119.

SOMMERVILLE, W. The effect of benzedrine on mental and physical fatigue in soldiers. *Canadian Medical Association Journal*, 1946, **55**, 470-476.

STONE, E.A. Swim—stress-induced inactivity: Relation to body temperature and brain norepinephrine, and effects of d-amphetamine. *Psychosomatic Medicine*, 1970, **32**, 51-59.

THORNTON, G.R., Holck, H.G.O., & Smith, E.L. The effect of Benzedrine and caffeine upon performance in certain psychomotor tasks. *Journal of Abnormal Social Psychology*, 1939, **34**, 96-113.

TYLER, D.B. The effect of amphetamine sulfate and some barbiturates on the fatigue produced by prolonged wakefulness. *American Journal of Physiology*, 1947, **150**, 253-262.

UYEDA, A.A., & Fuster, J.M. The effects of amphetamine on tachistoscopic performance in the monkey. *Psychopharmacologia*, 1962, **3**, 463-467.

UYENO, E.T. Hallucinogenic compounds and swimming response. *Journal of Pharmacology and Experimental Therapeutics*, 1968, **159**, 216-221.

VAN ROSSUM, J. Mode of action of psychomotor stimulant drugs. *International Review of Neurobiology*, 1970, **12**, 307-383.

VENERANDO, A., Gesmundo, F., & Dal Monte, A. Azione dell' amfetamina sul rendimento del lavoro muscolare nell' uomo. I. Osservazioni sul consumo di ossigeno. *Bollenttino Della Societa Italiana Di Biology*, 1966, **42**, 613-616.

WEISS, B., & Laties, V.G. Enhancement of human performance by caffeine and the amphetamines. *Pharmacological Review*, 1962, **14**, 1-36.

WENZEL, D., & Rutledge, C. Effects of centrally acting drugs on human motor and psychomotor performance. *Journal of Pharmaceutical Science*, 1962, **51**, 631-644.

WILLIAMS, M.H. *Drugs and athletic performance*. Springfield, IL: C.C. Thomas, 1974.

WILLIAMS, M.H., & Thompson, J. Effect of varient dosages of amphetamine upon endurance. *Research Quarterly*, 1973, **44**, 417-422.

WYNDHAM, C.H., Rogers, G.G., Benade, A.J.S., & Strydom, N.B. Physiological effects of the amphetamines during exercise. *South African Medical Journal*, 1971, **45**, 247-252.

5

Caffeine

Peter Van Handel

The compounds responsible for the stimulating action of coffee, tea, and cocoa are methyl derivatives of xanthine (2,6-dihydroxypurine). They are basically purines, compounds containing two condensed heterocyclic rings, and are naturally occurring chemicals found in leaves, seeds, and fruit of more than 60 species of plants (see Figure 1). Caffeine (1,3,7-trimethylxanthine, molecular weight 194.20) is found in tea, coffee (*Coffea arabica*), cola nuts (*Cola acuminata*), mate and many other plants. Theobramine is found in cocoa (*Theobroma cacao*) and theophylline in tea (*Thea sinensis*). Activity of the xanthines differs. For example, caffeine is most active, theobromine the least, on the central nervous system. General actions include stimulation of (a) the central nervous system; (b) the heart and skeletal muscles; (c) the kidneys, inducing diuresis; (d) respiratory rate and depth; and (e) possibly the adrenal glands. Xanthines may also induce relaxation of smooth muscle, stimulate gastric secretion, and elevate plasma-free fatty acid and glucose concentrations.

Peter Van Handel, Ph.D., F.A.C.S.M., is with the Sports Physiology Laboratory at the United States Olympic Training Center in Colorado Springs, Colorado.

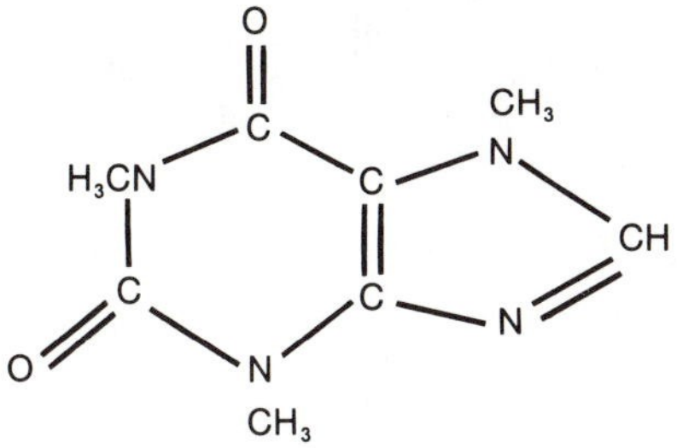

Figure 1—The structure of caffeine. Caffeine and the other xanthines and purine-based compounds consist of two heterocyclic rings containing various numbers of methyl groups.

Review of both *in vivo* and *in vitro* studies, however, would suggest that any ergogenic effects are often unclear and equivocal. That no clear pattern of work enhancement exists is likely due to the following: (a) There is a dose-response effect. (b) There are subject differences in the distribution, metabolism and/or excretion of the drug. (c) There are differences in response between habitual users and nonusers. (d) There are species differences that make extrapolation of animal data tenuous. (e) Studies may have been poorly controlled. (f) The natural sympathetic response to exercise may mask similar responses caused by the xanthine. (g) There may be conflicting responses due to both direct and indirect actions. Further complicating factors include the type of task, fitness level and nutritional status of the subjects, and the environmental conditions.

Regardless of the ability of the xanthines to induce a true ergogenic effect, caffeine has long been considered a doping agent (Venerando, 1963) that could enhance performance or physiological functions (Alles & Feigen, 1942, for review, Grollman, 1930; Pickering, 1893; Rivers & Webber, 1907; Schirlitz, 1930) and that led to suggestions that caffeine or caffeine preparations be prohibited in conjunction with athletic events (Boje, 1939). Although caffeine was reported to be one of the few drugs capable of enhancing athletic performance (Mustala, 1967), the Medical Commission of the British Commonwealth Games (1971) reported that the caffeine present in coffee was not regarded as a doping agent. In 1972 the International Olympic Committee removed caffeine from its list of doping agents. This is perhaps due to the equivocal nature of xanthine effects and to the fact that caffeine is a constituent of many common beverages and over-the-counter drugs (see Table 1).

In spite of questions concerning the ergogenic action (Perkins & Williams, 1975) and possible links to infarction (Jick, Mittinen,

Table 1
Caffeine Content of Some Common Items

Soft drinks		mg/12 oz	
Colas (in general)		46-53	
Coca Cola		33, 65[a]	
Diet Rite		32	
Dr. Pepper		38, 61	
Mellow Yellow		51	
Mountain Dew		54, 55	
Pepsi Cola		38, 43	
Tab		32, 49	
Royal Crown Cola		26, 33	

Coffee	mg/serving	per 6 oz	per cup
Drip	146	181	-
Instant	66	54	80-90
Percolated	110	125	150
"Decaffeinated"	-	-	15-25

Tea (depends upon brewing time)	weak	medium	strong
Red Rose	45	62	90
Tetley	18	48	70
English Breakfast	26	78	107

Cocoa/chocolate	
Chocolate candy	240-270 mg/12 oz
Chocolate milk	72 mg/12 oz
Cocoa	13 mg/serving

Over-the-counter drugs	(mg/tablet)		
Anacin	32.5	Empirin	32
Aqua-ban	100	Excedrine	64
Aspirin	15-30	Midol	32.4
Caffedrine	200	No Doz	100
Dexatrim	200	Vanquish	33
Dristan	16	Vivarin	200

Note: Taken from Bunker & McWilliams, 1976; Burg, 1975a; FDA Fact Sheet, 1971; Truitt, 1971; Wolman, 1955.

[a]Similar items are given different values for caffeine content by various authors.

Neff, Shapiro, Heinonen, & Slone, 1973); arrhythmias (Prineas, Jacobs, Crow, & Blackburn, 1980); and other deleterious effects such as diuresis, insomnia, withdrawal headache, diarrhea, anxiety, tremulousness, and irritability (Stephenson, 1977; Victor, Lubetsky, & Greden, 1981), use of caffeine as an aid to performance has increased in recent years. This is perhaps due to its popularization in the lay literature as an enhancer of endurance performance. Interestingly, the International Olympic Committee has again banned "high levels" of caffeine, those likely attained by injections or suppositories.

Mechanism of Xanthine Action

The ability of caffeine or the other xanthines to aid sports performance (more generally work output) is based upon direct action on the heart or skeletal muscles and/or indirect actions on these organs mediated through the nervous system, altered hormone activity, or shifts in the mobilization of substrates. There is also the possibility that the drug may alter the release, binding, or activity of neurotransmitters in the brain, thus affecting "perception" of work intensity.

More specifically, the xanthines may exert their effects (a) through antagonism of adenosine receptors (Fredholm, 1980); (b) by inhibition of enzyme activity such as that of phosphodiesterase (Beavo, Rogers, Crofford, Hardman, Sutherland, & Newman, 1970), catechol-O-methyltransferase (Kalsner, 1977) or phosphorylase (Kavinsky, Shechosky, & Fletterick, 1978; Steiner, Greer, Bhat, & Oton, 1980); (c) by altering the release (Fabiato & Fabiato, 1975; Weber & Herz, 1968) or uptake (Weber, 1968) of calcium by the sarcoplasmic reticulum; (d) by altering the calcium permeability of the sarcolemma (Kavaler, Anderson, & Fisher, 1978); or (e) by facilitating neuromuscular impulse transmission (Breckenridge, Burn, & Matshinsky, 1967; Varagic & Zugic, 1971).

Once absorbed, caffeine distributes in the tissues in approximate proportion to their water content, and the subsequent physiological response is proportional to the concentration (Axelrod & Reichenthal, 1953). Thus, dosage, body composition (fat content), and hydration state may be important factors related to the subjects' response(s). If one also considers the response differences between those who are "abstainers" versus chronic coffee/ caffeine drinkers (Goldstein, Kaizer, & Whitby, 1969; Goldstein, Warren, & Kaizer, 1965; Robertson, Wade, Workman, Woosley, & Oates, 1981) and that some subjects are intrinsically less sensitive to caffeine than others (Goldstein et al., 1965), it is easy to account for the large interindividual variations noted in many studies. Moreover, it may be possible to ascribe some of the adverse reactions (Costill, Dalsky, & Fink, 1978; Essig, Costill, & Van Handel, 1980; Fishbach, 1970, 1972; Victor et al., 1981) and observations of "susceptibility" (Little, Shanoff, Csima, & Yano, 1966) to these same factors. For these reasons, a careful evaluation of subject status and methodology must be made when comparing human and animal subjects.

Even more tenuous are attempts to relate *in vitro* data to *in vivo* observations. As an example, studies using oral ingestion in humans and administration by gavage for rats, guinea pigs, and rabbits indicate that there are species differences in the metabolism of the drug such that kinetic data allow calculation of equivalences only in terms of caffeine plasma levels (Second International Caffeine Workshop, 1980). There also appear to be differences between the muscle fiber types and species in the ability of caffeine to potentiate twitch responses (Bianchi, 1962; Chuck & Parmley, 1980; Fabiato & Fabiato, 1975; Henderson, Claes, & Brutsaert, 1973; Isaacson & Barany, 1973; Kavaler et al., 1978; MacIntosh, Barbee, & Stainsby, 1981; Ugol, Hammack, & Hays, 1981; Wood, 1978).

Absorption, Distribution, and Metabolism

In humans, caffeine solutions empty rapidly from the stomach and are absorbed from the gastrointestinal tract (Axelrod & Reichenthal, 1953). With ingestion of 250 mg, significant amounts appear in the plasma within 15 minutes (Robertson et al., 1981), and peak concentrations are reached at approximately 60 minutes regardless of the dose (Axelrod & Reichenthal, 1953; Bellet, Kershbaum, & Finch, 1968; Robertson et al., 1981). Robertson et al. (1981) have also noted that large interindividual variations exist in this time course. Similarly, Burg (1975b) has indicated that the half-life of caffeine in the blood is 2.0-2.8 hours, so no significant amount remains 24 hours after administration. Axelrod and Reichenthal (1953) described a half-life of 3.5 hours while Robertson et al. (1981) found a t½ for elimination of nearly 10 hours. Regardless of the estimated half-life, the rate appears to be fairly uniform with excretion as single methyl group xanthines and methyl-uric acids. Approximately 1% of the caffeine is excreted unchanged (Axelrod & Reichenthal, 1953). Caffeine and its by-products can be measured in body fluids by spectrophotometric methods so that detection is relatively easy.

Effects on the Central Nervous System

Caffeine is able to pass the blood brain barrier (Oldendorf, 1971) and, as a result, increases the percentage of spontaneously firing units in the sensorimotor cortex (Arushanyan, Belozertsev, & Arvazov, 1974) and the nature of cortical EEG recordings. Increases in locomotor activity in a dose-related manner are also cited as support for a central stimulating action (Thetapandha, Maling, & Gilette, 1972). It has also been suggested that caffeine may act directly on the medullary, vasomotor, and vagal centers (Syed, 1976). Reports of increased alertness and decreased drowsiness are common (Goldstein et al., 1965), and several recent projects have found a reduced perception of fatigue during work tasks (Costill et al., 1978; Essig et al., 1980; Ivy, Costill, Fink, & Lower, 1979). Waldeck (1973) noted that caffeine increases excitability, possibly by reducing neuron threshold. Perhaps this results in an "easier" recruitment of motor units, spreading the tension requirement over a larger muscle mass, thus reducing both the perception of exertion and, as a result, altering the pattern of substrate utilization in the working fibers.

On the other hand, caffeine acts as an antagonist to adenosine receptors in the brain (Second International Caffeine Workshop, 1980; Fredholm, 1980). Adenosine is a neurotransmitter or modulator with depressant, hypnotic, and anticonvulsant properties. These states are antagonized by caffeine. Other neurotransmitters, however, such as norepinephrine, histamine, and serotinin potentiate adenosine-elicited inhibition of central neurons. Therefore, their actions could also be influenced by caffeine. In this regard, the concentration of catecholamines in the blood and urine increases following caffeine administration (Atuk, Blaydes, Westerveldt, & Wood, 1967; Bellet et al., 1968; Bellet, Roman, DeCastro, Kim, & Kershbaum, 1969; Berkowitz & Spector, 1971; Patwardhan, Desmond, Johnson, Dunn, Robertson, Hoyumpa, & Schenker, 1980; Van Handel, Burke, Costill, & Cote, 1977). The increased blood and urinary catecholamine levels are consistent with a generalized stimulation of the sympathetic nervous system due to the direct effect of caffeine on the adrenal medulla (Berkowitz & Spector, 1971). These observations suggest a possible conflict between the direct effects of caffeine on adenosine receptors and the indirect potentiating effects of caffeine-induced catecholamine release.

There is a complex and confusing pattern of central nervous system activity in response to caffeine administration, not the least of which is a dose-response curve. Because the adenosine antagonist action occurs at much lower concentrations than are needed for inhibition of phosphodiesterase (Second International Caffeine Workshop, 1980) and there appears to be a dose-response relationship, it may be suggested that the direct effects of caffeine on perception are paramount over the indirect effects mediated by catecholamines. Indeed, Goldstein et al. have indicated that the autonomic and cardiovascular systems' tolerance to chronic caffeine administration likely originates within the central nervous system; that is, caffeine's stimulation of sympathetic function is mediated by higher brain centers (Goldstein et al., 1969).

Regardless of the mechanism (direct or indirect), caffeine is able to act upon the central nervous system and, at low doses, has marked effects on perception, alertness, and wakefulness (Goldstein et al., 1965) and on fatigue during muscular work (Costill et al., 1978; Ivy et al., 1979).

Effects on the Heart and Vasculature

Cardiovascular effects of xanthine administration are mediated through stimulation of the central nervous system and/or direct action on the heart and vessels. The overall action is to increase systemic pressure (Gould, Manoj Duman Goswami, Ramana, & Gomprecht, 1973; Grollman, 1930; Robertson et al., 1981) such that chronic use has been linked to coronary risk (Jick et al., 1973; Prineas et al., 1980). Epidemiological evidence, however, indicates that coffee as an independent risk factor does not increase the incidence of hypertension (Bertrand, Pomper, Hillman, Duffy, & Micheli, 1978) or myocardial infarction (Hennekens, Drolette, Jesse, Davies, & Hutchison, 1976). Furthermore, it has been found that there is no relationship between the amount of caffeine consumed and the level of serum lipids, that high caffeine doses are required to induce increased lipolysis concomitant with elevated serum triglyceride levels, and that lipolysis is inhibited by simultaneous food intake (Studlar, 1973). Perhaps these differences can be attributed, in part, to the fact that some subjects are intrinsically less sensitive to caffeine than others (Goldstein et al., 1965) and that administration of caffeine (acute or chronic) has different effects on users versus those who abstain from xanthine ingestion (Robertson et al., 1981).

Both the distribution pattern and volume of blood delivered are altered following xanthine administration (Goodman & Gilman, 1965). The former is mediated through a relaxant effect upon vascular smooth muscle tone (Somlyo & Somlyo, 1968) in the coronary, pulmonary, and systemic vessels. It should be noted, however, that similar doses cause vessel constriction in the brain, inducing a decrease in cerebral blood flow, and that there may be a constriction of systemic vessels due to stimulation of the medullary vasomotor center. The fact that the volume and/or the distribution of blood may be altered has interesting implications for the distribution of substrates and waste products during exercise.

As indicated previously, xanthine administration may have a pressor effect. Robertson et al. (1981) reported a significant increase in systolic and, to a lesser degree, diastolic pressures after oral administration of 250 mg caffeine. Van Handel et al. (1977), however, administered fasting adults 10 oz of cola-flavored soft drink containing either 0, 22.5, 35, or 150 mg caffeine and found that only the 150 mg caused a significant increase in mean arterial pressure over control (0 mg caffeine). Lesser, but nonsignificant increases were observed following ingestion of the 22.5- and 35.0-mg solutions. In light of the alterations seen in heart rate and pulse and systolic and diastolic blood pressures, the data suggested that the increases in mean arterial pressure were due to constriction of the vasculature (increased diastolic pressure) and not to an increased stroke output or heart rate. The data also suggested a dose-response relationship.

Several studies indicate that it is unlikely that either a direct effect of caffeine on vascular resistance or increased catecholamine levels can account for observed blood pressure increases (Berkowitz & Spector, 1971; Clutter, Bier, Shak, & Cryer, 1980; Fitzgerald, Hossmann, Hamilton, Reid, Davis, & Dollery, 1979; Robertson, Johnson, Robertson, Nies, Shand, & Oates, 1979). Indeed, caffeine has been reported to have a relaxant effect upon vascular smooth muscle (Somlyo & Somlyo, 1968). Rather, several older papers indicate a positive inotropic effect of methylxanthines on cardiac output (Grollman, 1930; Hess & Haugaard, 1958). Although there may be an increased heart rate, bradycardia is also possible because of the xanthine stimulation of medullary vagal nuclei that, in turn, decreases heart rate (Colton, Gosselin, & Smith, 1968). That cardiac and stroke indexes and oxygen pulse increase following cardiac output is due to enhanced contractility (Crass, 1973; Ivy et al., 1979; Pickering, 1893).

The latter is evidenced by a delayed onset of activation, increased time to peak force, and slower relaxation time (Henderson et al., 1973). The mechanism behind these effects has been related to (a) alterations in the activity or concentration of cyclic AMP (Crass, 1972; Hicks, Shigekawa, & Katz, 1979; Waldeck, 1973); (b) increased mobilization of calcium (Berkowitz, Tarver, & Spector, 1970); and (c) decreased stores of calcium due to increased permeability of the sarcoplasmic reticulum (Blayney, Thomas, Muir, &

Henderson, 1978). Kubovetz and Poch (1967) suggested that caffeine-mediated inhibition of phosphodiesterase concomitant with increases in cAMP activity may alter sarcolemmal permeability to calcium. Caffeine may also antagonize the cellular uptake or binding of adenosine. This compound can inhibit the formation of cAMP (Fain, 1977) and calcium exchange (Guthrie & Nayler, 1967). It is interesting that adenosine is thought to be one of the compounds responsible for inducing vasodilation during exercise stress.

It is important to note that the forecited studies on contractility have been done on *in vitro* isolated perfused hearts or papillary muscle/strip preparations. For example, caffeine has been used as a modulator in studies of the traditional length-tension status of contractile tissue. These studies have shown that caffeine is able to alter the slow response to length changes by acting upon both the sarcolemma and the sarcoplasmic reticulum. These observations have raised questions (Chuck & Parmley, 1980) concerning the traditional views of the independence of the Frank-Starling relationship (Gordon, Huxley, & Julian, 1966) and the positive inotropic effects of various agents on cardiac performance (Katz, 1970). Caffeine has been found to (a) reverse the direction of the length-dependent changes in both maximum dF/dt and force, (b) have concentration-dependent effects (> 10 mM), and (c) alter time to peak force at both L_{90} and L_{max}. Whether these alterations in the traditional Frank-Starling relationship occur with caffeine administration *in vivo* is, of course, unknown.

Effects on Skeletal Muscle

Caffeine distributes in the body water, and therefore the greatest amount is concentrated in the skeletal muscle mass (Burg, 1975b). Because tissue response is proportional to xanthine concentration (Axelrod & Reichenthal, 1953), significant effects on muscle could be expected and may include enhanced contractile status, altered patterns of fiber recruitment and substrate mobilization, and shifts in the rate of substrate use. As suggested previously, these actions are mediated by direct action of the xanthine on muscle or indirectly via alterations in hormone status (see Figure 2).

Contractile Status. The xanthines potentiate contractile activity of skeletal muscle in a manner analagous to that described for the heart. Effects described in the literature include (a) facilitation of neuromuscular impulse transmission, (b) potentiation of twitch response *in vitro* nerve-muscle preparations, (c) induction of "con-

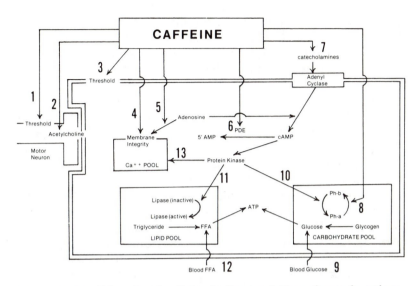

Figure 2—Possible role of caffeine in the regulation of muscle actions. These include both direct and indirect mechanisms (clockwise from the left): alteration of neuron threshold (1), stimulation of neurotransmitter release (2), alteration of sarcolemma threshold (3), alteration of membrane activity related to calcium storage (4), inhibition of adenosine binding (5) and phosphodiesterase activity (6), stimulation of catecholamine release (7), that, in turn, increases cAMP activity. The latter activates protein kinases that turn on glycogenolysis (10), lipolysis (11), and contractility (13). In addition, caffeine may inhibit glycogenolysis (8), increase blood glucose levels (9), and induce FFA mobilization from adipose tissue (12).

tractures" and loss of ability to respond to electrical stimulation with a twitch, (d) potentiation of the contractile capacity of both rested and fatigued muscle *in situ*, and (e) induction of waves of sarcomere contraction ("escalation") following twitches of cultured fibers. These phenomena are apparently related to alterations in the release, uptake, or storage capacity of the sarcoplasmic reticulum for calcium; follow a dose-response pattern; and may show both species and muscle fiber type differences. Again, it is important to note that whether or not these isolated events occur *in vivo* is unknown.

Both aminophylline and caffeine have been found to produce an augmentation of the twitch response of an isolated rodent phrenic nerve-diaphragm preparation caused by either direct or indirect stimulation (Varagic & Zugic, 1971). The data also confirm earlier suggestions that the xanthines may have an effect on neuromuscular impulse transmission (Breckenridge et al., 1967). Varagic and

Zugic (1971) suggested that this effect is perhaps due to a prejunctional action through which the amount of acetylcholine released by a nerve impulse is increased. It may also be true that the xanthines increase neuronal excitability by reducing the threshold of the neurons (Waldek, 1973).

Caffeine has also been used for *in vitro* muscle bath studies of tension development. Hartree added caffeine to normal Ringer's solution and observed enhanced tension production (Hartree & Hill, 1924). Subsequent studies found that caffeine rapidly penetrated the muscle fibers (Bianchi, 1962), inducing shortening from resting length and potentiating electrically induced twitches at low concentrations while causing "contractures" at high doses. Changes in length were independent of electrical activity at the sarcolemma (Bianchi, 1961; Isaacson & Sandow, 1967), yet were mediated by Ca^{++} release. This shortening from resting length has been found to be more pronounced in frog sartorius than gastrocnemius (Bianchi, 1962), suggesting fiber type differences in response to caffeine administration. Ugol, for example, noted that as with frog muscle, electrically induced twitches of rodent sartorius were potentiated by low doses of caffeine. Higher doses resulted in contracture and loss of ability to respond to electrical stimulation with a twitch. Unlike sartorius, however, soleus produced biphasic tension development and also was able to relax in the presence of caffeine. The speed of tension development and of relaxation were dependent upon the caffeine dose. Measurement of high energy phosphate content and calcium indicated that relaxation was not caused by loss of either of these compounds from the cell (Ugol et al., 1981).

Methylxanthines are also able to induce, in cultured fibers, a phenomenon known as "escalation" (Coleman & Coleman, 1980). Whether these events occur *in situ* or *in vivo* is unknown, but it is reasonable to suggest that escalation, if it does occur, may be responsible, in part, for observed changes in resting length or rate changes in relaxation following twitch. As previously indicated, addition of an appropriate amount of methylxanthine induces twitches or contractures within a second or two after it reaches the fibers. With cultured fibers, this is followed by a brief period of quiescence (15-30 seconds) before waves of escalation occur. A wave is detected as a local change in the appearance of the fiber; a band of brightness covering about five sarcomeres. It starts at one point (labeled the indicator site), and there may be a "twitch" involving the A and I bands of only two or three of the affected sarcomeres. Each of these localized twitches results in the generation of a wave that spreads in all directions. Waves equidistant from the initiation point spread in opposite directions along the fiber. If the initiator repeatedly fires in rhythmic fashion, a series of waves moves in opposite directions. A single fiber can have numerous sites initiating waves at the same time, and active sites may become quiescent while an adjacent site becomes active. The waves do not usually diminish in intensity but continue for hundreds of microns until they collide with a wave moving in the opposite direction. All "escalation" ceases instantly with initiation of a normal twitch and resumes one or two seconds after relaxation has occurred.

Other compounds that can induce escalation resemble the xanthines in their twitch potentiating properties or their ability to block the activity of the enzyme phosphodiesterase. Other observations include: (a) There are species and fiber type differences. (b) Escalation activity increases with increasing external calcium concentration. (c) Though there is a need for the presence of divalent cations, activity doesn't depend upon the membrane resting potential. (d) The phenomenon is related to caffeine-induced local release of calcium from sarcoplasmic reticulum that, in turn, induces further release along the sarcoplasmic reticulum but not enough to induce a full twitch. The actual mechanism of this effect, however, has not been elucidated (Coleman & Coleman, 1980). The fact that escalation is related to the caffeine-induced local release of calcium provides insight into caffeine's ability to alter the state of "fatigue" that recently has been suggested to be due to altered ability to sequester calcium (Bianchi & Narayan, 1982). These studies suggest four possible intracellular mechanisms by which caffeine directly alters length dependence and twitch characteristics of the contractile state. Caffeine may (a) rapidly release calcium from the sarcoplasmic reticulum (Fabiato & Fabiato, 1975; Weber & Herz, 1968); (b) decrease the rate of calcium uptake by the sarcoplasmic reticulum (Weber, 1968); (c) increase the calcium permeability of the sarcolemma (Kavaler et al., 1978) and/or vesicles (Blayney et al., 1978); and (d) as a phosphodiesterase inhibitor, increase intracellular cyclic AMP levels (Butcher & Sutherland, 1962). The last, in turn, may induce protein kinase catalyzed phosphorylation and increase Ca^{++} uptake by the reticulum calcium pump (Hicks et al., 1979). Recently it has been suggested that caffeine's effects on skeletal muscle contractility may be mediated by all four of the above cited events (Chuck & Parmley, 1980).

Caffeine has also been used to study the contractile response of fatigued muscle in that fatigue may be due to a redistribution of calcium within the cell (Bianchi & Narayan, 1982), making less available for release. Stainsby and co-workers have recently found that caffeine potentiates the contractile capacity of both fatigued and rested skeletal muscle stimulated *in situ* (MacIntosh et al., 1981). Addition of caffeine to the muscle perfusate (20 to 40 ng/liter) increased the isometric twitch response of stimulated dog gastrocnemius-plantaris. The increase (absolute or relative value) was always greater for the fatigued versus the rested muscles. The authors concluded that either muscle fatigue due to repeated stimulation was not due to redistribution of Ca^{++} within the cell or that caffeine makes available additional calcium not normally available (i.e., bound in sarcoplasmic reticulum or sequestered in mitochondria).

What is clear from the forecited studies is that caffeine directly induces changes in the capacity for storage, uptake, or release of intracellular calcium, the last a known modulator of contractility. The question is, however, how does caffeine exert these effects? At least two studies suggest that caffeine may induce a loss of membrane integrity resulting in permeability changes. Electronmicroscopy studies have found that exposure to 10 mM caffeine disrupts the sarcoplasmic reticulum (Huddart & Oates, 1970), whereas frog muscle exposed to 5 mM caffeine has a greater space accessible to ^{14}C-sucrose (normally a membrane-impermeant compound) used as a probe for whole muscle extracellular space (Isaacson & Barany, 1973).

As a final note on contractility, it should be mentioned that caffeine and other methylxanthines can increase glycogenolysis (Mac-Cornack, 1977; Strubelt, 1969; Syed, 1976) due to alterations in cyclic AMP levels. There may also be a potentiating effect with epinephrine to increase glucose-6-phosphate levels. The increases in the latter compound have been shown to increase contractility (Bowman & Raper, 1964). As a consequence of the increased contractility there is an increased oxygen pulse (Ivy et al., 1979), increased tissue oxygen consumption (Hoffman, 1976; Manchester, Bullock, & Roetzscher, 1973; Novotony & Bianchi, 1967), and an increased a-v0_2 difference (Grollman, 1930).

Substrate Mobilization and Use. The second major area of caffeine effects is on muscle substrate mobilization and use and includes alterations in the major lipid and carbohydrate storage pools (adipose and liver tissues, respectively) as well as direct actions on muscle itself. Potentially these actions may provide the most dramatic effects on work output under *in vivo* conditions. The mechanism is dependent upon altering the concentration or activity of cyclic AMP or of several regulating enzymes. Again, it is important to note that many of the reported effects of xanthine administration in *in vitro*, isolated preparations are contradictory when considered in intact systems or as factors in total body home-ostasis.

Glucose Homeostasis. Caffeine alters glucose homeostasis, reportedly having a hyperglycemic action (Cheraskin, Ringsdorf, Setyaadmadja, & Barrett, 1967; MacCornack, 1977; Syed, 1976) via activation of phosphorylase in liver tissue (Berthet, Sutherland, & Rall, 1957). The likely mechanism is dependent upon either caffeine-induced increases in blood catecholamine levels (Bellet et al., 1969; Berkowitz & Spector, 1971; Berkowitz et al., 1970; Van Handel et al., 1977) or a direct inhibition of phosphodiesterase (Butcher, Ho, Meng, & Sutherland, 1965; Butcher & Sutherland, 1962). Both lead to an increase in the intracellular concentration or activity of cyclic AMP. Cyclic AMP, in turn, activates a protein kinase which accelerates phosphorylase activity stimulating hepatic glycogenolysis (Strubelt, 1969; Syed, 1976). Interestingly, caffeine, via direct actions in muscle, may exert the opposite effects resulting in glycogen "sparing." As a result of the stimulation of hepatic glycogenolysis, there appears to be a release of glucose into the peripheral system that concurrently induces insulin secretion (Studlar, 1973), thus potentially making the glucose available for peripheral uptake and metabolism.

Whether this sequence of events occurs *in vivo* is unclear, however, since the adipokinetic effects (see below) of caffeine (Anderson, Hollefiedl, & Owen, 1966; Bellet et al., 1968; Butcher & Baird, 1969; Butcher et al., 1965; Butcher & Sutherland, 1962; Cheung, 1967; Davis, 1968; Dole, 1961) are well established and would likely suppress peripheral glucose uptake and oxidation via the glucose-free fatty acid cycle (Randle, Newsholme, & Garland, 1964). Recent *in vivo* studies on muscle (Essig et al., 1980; Essig & White, 1981) in fact suggest reduced carbohydrate use following caffeine administration. Thus, the observed hyperglycemia may be due to a reduced peripheral glucose uptake rather than to an increased hepatic output (Van Handel et al., 1977). Caffeine added to the incubation media of *in vitro* adipose tissue preparations has also resulted in a reduced glucose uptake and inhibited lipogenesis (El-Nady, Halfez, Lotfy, & El-banna, 1976) and to an increased lipolysis and oxygen consumption (Anderson et al., 1966). Moreover, small amounts of insulin would inhibit free fatty acid mobilization, and norepinephrine is a potent inhibitor of insulin release (Porte, Graber, Kuzuya, & Williams, 1966). The plasma concentration of both free fatty acids and catecholamines increase following caffeine administration. Increased lipolysis following caffeine ingestion has been related to retarded insulin secretion (Wachman, Hattner, George, & Bernstein, 1970). Low insulin levels act as a barrier to muscle glucose uptake, preserving hepatic glycogen stores (Pruett, 1970).

Blood Lipids. Caffeine stimulates lipolysis in *in vitro* and *in situ* adipose tissue preparations as well as *in vivo* following absorption of ingested xanthine solutions (Bellet et al., 1968; Bellet, Kershbaum, & Aspe, 1965; Anderson et al., 1966; Butcher & Baird, 1969; Butcher et al., 1965; Costill et al., 1978; Davis, 1968; Dole, 1961; El-Nady et al., 1976; Essig et al., 1980; Essig & White, 1981; Fain, 1977; Ivy et al., 1979; Patwardhan, et al., 1980; Stephenson, 1977; Syed, 1976; Wilcox, 1981). The enhanced lipolysis is mediated through the activation of lipase (Davis, 1968; Dole, 1961). Lipase activity is increased by two possible caffeine effects. On the one hand, catecholamines acting at the cell membrane activate adenyl cyclase which, in turn, increases intracellular cyclic AMP levels. The latter activates a protein kinase that accelerates phosphorylation of inactive triglyceride lipase. The activated form increases the hydrolysis of stored triglyceride, in turn increasing the release of free fatty acids and glycerol.

On the other hand, there may be a direct xanthine inhibition of phosphodiesterase (Butcher et al., 1965; Davis, 1968), the enzyme that controls the degradation of cyclic AMP to $5'$-AMP and, as such, also increases the activity of cyclic AMP. The *in vitro* concentration of caffeine needed to inhibit phosphodiesterase such that cyclic AMP levels increase, however, is 10-20 mM (Butcher & Sutherland, 1962; Cheung, 1967). Considering the gastric emptying, absorption, and distribution characteristics of ingested solutions (Axelrod & Reichenthal, 1953; Bellet et al., 1968), it is unlikely that this concentration range is achieved in most *in vivo* studies (Costill et al., 1978; Essig, et al., 1980; Essig & White, 1981; Ivy et al., 1979; Perkins, & Williams, 1975; Van Handel et al., 1977). It should also be noted that significantly less caffeine (1.0 mM) in combination with epinephrine stimulates lipolysis to a much greater degree than does caffeine alone (Butcher & Baird, 1969).

The time course for, and the magnitude of elevation of, plasma free fatty acid levels appears to be related to the dose ingested and perhaps to the nature of the solution. A cola-flavored drink (150 mg caffeine) significantly increased levels (22%) within 15 minutes following ingestion. Values progressively increased during the next 5 hours in resting subjects (Van Handel et al., 1977). Lesser concentrated solutions induced proportionally lower (and nonsignificant) increases over control conditions (0 mg caffeine). Bellet et al. found that plasma free fatty acid levels peaked 3-4 hours after administration (Bellet et al., 1965; Bellet et al., 1968), and Patwardhan recently found a 100% increase after 1 hour following a 250-mg oral dose. Values remained elevated for 4 hours (Patwardhan et al., 1980). Ivy observed that serum free fatty acids were significantly elevated relative to control only after 90 minutes of isokinetic cycling (Ivy et al., 1979), and Essig recently showed that the magnitude of free fatty acid increase with ingestion of 5 mg caffeine/kg body wt (mean approximately 385 mg) was 63% greater than control after 1 hour rest. Values fell substantially at the start of exercise and were not significantly different from control during the exercise task (Essig et al., 1980).

The blood fatty acid profile may change in response to caffeine administration. Patwardhan et al. (1980) found that while each individual free fatty acid rose following oral ingestion of 250 mg caffeine, the relative composition in the blood was altered. For example, 16:0 palmitic acid and 18:0 steric acid decreased from 31.6% and 14% to 27.0% and 12.3%, respectively, while 18:1 oleic increased from 31.6% to 37.8% of the total.

Both the time course for, and the magnitude of, increase in plasma free fatty acids following caffeine ingestion are important considerations for the interpretation of ergogenic effects; that is, the suggestions that increased mobilization from adipose tissue stores and subsequently an increased uptake and oxidation by skeletal muscle "spares" carbohydrate and thus provides for a greater work output and/or time to exhaustion (Costill et al., 1978; Ivy et al., 1979).

Availability of fuels is not considered to be a factor for short-term intense work tasks. Lack of carbohydrate in recruited muscle fibers, however, is acknowledged to be related to exhaustion during endurance exercise (Costill, Jansson, Gollnick, & Saltin, 1974; Gollnick, Armstrong, Saubert, Sembrowich, Shephard, & Saltin, 1973). Although both free fatty acid mobilization and peripheral utilization of lipid progressively increase with time during submaximal work (Carlson, Liljedahl, & Wirsen, 1965; Costill, Coyle, Dalsky, Evans, Fink, & Hoopes, 1977; Froberg, Rossner, & Ericsson, 1978; Hagenfeldt & Wahren, 1971; Hickson, Rennie, Conlee, Winder, & Holloszy, 1977; Ivy et al., 1979; Paul, Issekutz, & Miller, 1966; Rennie, Winder, & Holloszy, 1976; Spitzer & Gold, 1964), carbohydrate remains a necessary carbon source for muscle metabolism. As has been indicated previously, caffeine may have a hyperglycemic action, possibly providing additional glucose for muscle uptake and oxidation. High rates of fatty acid oxidation, however, suppress carbohydrate utilization (Paul et al., 1966) by altering the phosphofructokinase and pyruvate dehydrogenase reactions (Bremer, 1965; Neely, Bowman, & Morgan, 1968; Randle, 1963; Randle et al., 1964). Because increasing blood free fatty acid levels result in an increased uptake by the muscle (Hagenfeldt & Wahren, 1971; Spitzer & Gold, 1964), it has been proposed (Costill et al., 1978; Ivy et al., 1979) that the caffeine-induced increases in blood free fatty acids would induce shifts in substrate utilization, slowing glycolysis, "sparing" carbohydrate, and thus enhancing endurance performance.

This view is, in part, based upon earlier observations using a heparin treatment to induce increases in blood free fatty acid levels. This action is secondary to activation of lipoprotein lipase in capillary endothelium (Olivecrona, Hernell, & Egelrud, 1975) and the rise is rapid and short-lived in contrast to the effects of caffeine. Rennie, for example, subjected rodents to a fatty meal/heparin treatment that increased plasma free fatty acids 200% above controls at rest and 100% during prolonged exhaustive exercise (Rennie et al., 1976). These differences were associated with a "sparing" of glycogen in red muscle (50% depletion vs. 75% in controls) and liver (23% vs. 83%) and higher blood glucose levels following exhaustive exercise. There were no effects in fast-twitch white muscle, probably due to the low ability for fatty acid oxidation (Baldwin, Klinkerfuss, Terjung, Molé, & Holloszy, 1972). Similar observations have been made on human subjects in which, relative to controls, plasma free fatty acids were elevated 323% concomitant with a 40% decrease in muscle glycogen utilization during 30 minutes of work at approximately 70% $\dot{V}O_2$ max (Costill et al., 1977).

There are several important aspects to the forecited observations that need to be considered. First, it should be noted that although Costill and co-workers (1977) reported significant shifts to fat oxidation based upon respiratory exchange, plasma free fatty acids were not significantly elevated prior to, or during the time period when, glycogen "sparing" was suggested to occur in the caffeine studies. Moreover, the absolute free fatty acid levels were considerably lower than those reported for the diet/heparin studies (approximately 0.35 mM vs. 1.01 mM) at the start of exercise. In light of suggestions that uptake and oxidation of free fatty acids is roughly proportional to delivery rate to the muscle (Hagenfeldt & Wahren, 1971), it is unclear how the estimated lipid utilization (based upon $\dot{V}O_2$ and respiratory exchange) averaged 1.30 g/min and 0.72 g/min in the caffeine and heparin studies, respectively. Exercise intensities were nearly equivalent (80% max, 3.3 liter O_2/min and 70% max, 3.0 liter O_2/min). Equivalent amounts of fatty acid could only be delivered if flow patterns were markedly altered with caffeine administration, a possible (Goodman & Gillman, 1965) though unlikely event.

Secondly, blood lactic acid levels were reported to be slightly higher in the caffeine versus the placebo trials (Costill et al., 1978; Essig et al., 1980). This is in spite of significantly lower respiratory exchange and carbohydrate utilization data in the caffeine trials. These observations clearly suggest differences between the caffeine and heparin protocols for inducing carbohydrate "sparing."

Direct Measures of Muscle Lipid and Carbohydrate Use. Indirect estimates of *in vivo* carbohydrate and lipid utilization during exercise have implicated caffeine as a modulator of substrate mobilization, uptake, and metabolism. Essig et al. have recently provided information suggesting that although caffeine may increase use of blood-borne free fatty acids, it also affects muscle triglyceride use as well.

In one project, subjects cycled for 30 minutes at 70% of VO_2 max. Five mg caffeine/kg body wt was ingested 1 hour prior to exercise. Although there was an 18% increase in plasma free fatty acids by the start of exercise, glycogen use in the vastus lateralis was decreased by 42% and triglyceride use increased by 60% over control conditions. There was a large degree of subject variability in response to the caffeine dose. Estimates of substrate oxidation based upon respiratory exchange indicated that the subjects utilized 22% less carbohydrate during the 30 minutes of exercise following the caffeine ingestion. It was clear that caffeine altered use of endogenous muscle triglyceride (Essig et al., 1980).

In a second study (Essig & White, 1981), rats were administered isovolumic gavages of caffeine in 5, 10, or 15 $\mu g/g$ body wt doses 1 hour prior to beginning a treadmill exercise task (1 hr at 0.7 mph, 15% slope). At the start of exercise, no changes were found in the glycogen or triglyceride content of the plantaris muscle. Following exercise, the glycogen content was 81, 60, and 54% of pre-exercise values for the 5, 10, and 15 $\mu g/g$ groups, respectively. Control animals administered 0.9% NaCl had postexercise glycogens averaging 83% of initial values. Caffeine, in a dose-related manner, induced a greater glycogen use during exercise in this muscle. Triglyceride values were 240% greater postexercise for all experimental groups.

In contrast, any caffeine dose was related with lowered soleus glycogen content (50%) and increased triglyceride stores (40%) in the 1 hour following administration of the drug. Exercise further reduced glycogen by 56, 80, and 58% of pre values for the caffeine-treated animals (5, 10, and 15 $\mu g/g$, respectively) and 52% for controls. The absolute reduction in glycogen resulting from exercise, however, was 1.8, 0.8, 2.0, and 3.8 mg/g respectively. Following exercise, triglyceride contents were 69, 67, 59, and 140% of pre values. The authors concluded that in the soleus, the caffeine-induced reduction in absolute glycogen use during exercise is, in part, due to the initial decrease prior to exercise. In other words, the more glycogen available, the more was used, but caffeine was able to induce some sparing. They also suggested that the difference in response of the muscles was likely due to recruitment patterns and that there were dose-response and saturation effects.

An *in vitro* study supports the forecited observations on muscle lipid use. Crass (1972) found that theophyline produced a concentration-dependent stimulation of lipolysis and triglyceride fatty acid oxidation in working hearts. The effect was due to the inhibition of phosphodiesterase that was secondary to the release of tissue catecholamines. There was also a concomitant enhancement of contractile performance and glycogenolysis. Addition of exogenous free fatty acids to the perfusing media inhibited theophyline-stimulated lipolysis of endogenous triglyceride. In another related study, Bellet et al. (1965) have observed that caffeine administered intramuscularly increased plasma free fatty acid levels.

These data clearly support the suggestion that the "sparing" of carbohydrate and improved endurance performance following caffeine administration are, at least in part, due to the altered rates of metabolism of intracellular substrate as opposed to increased uptake and oxidation of mobilized free fatty acids. The latter may contribute to the modulation of muscle triglyceride pools (Dagenais, Tancredi, & Zierler, 1976; Froberg et al., 1978; Stankiewicz-Choroszucka & Gorski, 1978; Zierler, 1976).

These effects on carbohydrate and fat metabolism may be mediated through either direct or indirect mechanisms. Indirectly, enhanced uptake and oxidation of free fatty acids mobilized from adipose tissue depots (Hagenfeldt & Wahren, 1971; Spitzer & Gold, 1964) or the use of endogenous muscle triglyceride free fatty acids (Essig et al., 1980; Essig & White, 1981) may result in the accumulation of citrate. The latter has been shown, in *in vitro* kinetic enzyme studies, to act on both the pyruvate dehydrogenase (Taylor & Halperin, 1973) and phosphofructokinase (Mansour, 1972a) reactions, slowing glycolysis.

This theory, however, fails to consider compartmentation of metabolites within the cell. Cheema-Dhadli and Halperin (1976) have shown that increased levels of long-chain fatty acyl-CoA and/or increased beta oxidation results in a higher Km for the mitochondrial citrate transporter. As a consequence, mitochondrial citrate concentration increases, in turn decreasing the relative proportion of active pyruvate dehydrogenase (Taylor & Halperin, 1973) and the influx of pyruvate carbon into the mitochondria. Assuming a constant glycolytic flux, there is a channeling of pyruvate carbon into alanine or lactic acid (Mole, Baldwin, Terjung, & Holloszy, 1973). As the Km for the citrate transporter increases, cytosolic citrate concentration decreases, potentially increasing glycolytic flux (Cheema-Dhadli & Halperin, 1976). It is important to note that the aforementioned caffeine and diet/heparin studies (Costill et al., 1977; Costill et al., 1978; Hickson et al., 1977; Ivy et al., 1979; Rennie et al., 1976) have suggested that it is the increased cystosolic citrate inhibiting phosphofructokinase activity that is responsible for slowing carbohydrate use. Williamson et al. have indicated that the total tissue content of a metabolite provides a poor estimate of its concentration in a particular cellular compartment (Williamson, Ford, Illingworth, & Safer, 1976). If, using citrate as an example, there are large concentration gradients across the mitochondrial membrane, one can misinterpret data based upon measures of total tissue levels of the metabolite. It is interesting to note in this regard that the two recent caffeine studies involving human subjects have reported that blood lactic acid levels were elevated relative to control, suggesting increased rather than decreased glycolytic flux following caffeine administration (Costill et al., 1978; Essig et al., 1980). It may also be that as mitochondrial acetyl CoA levels increase due to enhanced lipid oxidation and a new steady state for the Krebs Cycle intermediates is achieved, there is an increased removal of intermediates and the flux goes directly to three carbon acids alanine and lactate (Lee & Davis, 1979). In light of the rodent data of Essig and White (1981), it may be suggested that there are fiber type and recruitment pattern differences involved such that blood lactic acid levels do not necessarily reflect the metabolic picture in the various exercising muscles. Depending upon the fiber type, tension requirements, and recruitment patterns, caffeine administration may have different overall effects.

Caffeine may also act directly in muscle to inhibit glycogenolysis. Kavinsky et al. (1978) in a series of kinetic and x-ray crystallographic studies, found that 1 mM caffeine induced a synergistic inhibition of phosphorylase a with both glucose or glucose-1-phosphate. While phosphorylase can be noncovalently activated by the binding of AMP, the negative allosteric effector glucose binds to a site nearby. Near this latter site is a second effector site that preferentially binds nucleotides including caffeine and adenosine. Thus there is synergistic inhibition by glucose (or glucose-1-phosphate) and the second ligand that binds at the nucleotide site. The combined action of the two promotes an inactive conformation that is susceptible to the activity of phosphorylase phosphatase. The phosphatase converts the active (a) form to phosphorylase b that releases the bound phosphatase. The latter, in turn, subsequently dephosphorylates and activates glycogen synthetase. Caffeine appears to induce a similar conformational changes in phosphorylase b (Steiner et al., 1980) and may also act in a like manner on the phosphofructokinase reaction (Mansour, 1972b). Interestingly, it has also been reported that caffeine induces and promotes glycogenolysis in skeletal muscle through the activation of phosphorylase (Gemmill, 1947). The recent data of Essig & White (1981) tend to support this observation. Whether the latter effect is due to the direct effect of caffeine upon phosphorylase b or mediated indirectly through catecholamine effects on the adenyl cyclase system producing cyclic AMP that, in turn, stimulates glycogenolysis (Himms-Hagen, 1967) is unknown (Bowman & Nott, 1969; Varagic & Zugic, 1971).

Research Findings on the Ergogenic Effects of the Xanthines

Two factors need to be considered when discussing the ergogenic effects of the xanthines. First, and perhaps not so obvious, is the question of what is an "ergogenic" effect? Strictly speaking, *ergogenic* has been defined as improving work or exercise performance (Fox, 1979) and an ergogenic aid is any factor that improves work performance (Fox & Mathews, 1981). As an example, if work is considered to be the application of force through distance, it is difficult to see how a reduction in reaction time (a caffeine effect) can be considered as ergogenic in nature unless power is affected and is an important factor in the movement.

Secondly, there are methodological considerations that make interpretation of the data difficult. These include (a) use of different xanthine doses and compounds, (b) too few subjects, (c) uncontrolled extraneous variables that could affect performance, and (d) use of questionable protocols to answer the proposed question. As an example, even two of the most recent studies involving human subjects (Costill et al., 1978; Ivy et al., 1979) gave male and female subjects of considerably different body weights and of reportedly different normal daily caffeine intakes absolute caffeine doses that, when expressed in relative terms to body weight, are some 50% greater for the lighter individuals as compared to the heavier subjects. Moreover, the former study administered the caffeine in a solution that also contained 5 g of decaffeinated coffee. Five grams decaffeinated coffee was also present in the control drink. Decaffeinated coffee has been reported to contain 15-25 mg caffeine/cup (Wolman, 1955) as well as trigonelline and chlorogenic, tanic, caffeic, quinic, acetic, propionic, butyric, and valeric acids; ketones; acetonin; furfural; and a variety of other acidic carbonyl compounds (Merritt & Proctor, 1959; Clements & Deatherage, 1957). What effects these substances may have had cannot be determined.

It should also be noted that there are individual differences in sensitivity and tolerance to the drug (Colton et al., 1968; Goldstein et al., 1969; Goldstein et al., 1965; Robertson et al., 1981) such that a wide variation in response to a given dose can be observed. This makes the ability to achieve statistical significance more difficult. The fact that this significance is not obtained, however, does not mean that for a number of subjects there is no ergogenic effect. Indeed, interpretation of nearly all reported studies is difficult since both positive and negative effects can be related to xanthine administration. For these reasons, the following discussion generalizes the results of the ergogenic effects of caffeine.

Indifferent or Negative Effects

When caffeine is used to modify performance in large-muscle short-term intense exercise requiring strength and power, the studies show essentially no effect. Apparently caffeine's ability to enhance contractility under *in vitro* or *in situ* conditions (Bianchi, 1961, 1962; Chuck & Parmley, 1980; Isaacson & Sandow, 1967; MacIntosh et al., 1981; Varagic & Zugic, 1971) or to alter neuromuscular thresholds (Breckenridge et al., 1967; Varagic & Zugic, 1971; Waldeck, 1973) cannot be translated into improved performance requiring maximal efforts. Caffeine has had no effect on a 100 yd-swim for speed (Haldi & Wynn, 1946), maximal oxygen consumption, or performance time for a treadmill run to exhaustion (Margaria, Aghemo, & Rovelli, 1964); work capacity on the Balke Test (Ganslen, Balke, Nagle, & Phillips, 1964); or maximal heart rate, perceived exertion, and cycling time to exhaustion (Perkins & Williams, 1975). Under these conditions, it is possible that the sympathetic response to work stress is of such a magnitude that it masks the caffeine-induced alterations seen in *in vitro, in situ,* or resting *in vivo* studies, the homeostatic adjustments *in vivo* preclude effects on contractility seen *in vitro* or *in situ*, or that the dose relative to the muscle mass involved is too small.

Positive Effects

There are two types of activities where caffeine may have positive effects upon sports performance. The first is in endurance events, the second in areas requiring increased alertness, decreased reaction time, and lowered anxiety levels. The latter has implications for performance in events such as shooting or archery, where control, concentration, and perception are important.

Bradycardia (Colton et al., 1968) and decreased reaction time can occur following administration of coffee or caffeine (Cheney, 1935; Hawk, 1929; Horst & Jenkins, 1935; Thornton, 1939; Wenzel & Rutledge, 1962; White, Lincoln, Pearce, Reeb, & Vaida, 1980), both of which could be of benefit in events requiring quick discriminative reactions and muscle control. Moreover, as Goldstein and co-workers have indicated, subjects feel more alert and active and have a decreased sensation of drowsiness (Goldstein et al., 1965; Goldstein et al., 1969). In addition, there can be a reduction in tremor or muscle tension as evidenced by altered EMG activity (White et al., 1980).

These positive effects, however, appear to be both dose-related and affected by the amount of caffeine normally consumed by the subject. Several early studies indicated that low caffeine doses had no effects upon reaction time but that higher doses were required. Cheney (1935) noted that reaction time was not affected unless the dose exceeded 3.0 mg/kg body wt and that higher doses impaired performance. Hollingsworth (1912) found that beneficial motor and mental effects occurred when subjects were administered 65-130 mg caffeine, though tremor and poor motor performance were obtained when the dose was 390 mg. In contrast, Thornton (1939) found that, in general, 300 mg caffeine improved reaction time. Wenzel and Rutledge (1962) studied the effects of various doses of caffeine (100-300 mg) on various psychomotor and motor tasks and noted dose-related improvement in simple reaction time and an inverse relationship on complex reaction time. The highest dose tended to result in a general (nonsignificant) decrement in performance. White et al. noted that while there were positive effects of caffeine on a discriminative reaction time test, EMG activity of the volar portion of the right forearm (reflecting muscle tension) was reduced only in individuals labeled as high caffeine consumers (White et al., 1980). They also noted that recent abstinence from caffeine caused an increase in anxiety and muscle tension reactivity in regular caffeine users. Hawk (1929) had observed that withdrawal from coffee drinking (2-6 cups/day) increased reaction time. Administration of caffeine to the high consumer subjects (White et al., 1980) decreased the reaction time and relieved anxiety. Victor et al. (1981) noted that somatic manifestations including diuresis, insommnia, anxiety, tachycardia, tremulousness, headache, and light-headedness varied with the normal amount of caffeine ingested on a daily basis and with the dose given. Most symptom associations were reported by low or high consumers, low being a consumption of 0-249 mg/day, moderate 250-749 mg/day, and high 750+ mg/day.

These observations suggest that although positive effects of caffeine administration may occur for parameters associated with general perception of well-being or reaction time, it is perhaps equally likely that negative effects may occur depending upon the current caffeine status of the subject. It may also be true that administration of caffeine after a period of forced abstinence may be of benefit to an athlete considered a regular user.

Although caffeine does not enhance maximal work capacity, investigations have indicated that the drug may be of benefit during work of longer duration. It has been reported (Alles & Feigen, 1942) that as far back as the late 1800s caffeine was recognized as an aid to endurance activities. Rivers and Webber (1907) found that caffeine increased the capacity for muscular work as measured by ergographic techniques. Asmussen and Boje (1948) found that 300 mg of caffeine could overcome the effects of fatigue when cycling to exhaustion on the ergometer if the task was of "longer" rather than of "shorter" duration. Schirlitz (1930) and Herxheimer (1960) found that caffeine increased the work output on a cycle ergometer. In their review, Weiss and Laties (1962) suggested that caffeine could prolong work time to exhaustion. Two more recent studies provide further support for these observations.

Ivy et al. (1979) found that during isokinetic cycling for a 2-hour duration, administration of a total of 500 mg caffeine significantly (7.4%) increased work production by trained cyclists. Oxygen consumption showed a parallel increase while perception of exertion remained unchanged. Because heart rates were also unaffected, the oxygen pulse was elevated during the caffeine trial, suggesting a greater stroke volume and/or an enhanced a-v O_2 difference. Estimates of substrate utilization based upon oxygen consumption and respiratory exchange data suggested that caffeine enhanced the use of lipids during the last half of the exercise task. In a companion study, cyclists were asked to ride at 80% of $\dot{V}O_2$ max until voluntary exhaustion. The subjects were able to continue for 90+ minutes in the caffeine trial as opposed to 75 minutes in a control trial. There were no differences between trials for heart rate or $\dot{V}O_2$, but the perceived exertion was lower in the caffeine trial. This suggested to the authors that under some conditions perceived exertion scales may not serve as an accurate index of metabolic stress (Costill et al., 1978). The mechanism behind the increased rate of work production and total work output was suggested to be due to an enhanced lipid utilization.

Studies on animals have confirmed these observations and have demonstrated that performance is enhanced and that both uptake of free fatty acids and the use of muscle triglyceride may be responsible for the "carbohydrate sparing" (Essig & White, 1981; Rennie et al., 1976; Villa & Panceri, 1973).

As an interesting sidelight, caffeine has also been used in diet preparations formulated to promote weight loss. Means et al. demonstrated that the basal metabolic rate increases substantially with caffeine administration (Means, Aub, & DuBois, 1947). Indeed, overconsumption can lead to a continued low-grade fever (Reimann, 1967). As a result of its negligible energy values and the forecited thermogenic properties, it has been suggested that caffeine may be of value in weight-reducing regimens. Two recent animal studies support these suggestions. Compared to saline-treated control rats, caffeine administered prior to exercise increased the extent to which fat was utilized from epididymal and retroperitoneal fat pads. The author concluded that fat loss with exercise is increased when caffeine (2.5 mg/kg body wt) is ingested prior to exercise (Wilcox, 1981). Merkel et al. noted that, depending upon the experimental condition, caffeine may both enhance or decrease both food and water intake, as a result lowering caloric consumption (Merkel, Wayner, Jolicoeur, & Mintz, 1981).

Summary

In vitro and *in situ* studies have demonstrated that a wide variety of physiological effects can be linked to xanthine administration. These include a general stimulation of the central nervous system, mobilization of hormones and various tissue substrates and metabolites, and a potentiation of muscle contractile status. That these events occur *in vivo* is less clear, likely due to the fact that homeostatic mechanisms may modulate the response as seen in isolated tissues. This is perhaps even more true during exercise when the natural sympathetic response may mask those due to xanthine administration.

In spite of these problems, caffeine administration has been found to enhance performance, especially of an endurance nature. This is due to alterations in the mobilization and rate of utilization of carbohydrate and fat. There may also be increases in neuronal excitability, possibly reducing the threshold of motor neurons and thereby altering fiber recruitment patterns and/or the perception of work.

Several final points regarding these research studies should be emphasized. (a) There are species differences in the response to xanthine administration. (b) There are both dose and susceptibility considerations. For the latter, the extent of caffeine normally consumed and the length of abstinence play a role in the nature of the response. (c) Oral ingestion is markedly different from perfusion or other forms of administration, making distribution and concentration considerations important. In this regard, the nature of the media in which caffeine is given should be considered. For example, decaffeinated coffee contains many other chemicals, the effects of which have not been ascertained. Lastly, whole body homeostasis needs to be considered as opposed to isolated tissue effects obtained under *in vitro* or *in situ* conditions.

References

ALLES, G., & Feigen, G. The influence of benzedrine on work decrement and patellar reflex. *American Journal of Physiology*, 1942, **136**, 392-400.

ANDERSON, J., Hollefiedl, G., & Owen, J.A. Effects of caffeine on the epididymal fat pad in vitro. *Clinical Research*, 1966, **14**, 60-67.

ARUSHANYAN, E.B., Belozertsev, A.Y., & Arvazov, K.G. Comparative effect of amphetamine and caffeine on spontaneous activity of sensorimotor cortical units and their responses to stimulation of the caudate nucleus. *Bulletin of Experimental Biology and Medicine*, 1974, **78**, 776-779.

ASMUSSEN, E., & Boje, O. The effects of alcohol and some drugs on the capacity to work. *Acta Physiologica Scandinavica*, 1948, **15**, 109-118.

ATUK, N.O., Blaydes, M.C., Westerveldt, P.O., & Wood, J.E. Effect of aminophylline on urinary excretion of epinephrine and norepinephrine in man. *Circulation*, 1967, **35**, 745-753.

AXELROD, J., & Reichenthal, J. The fate of caffeine in man and a method for its estimation in biological material. *Journal of Pharmacology and Experimental Therapeutics*, 1953, **107**, 519-523.

BALDWIN, K.M., Klinkerfuss, G.H., Terjung, R.L., Mole, P.A., & Holloszy, J.O. Respiratory capacity of red, white and intermediate muscle: Adaptive response to exercise. *American Journal of Physiology*, 1972, **222**, 373-378.

BEAVO, J.A., Rogers, N.L., Crofford, O.B., Hardman, J.G., Sutherland, E.W., & Newman, E.V. Effects of xanthine derivatives on lipolysis and on adenosine $3'5'$-monophosphate phosphodiesterase activity. *Molecular Pharmacology*, 1970, **6**, 597-603.

BELLET, S., Kershbaum, A., & Aspe, J. The effect of caffeine on free fatty acids. *Archives of Internal Medicine*, 1965, **116**, 750-752.

BELLET, S., Kershbaum, A., & Finch, E. Response of free fatty acids to coffee and caffeine. *Metabolism*, 1968, **17**, 702-707.

BELLET, S., Roman, L., DeCastro, O., Kim, K.E., & Kershbaum, A. Effect of coffee ingestion on catecholamine release. *Metabolism*, 1969, **18**, 288-291.

BERKOWITZ, B., & Spector, S. Effect of caffeine and theophylline on peripheral catecholamines. *European Journal of Pharmacology*, 1971, **13**, 193-196.

BERKOWITZ, B., Tarver, J.H., & Spector, S. Release of norepinephrine in the central nervous system by theophylline and caffeine. *European Journal of Pharmacology*, 1970, **10**, 64-71.

BERTHET, J., Sutherland, E.W., & Rall, T.W. The assay of glucagon and epinephrine with use of liver homogenates. *Journal of Biological Chemistry*, 1957, **229**, 351-354.

BERTRAND, C.A., Pomper, I., Hillman, G., Duffy, J.G., & Micheli, I. No relation between coffee and blood pressure. *New England Journal of Medicine*, 1978, **299**, 315-316.

BIANCHI, C.P. Effect of caffeine on radiocalcium movement in frog sartorius. *Journal of General Physiology*, 1961, **44**, 845-858.

BIANCHI, C.P. Kinetics of radiocaffeine uptake and release in frog sartorius. *Journal de Pharmacologie*, 1962, **138**, 41-47.

BIANCHI, C.P., & Narayan, S. Muscle fatigue and the role of transverse tubules. *Science*, 1982, **215**, 295-296.

BLAYNEY, L., Thomas, H., Muir, J., & Henderson, A. Action of caffeine on calcium transport by isolated fractions of myofibrils, mitochondria, and sarcoplasmic reticulum from rabbit heart. *Circulation Research*, 1978, **43**, 520-526.

BOJE, O. Doping. *Bulletin of the Health Organization of the League of Nations*, 1939, **8**, 439-469.

BOWMAN, W.C., & Nott, M.W. Actions of sympathomimetic amines and their antagonists on skeletal muscle. *Pharmacological Reviews*, 1969, **21**, 27-72.

BOWMAN, W.C., & Raper, C. The effects of adrenalin and other drugs affecting carbohydrate metabolism on contractions of the rat diaphragm. *British Journal of Pharmacology*, 1964, **23**, 184-200.

BRECKENRIDGE, B.M., Burn, J.H., & Matshinsky, F.M. Theophylline, epinephrine and neostigmine facilitation on neuromuscular transmission. *Proceedings of the National Academy of Science (Washington)*, 1967, **57**, 1893-1897.

BREMER, J. The effect of acylcarnitines on the metabolism of pyruvate in rat heart mitochondria. *Biochimica et Biophysica Acta*, 1965, **104**, 581-590.

BUNKER, M.I., & McWilliams, M.E. Caffeine content of common beverages. *Journal of the American Dietetic Association*, 1979, **74**, 28.

BURG, A.W. Effects of caffeine on the human system. *Tea and Coffee Trade Journal*, 1975, **147**, 40. (a)

BURG, A.W. Physiological disposition of caffeine. *Drug Metabolism Reviews*, 1975, **4**, 199-228. (b)

BUTCHER, R.W., & Baird, C.E. The regulation of cAMP and lipolysis in adipose tissue by hormones and other agents. In W. Holmes, L.A. Carlson, & R. Paoletti (Eds.), *Drugs Affecting Lipid Metabolism*. New York: Plenum, 1969.

BUTCHER, R.W., Ho, R.J., Meng, H.C., & Sutherland, E.W. Adenosine $3',5'$-monophosphate in biological materials. II. The measurement of adenosine $3',5'$-monophosphate in tissues and the role of the cyclic nucleotide in the lipolytic response of fat to epinephrine. *Journal of Biological Chemistry*, 1965, **240**, 4515-4523.

BUTCHER, R.W., & Sutherland, E.W. Adenosine $3',5'$phosphate in biological materials. *Journal of Biological Chemistry*, 1962, **237**, 1244-1255.

CARLSON, L.A., Liljedahl, S.W., & Wirsen, C. Blood and tissue changes in the dog during and after excessive free fatty acid mobilization: A biochemical and morphological study. *Acta Medica Scandinavica*, 1965, **178**, 81-107.

CHEEMA-DHADLI, S., & Halperin, M.L. The effect of palmitoyl-CoA and β oxidation of fatty acids on the kinetics of mitochondrial citrate transporter. *Canadian Journal of Biochemistry*, 1976, **54**, 171-177.

CHENEY, R. Comparative effect of caffeine per se and a caffeine beverage (coffee) upon the reaction time in normal young adults. *Journal de Pharmacologie*, 1935, **53**, 304-313.

CHERASKIN, E., Ringsdorf, W.H., Setyaadmadja, A., & Barrett, R. Effect of caffeine versus placebo supplementation on blood glucose concentration. *Lancet*, 1967, **i**, 1299-1300.

CHEUNG, W.Y. Properties of cyclic $3',5'$ nucleotide phosphodiesterase from rat brain. *Biochemistry*, 1967, **6**, 1079-1087.

CHUCK, L.H.S., & Parmley, W.W. Caffeine reversal of length-dependent changes in myocardial contractile state in the cat. *Circulation Research*, 1980, **47**, 592-598.

CLEMENTS, R.L., & Deatherage, F.E. A chromatographic study of some of the compounds in roasted coffee. *Food Research*, 1957, **22**, 222-225.

CLUTTER, W.E., Bier, D.M., Shak, S.D., & Cryer, P.E. Epinephrine plasma metabolic clearance rates and physiologic thresholds for metabolic and hemodynamic actions in man. *Journal of Clinical Investigation*, 1980, **66**, 94-101.

COLEMAN, A.W., & Coleman, J.R. Characterization of the methylxanthine-induced propagated wave phenomenon in striated muscle. *The Journal of Experimental Zoology*, 1980, **212**, 403-413.

COLTON, T., Gosselin, R.E., & Smith, R.P. The tolerance of coffee drinkers to caffeine. *Clinical Pharmacology and Therapeutics*, 1968, **9**, 31-39.

COSTILL, D.L., Coyle, E., Dalsky, G., Evans, W., Fink, W., & Hoopes, D. Effects of elevated plasma FFA and insulin on muscle glycogen usage during exercise. *Journal of Applied Physiology*, 1977, **43**, 695-699.

COSTILL, D.L., Dalsky, G., & Fink, W. Effects of caffeine ingestion on metabolism and exercise performance. *Medicine and Science in Sports*, 1978, **10**, 155-158.

COSTILL, D.L., Jansson, E., Gollnick, P.D., & Saltin, B. Glycogen utilization in leg muscles of men during level and uphill running. *Acta Physiologica Scandinavica, 1974*, **91**, 475-481.

CRASS, M.F. Exogenous substrate effects of endogenous lipid metabolism in the working rat heart. *Biochimica et Biophysica Acta*, 1972, **280**, 71-81.

CRASS, M.F. Heart triglyceride and glycogen metabolism: Effects of catecholamines, dibutyrl cAMP, theophylline and fatty acids. *Recent Advances in the Study of Cardiac Structure and Metabolism*, 1973, **3**, 275-290.

DAGENAIS, G.R., Tancredi, R.G., & Zierler, K.I. Free fatty acid oxidation by forearm muscle at rest, and evidence for an intramuscular lipid pool in the human forearm. *Journal of Clinical Investigation*, 1976, **58**, 421-431.

DAVIS, I. In vitro regulation of the lipolysis of adipose tissue. *Nature*, 1968, **218**, 349-352.

DOLE, V.P. Effect of nucleic acid metabolites on lipolysis in adipose tissue. *Journal of Biological Chemistry*, 1961, **236**, 3125-3128.

EL-NADY, A., Halfez, T.A., Lotfy, R.A., & El-banna, M. Interrelationship between the stimulant effect of caffeine on lipolysis and its effect on glucose utilization and respiration of adipose tissue. *Egyptian Journal of Physiological Sciences*, 1976, **3**, 105-110.

ESSIG, D., Costill, D.L., & Van Handel, P.J. Effects of caffeine injestion on utilization of muscle glycogen and lipid during leg ergometer cycling. *International Journal of Sports Medicine*, 1980, **1**, 86-90.

ESSIG, D.A., & White, T.P. Effects of caffeine on glycogen and triglyceride concentration in the soleus and plantaris muscles of the exercising rat. *Federation Proceedings*, 1981, 513. (Abstract)

FABIATO, A., & Fabiato, F. Dependence of the contractile activation of skinned cardiac cells on the sarcomere length. *Nature (London)*, 1975, **256**, 54-56.

FAIN, J.N. Cyclic nucleotides in adipose tissue. In H. Cramer & J. Schultz (Eds.), *Cyclic 3′,5′ nucleotides: Mechanisms of action*. London: J. Wiley and Sons, 1977.

FDA Fact Sheet. Rockville, MD: U.S. Dept. HEW (PHS), Food and Drug Administration, July 1971. (FDA)72-3003.

FISCHBACH, E. Coffee and sports. *Minerva Medica*, 1970, **61**, 4367-4369.

FISCHBACH, E. Problems of doping. *Medizinische Monatsschrift für Pharmazeuten*, 1972, **26**, 377-381.

FITZGERALD, G.A., Hossmann, V., Hamilton, C.A., Reid, J.L., Davis, D.S., & Dollery, C.T. Interindividual differences in the kinetics of infused norepinephrine in man. *Clinical Pharmacology and Therapeutics*, 1979, **26**, 669-675.

FOX, E.L. *Sports physiology*. Philadelphia: W.B. Saunders, 1979.

FOX, E.L., & Mathews, D.K. *The Physiological Basis of Physical Education and Athletics*. Philadelphia: Saunders College Publishing, 1981.

FREDHOLM, B.B. Are methylxanthine effects due to antagonism of endogenous adenosine? *Trends in Pharmacological Research*, 1980, **1**, 129-132.

FROBERG, S.O., Rossner, S., & Ericsson, M. Relation between triglycerides in human skeletal muscle and serum and the fractional elimination rate of exogenous plasma triglycerides. *European Journal of Clinical Investigation*, 1978, **8**, 93-97.

GANSLEN, R.V., Balke, B., Nagle, F., & Phillips, E. Effects of some tranquilizing analeptic and vasodilating drugs on physical work capacity and orthostatic tolerance. *Aerospace Medicine*, 1964, **35**, 630-633.

GEMMILL, C.L. The effects of caffeine and theobromine derivatives on glycolysis in muscle. *Journal of Pharmacology and Experimental Therapeutics*, 1947, **91**, 292-296.

GOLDSTEIN, A., Kaizer, S., & Whitby, O. Psychotropic effects of caffeine in man. IV. Quantitative and qualitative differences associated with habituation to coffee. *Clinical Pharmacology and Therapeutics*, 1969, **10**, 489-497.

GOLDSTEIN, A., Warren, R., & Kaizer, S. Psychotropic effects of caffeine in man. I. Interindividual differences in sensitivity to caffeine-induced wakefulness. *Journal of Pharmacology and Experimental Therapeutics*, 1965, **149**, 156-159.

GOLLNICK, P.D., Armstrong, R.B., Saubert, C.W., Sembrowich, W.L., Shephard, R.E., & Saltin, B. Glycogen depletion patterns in human skeletal muscle fibers during prolonged work. *Pfluegers Archiv. European Journal of Physiology*, 1973, **344**, 1-12.

GOODMAN, L.S., & Gilman, A. *The pharmcological basis of therapeutics*. New York: Macmillan, 1965.

GORDON, A.M., Huxley, A.F., & Julian, F.J. The variation in isometric tension with sarcomere length in vertebrate muscle fibers. *Journal of Physiology*, 1966, **184**, 170-192.

GOULD, L., Manoj Duman Goswami, C.V., Ramana, R., & Gomprecht, R. The cardiac effects of tea. *Journal of Clinical Pharmacology*, 1973, **13**, 469-474.

GROLLMAN, A. The action of alcohol, caffeine and tobacco on the cardiac output (and its related functions) of normal man. *Journal of Pharmacology and Experimental Therapeutics*, 1930, **39**, 313-327.

GUTHRIE, J.R., & Nayler, W.G. Interaction between caffeine and adenosine on calcium exchangeability in mammalian atria. *Archives of International Pharmacology and Therapeutics*, 1967, **170**, 249-255.

HAGENFELDT, L., & Wahren, J. Metabolism of free fatty acids and ketone bodies in skeletal muscle. In B. Pernow & B. Saltin (Eds.), *Muscle metabolism during exercise*. New York: Plenum, 1971.

HALDI, J., & Wynn, W. Action of drugs on the efficiency of swimmers. *Research Quarterly*, 1946, **17**, 96-101.

HARTREE, W., & Hill, A.V. The heat production of muscles treated with caffeine or subjected to prolonged discontinuous stimulation. *Journal of Physiology*, 1924, **58**, 441-454.

HAWK, P. A study of the physiological and psychological reactions of the human organism to caffeine drinking. *American Journal of Physiology*, 1929, **90**, 380-381.

HENDERSON, A.H., Claes, V.A., & Brutsaert, D.I. Influence of caffeine and other inotropic interventions on the onset of unloaded shortening velocity in mammalian heart muscle. *Circulation Research*, 1973, **33**, 291-302.

HENNEKENS, C.H., Drolette, M.E., Jesse, M.J., Davies, J., & Hutchison, G. Coffee drinking and death due to coronary heart disease. *New England Journal of Medicine*, 1976, **294**, 633-636.

HERXHEIMER, H. Zur Wirkung des Koffeins auf die Sportliche Leistung. *Moenchen Medizinische Wochenschrift*, 1960, **21**, 140-149.

HESS, M.E., & Haugaard, N. The effects of epinephrine and aminophylline on phosphorylase activity of perfused, contracting heart muscle. *Journal of Pharmacology and Experimental Therapeutics*, 1958, **122**, 169-175.

HICKS, M.J., Shigekawa, M., & Katz, A.M. Mechanism by which cyclic adenosine 3'5'-monophosphate-dependent protein kinase stimulates calcium transport in cardiac sarcoplasmic reticulum. *Circulation Research*, 1979, **44**, 384-391.

HICKSON, R.C., Rennie, M.J., Conlee, R.K., Winder, W.W., & Holloszy, J.O. Effects of increased plasma free fatty acids on glycogen utilization and endurance. *Journal of Applied Physiology: Respiratory, Environmental and Exercise Physiology*, 1977, **43**, 829-833.

HIMMS-HAGEN, J. Sympathetic regulation of metabolism. *Pharmacological Reviews*, 1967, **19**, 367-461.

HOFFMAN, W.W. Oxygen consumption by human and rodent striated muscle in vitro. *American Journal of Physiology*, 1976, **230**, 34-40.

HOLLINGSWORTH, H. The influence of caffeine on mental and motor efficiency. *Archiv für Psychologie (Frankfurt am Main)*, 1912, **3**, 1-166.

HORST, K., & Jenkins, W.L. The effect of caffeine, coffee and decaffeinated coffee upon blood pressure, pulse rate and simple reaction time of men of various ages. *Journal of Pharmacology and Experimental Therapeutics*, 1935, **53**, 385-400.

HUDDART, H., & Oates, K. Localization of the intracellular site of caffeine on skeletal muscle. *Comparative Biochemistry and Physiology*, 1970, **36**, 677-682.

ISAACSON, A., & Barany, M. Effects of caffeine on water content, sucrose space and 3-0-methyl glucose uptake of frog semitendinosus muscle. *Federation Proceedings*, 1973, **32**, 346.

ISAACSON, A., & Sandow, A. Quinine and caffeine effects on 45 Ca movements in frog sartorius muscle. *Journal of Physiology*, 1967, **50**, 2109-2128.

IVY, J.L., Costill, D.L., Fink, W.J., & Lower, R.W. Influence of caffeine and carbohydrate feedings on endurance performance. *Medicine and Science in Sports and Exercise*, 1979, **11**, 6-11.

JICK, H., Mittinen, O.S., Neff, R.K., Shapiro, S., Heinonen, O., & Slone, D. Coffee and myocardial infarction. *New England Journal of Medicine*, 1973, **289**, 63-67.

KALSNER, S. Mechanism of potentiation of contractor responses to cate-cholamines in aortic strips. *British Journal of Pharmacology*, 1977, **43**, 379-388.

KATZ, A. Contractile proteins of the heart. *Physiological Reviews*, 1970, **50**, 63-158.

KAVALER, F., Anderson, T.W., & Fisher, V.J. Sarcolemmal site of caffeine's inotropic action on ventricular muscle of the frog. *Circulation Research*, 1978, **42**, 285-290.

KAVINSKY, P.J., Shechosky, S., & Fletterick, R.J. Synergistic regulation of phosphorylase a by glucose and caffeine. *Journal of Biological Chemistry*, 1978, **253**, 9102-9106.

KUBOVETZ, W.R., & Poch, G. The action of imidazole on the effects of methylxanthines and catecholamines on cardiac contraction and phosphorylase activity. *Journal of Pharmacology and Experimental Therapeutics*, 1967, **156**, 514-521.

LEE, S.H., & Davis, E.J. Carboxylation and decarboxylation reactions. Anaplerotic flux and removal of citric acid cycle intermediates in skeletal muscle. *Journal of Biological Chemistry*, 1979, **254**, 420-430.

LITTLE, J.A., Chanoff, H.M., Csima, A., & Yano, R. Coffee and serum-lipids in coronary heart disease. *Lancet*, 1966, **i**, 732-734.

MACCORNACK, R.A. The effects of coffee drinking on the cadiovascular system; Experimental and epidemiological research. *Preventive Medicine*, 1977, **6**, 104-119.

MACINTOSH, B.R., Barbee, R.W., & Stainsby, W.N. Contractile response to caffeine of rested and fatigued skeletal muscle. *Medicine and Science in Sports and Exercise*, 1981, **13**, 95.

MANCHESTER, K.L., Bullock, G., & Roetzscher, U.M. Influence of methylxanthines and local anesthetics on the metabolism of muscle and associated changes in mitochondrial morphology. *Chemical-Biological Interactions*, 1973, **6**, 273-296.

MANSOUR, T.E., Phosphofructokinase. *Current Topics in Cellular Regulation*, 1972, **5**, 1-46. (a)

MANSOUR, T.E. Phosphofructokinase activity in skeletal muscle extracts following administraction of epinephrine. *Journal of Biological Chemistry*, 1972, **247**, 6059-6066. (b)

MARGARIA, R., Aghemo, P., & Rovelli, E. The effect of some drugs on the maximal capacity of athletic performance in men. *Internationale Zeitschrift für Angewandte Physiologie Einschliesslich Arbeitsphysiologie*, 1964, **20**, 281-287.

MEANS, J.H., Aub, J.C., & DuBois, E.F. The effect of caffeine on the heat production. *Archives of Internal Medicine*, 1947, **19**, 832-839.

MEDICAL Commission of the British Commonwealth Games. Prevention and detection of drug taking (doping) at the IX British Commonwealth Games. *Scottish Medical Journal*, 1971, **16**, 364-368.

MERKEL, A.D., Wayner, M.J., Jolicoeur, F.B., & Mintz, R. Effects of caffeine administration on food and water consumption under various experimental conditions. *Pharmacology, Biochemistry & Behavior*, 1981, **14**, 235-240.

MERRITT, M.C., & Proctor, B.E. Effects of temperature during the roasting cycle on selected components of different types of whole bean coffee. *Food Research*, 1959, **24**, 672-676.

MOLÉ, P.A., Baldwin, K.M., Terjung, R.L., & Holloszy, J.O. Enzymatic pathways of pyruvate metabolism in skeletal muscle: Adaptations to exercise. *American Journal of Physiology*, 1973, **224**, 50-54.

MUSTALA, O. Improvement of athletic performance by drugs. *Suomen Laakarilehti*, 1967, **22**, 690-695.

NEELY, J.R., Bowman, R.H., & Morgan, H.E. Conservation of glycogen in the perfused rat heart developing intraventricular pressure. In W.J.Whelan (Ed.), *Control of Glycogen Metabolism*. New York: Academic Press, 1968.

NOVOTONY, I., & Bianchi, C.P. The effect of xylocaine on oxygen consumption in the frog sartorius. *Journal of Pharmacological and Experimental Therapeutics*, 1967, **155**, 450-462.

OLDENDORF, W.H. Brain uptake of metabolites and drugs following carotid arterial injections. *Transactions of the American Neurological Association*, 1971, **96**, 46-50.

OLIVECRONA, T., Hernell, O., & Egelrud, T. Lipoprotein lipase. *Advances in Experimental Medicine and Biology*, 1975, **52**, 269-279.

PATWARDHAN, R.V., Desmond, P.V., Johnson, R.F., Dunn, G.D., Robertson, D.H., Hoyumpa, A.M., & Schenker, S. Effects of caffeine on plasma free fatty acids, urinary catecholamines and drug binding. *Clinical Pharmacology and Therapeutics*, 1980, **28**, 398-403.

PAUL, P., Issekutz, B., & Miller, H.I. Interrelationship of free fatty acids and glucose metabolism in dogs. *American Journal of Physiology*, 1966, **211**, 1313-1320.

PERKINS, R., & Williams, M.H. Effect of caffeine upon maximum muscular endurance of females. *Medicine and Science in Sports*, 1975, **7**, 221-224.

PICKERING, J.W. Observations on the physiology of the embryonic heart. *Journal of Physiology (London)*, 1893, **14**, 383-466.

PORTE, D., Graber, A., Kuzuya, T., & Williams, R. The effect of epinephrine on immunoreactive insulin levels in man. *Journal of Clinical Investigation*, 1966, **45**, 228-236.

PRINEAS, R.J., Jacobs, D.R., Crow, R.S., & Blackburn, H. Coffee, tea and VPB. *Journal of Chronic Diseases*, 1980, **33**, 67-72.

PRUETT, E.D.R. Glucose and insulin during prolonged work stress in men living on different diets. *Journal of Applied Physiology*, 1970, **28**, 199-208.

RANDLE, P.J. Endocrine control of metabolism. *Annual Reviews of Physiology*, 1963, **25**, 291-324.

RANDLE, P.J., Newsholme, E.A., & Garland, P.B. Regulation of glucose uptake by muscle: Effects of fatty acids, ketone bodies and pyruvate and of alloxan diabetes and starvation on the uptake and metabolic rate of glucose in rat heart and diaphragm muscles. *Biochemical Journal*, 1964, **93**, 652-665.

REIMANN, H.A. Caffeinism: A cause of long-continued, low-grade fever. *Journal of the American Medical Association*, 1967, **202**, 131-132. (December 18, 1967)

RENNIE, M., Winder, W.W., & Holloszy, J.O. A sparing effect of increased free fatty acids on muscle glycogen content in exercising rat. *Biochemical Journal*, 1976, **156**, 647-655.

RIVERS, W., & Webber, H. The action of caffeine on the capacity for muscular work. *Journal of Physiology*, 1907, **36**, 33-47.

ROBERTSON, D., Johnson, G.A., Robertson, R.M., Nies, A.S., Shand, D.G., & Oates, J.A. Comparative assessment of stimuli that release neuronal and adrenomedullary catecholamines in man. *Circulation*, 1979, **59**, 637-643.

ROBERTSON, D., Wade, D., Workman, R., Woosley, R.L., & Oates, J.A. Tolerance to the humoral and hemodynamic effects of caffeine in man. *Journal of Clinical Investigation*, 1981, **67**, 1111-1117.

SCHIRLITZ, K. Über caffein bei ermüdender Muskelarbeit. *Internationale Zeitschrift für Angewandte Physiologie Einschliesslich Arbeitsphysiologie*, 1930, **2**, 273-277.

SECOND International Caffeine Workshop. Special Report. *Nutrition Reviews*, 1980, **38**, 196-200.

SOMLYO, A.V., & Somlyo, A.P. Electromechanical and pharmacomechanical coupling in vascular smooth muscle. *Journal of Pharmacology and Experimental Therapeutics*, 1968, **159**, 129-145.

SPITZER, J.J., & Gold, M. Free fatty acid metabolism by skeletal muscle. *American Journal of Physiology*, 1964, **206**, 159-163.

STANKIEWICZ-CHOROSZUCHA, B., & Gorski, J. Effect of decreased availability of substrates on intramuscular triglyceride utilization during exercise. *European Journal of Applied Physiology and Occupational Physiology*, 1978, **40**, 27-35.

STEINER, R.F., Greer, L., Bhat, R., & Oton, J. Structural changes induced in glycogen phosphorylase b by the binding of glucose and caffeine. *Biochimica et Biophysica Acta*, 1980, **611**, 269-279.

STEPHENSON, P.E. Physiologic and psychotropic effects of caffeine on man. *Journal of the American Dietic Association*, 1977, **71**, 240-247.

STRUBELT, O. The influence of respirine, propanolol and adrenal medullectomy on the hyperglycemic actions of theophylline and caffeine. *Archives Internationales de Pharmacodynamie et de Therapie*, 1969, **179**, 215-224.

STUDLAR, M. Über den Einfluss von Caffein auf den Fett-und Kohlenhydratestoffwechsel des Menschen. *Zeitschrift für Ernaehrungswissenschaft*, 1973, **12**, 109-120.

SYED, I.B. The effects of caffeine. *Journal of the American Pharmaceutical Association*, 1976, **16**, 568-572.

TAYLOR, W.A., & Halperin, M.L. Regulation of pyruvate dehydrogenase in muscle: inhibition by citrate. *Journal of Biological Chemistry*, 1973, **248**, 6080-6083.

THETAPANDHA, A., Maling, H.M., & Gilette, J.R. Effects of caffeine and Theophylline on activity of rats in relation to brain xanthine concentrations. *Proceedings for Experimental Biology and Medicine*, 1972, **139**, 582-586.

THORNTON, G. The effects of benzedrine and caffeine upon performance in certain psychomotor tasks. *Journal of Abnormal and Social Psychology*, 1939, **34**, 96-113.

TRUITT, E.B. The xanthines. In J.R. DePalma (Ed.), *Drill's pharmacology in medicine*. New York: McGraw-Hill, 1971.

UGOL, L.M., Hammack, M.J., & Hays, E.T. Caffeine contractures in rat soleus muscle. *Federation Proceedings*, 1981, **40** (3 part 1), 513.

VAN HANDEL, P.J., Burke, E., Costill, D.L., & Cote, R. Physiological responses to cola ingestion. *Research Quarterly*, 1977, **48**, 436-444.

VARAGIC, V.M., & Zugic, M. Interactions of xanthine derivatives, catecholamines and glucose-6-phosphate on the isolated phrenic nerve diaphragm preparation of the rat. *Pharmacology*, 1971, **5**, 275-286.

VENERANDO, A. Doping: Pathology and ways to control it. *Medicine dello Sport*, 1963, **3**, 972-993.

VICTOR, B.S., Lubetsky, M., & Greden, J.F. Somatic manifestations of caffeinism. *Journal of Clinical Psychiatry*, 1981, **42**, 185-188.

VILLA, R., & Panceri, P. Action of some drugs on performance time in mice. Farmaco, *Edizione Pratica*, 1973, **28**, 43-48.

WACHMAN, A., Hattner, R.S., George, B., & Bernstein, D.S. Effects of decaffeinated and nondecaffeinated coffee ingestion on blood glucose and plasma radioimmunoreactive insulin responses to rapid intravenous infusion of glucose in normal men. *Metabolism*, 1970, **19**, 539-546.

WALDECK, B. Sensitization by caffeine of central catecholamine receptors. *Journal of Neural Transmission*, 1973, **34**, 61-72.

WEBER, A. The mechanism of the action of caffeine on sarcoplasmic reticulum. *Journal of General Physiology*, 1968, **52**, 760-772.

WEBER, A., & Herz, R. The relationship between caffeine contracture of intact muscle and the effect of caffeine on reticulum. *Journal of General Physiology*, 1968, **52**, 750-759.

WEISS, B., & Laties, V. Enhancement of human performance by caffeine and the amphetamines. *Pharmacological Reviews*, 1962, **14**, 1-36.

WENZEL, D., & Rutledge, C. Effects of centrally acting drugs on human motor and psychomotor performance. *Journal of Pharmaceutical Science*, 1962, **51**, 631-644.

WHITE, B.C., Lincoln, C.A., Pearce, N.W., Reeb, R., & Vaida, C. Anxiety and muscle tension as consequences of caffeine withdrawal. *Science*, 1980, **209** (4464), 1547-1548.

WILCOX, A. The effects of caffeine and exercise on body weight and adiposity in the rat. *Medicine and Science in Sports and Exercise*, 1981, **13**, 122.

WILLIAMSON, J.R., Ford, C., Illingsworth, J., & Safer, B. Coordination of citric acid cycle activity with electron transport flux. *Circulation Research*, 1976, **38**, 139-151. (Supplement 1)

WOLMAN, W. Instant and decaffeinated coffee. *Journal of the American Medical Association*, 1955, **159**, 250.

WOOD, D.S. Human skeletal muscle: Analysis of Ca^{++} regulation in skinned fibers using caffeine. *Experimental Neurology*, 1978, **58**, 218-230.

ZIERLER, K.L. Fatty acids as substrates for heart and skeletal muscle. *Circulation Research*, 1976, **38**, 459-463.

6

Anabolic Steroids

David R. Lamb

Anabolic steroids are chemical compounds whose structures are similar to those of naturally occurring male and female sex hormones, for example, testosterone and estradiol, respectively. Such compounds can, under certain conditions, promote the synthesis of proteins used to build tissues in the reproductive system and in skeletal muscles. The steroids used in athletics are almost universally those with structures related to male sex hormones, that is, steroids that have androgenic (Gk: "male-producing") properties in addition to their anabolic properties. Accordingly, these substances are also known as androgenic-anabolic steroids. In World War II it was found that anabolic steroids were useful in helping malnourished persons regain body weight; since that time anabolic steroids have been promoted as an aid to the development of muscle mass and strength to enhance athletic performance (Ryan, 1976). Reports are abundant in the scientific and popular literature that many athletes, both males and females, regularly

David R. Lamb, Ph.D., F.A.C.S.M., is with the Department of Physical Education, Health and Recreation Studies at Purdue University in West Lafayette, Indiana.

treat themselves with large doses of anabolic steroids in hopes of achieving a competitive edge (Freed, Banks, Longson, & Burley, 1975; Golding, Freydinger, & Fishel, 1974; Ryan, 1976). Dramatic evidence that anabolic steroids are abused at the highest levels of competition was provided in 1981, when the world record holder in the discus throw was suspended indefinitely from international competition by the International Amateur Athletic Federation after a urine analysis showed evidence that the athlete had used anabolic steroids prior to a major competition (Steroid Bust, 1981).

Questions raised by the continuing abuse of steroids by athletes include the following: (a) What is the scientific basis for believing that anabolic steroids might affect athletic performance positively? (b) Are naturally secreted anabolic steroids responsible for some of the known responses and adaptations of the organism to physical activity? (c) Can the administration of supplementary anabolic steroids improve athletic performance? (d) Is there any potential for harm from the chronic use of anabolic steroids? These questions will now be addressed.

Theoretical Benefits

Accelerated Muscular Growth

Laboratory and Domestic Animals. There is evidence from studies on laboratory rats that anabolic hormones have a limited potential to bind to receptors in the cytoplasm of skeletal muscle fibers and then move to the cell nuclei where they can stimulate the protein synthesis apparatus of the cells (Michel & Baulieu, 1980; Rogozkin, 1979). However, Dohm, Tapscott, and Louis (1979) were unable to detect any effect of testosterone treatment for 7 days on protein synthesis or degradation in hind limb muscles of the rat. *Small doses* of androgenic-anabolic steroids usually cause increased nitrogen retention, increased lean body weight, and enhanced musular growth in *castrated* male rats (Kochakian, 1976; Krotkiewski, Kral, & Karlsson, 1980), in castrated male cattle (Heitzman, 1976), in normal male rats forced to eat a constant diet (Kochakian & Endahl, 1959), in normal female cattle (Heitzman, 1976), in normal female chickens and turkeys (Nesheim, 1976), and in normal female rats (Kochakian, 1976).

Large doses of testosterone-like drugs in *castrated* male rats cause a brief rise in body weight followed by a sharp *drop* in weight to levels below those observed in nontreated castrated control rats (Kochakian & Endahl, 1959). In *normal* male rats allowed to eat freely, androgenic steroids depress appetite and cause a marked *reduction* in body weight (Hervey & Hutchinson, 1973; Kochakian & Endahl, 1959). Androgens have no substantial effect on weight gain in normal male cattle (Heitzman, 1976; VanderWal, 1976), in normal male chickens and turkeys (Nesheim, 1976), or in pigs (Fowler, 1976). In fact, in normal male cattle and sheep, *estrogenic* compounds such as estradiol and diethylstilbesterol are used to enhance meat production; androgens have little or no effect (Heitzman, 1976; Trenkle, 1976; VanderWal, 1976). (It is curious that there are no reports of studies where human male athletes attempted to gain body mass with estrogen treatment.) Neither androgens nor estrogens are effective in producing weight gain in normal male pigs (Fowler, 1976).

It can be concluded from studies of laboratory and domestic animals that, in those species where a positive effect of steroids on lean body mass is observed, such an effect is unlikely unless the animal has low levels of naturally occurring androgenic hormones, for example, castrated males or female animals. Androgenic supplements to sexually intact male animals generally have little or no effect on lean body mass.

Anabolic steroids are said to have a "myotrophic" effect; that is, they stimulate growth of skeletal muscles. However, the early studies that established the myotrophic effect of steroids were performed with specialized sex-related skeletal muscles, especially the levator ani muscle of the male rat (Kochakian, 1976). It has since become clear that skeletal muscles related to sexual function are much more dramatically affected by steroids than are more typical skeletal muscles (Dohm et al., 1979; Hervey & Hutchinson, 1973). Thus, most of the reports of marked beneficial effects of steroids on the growth of rat muscles apply only to sex-linked muscles; growth of skeletal muscles of the legs and arms is at the most only slightly affected.

Advocates of steroid use by power athletes have cited the results of animal studies in support of a positive effect of steroids on muscle growth. As has been pointed out, the vast majority of the positive results have been obtained in castrated animals and in sex-linked muscles. Little support can be cited in the literature for positive effects of anabolic steroids on growth of typical skeletal muscles in sexually intact male animals.

Human Beings. Before the age of puberty, plasma androgen concentrations and muscular strength levels of male and female children are similar. However, at puberty, males show tremendous increases in muscle mass and strength (Hettinger, 1961) that are associated with a 20-fold increase in circulating testosterone

(Vermeulen, 1976). There can be little argument that secretions of the testes are responsible for the male's increase in strength upon sexual maturation; hypogonadal males or males castrated before puberty do not demonstrate the pubertal effect on strength. It does not necessarily follow that supplementary androgens will stimulate further strength development in sexually mature males, but clinical studies have shown that testosterone injections can increase nitrogen retention, salt retention, and lean body weight in both hypogonadal males and in normal males and females of all ages (Landau, 1976). However, the nitrogen retention responses of sexually intact persons to testosterone injections is less than half that observed in males without functioning testes, and this anabolic effect tends to decline toward control levels upon repeated administration of the drug (Landau, 1976). On average, short-term testosterone injections of 25 mg/day produce body weight increases of about 2 kg in normal adult men (Landau, 1976). The extent to which this rather small increase in weight is caused by growth of muscle mass as opposed to growth of the prostate and other organs of the reproductive system is unknown. Simply not enough information on humans is available to predict accurately the effect of prolonged administration of large doses of oral androgenic-anabolic steroids on body weight, lean body mass, and muscular strength.

Accelerated Red Blood Cell Production

Another theoretical advantage of increased circulating levels of androgenic steroids is that of enhanced red blood cell production (erythropoiesis). Presumably, the principal explanation for the difference in red blood cell production between men and women is the effect of androgens on stimulating the production of erythropoietin, a hormone activated by the kidneys. Erythropoietin accelerates the maturation of red blood cells. If supplements of anabolic steroids could stimulate an increase in red cell mass, it might be possible to improve oxygen transport to enhance performance in athletic events requiring high levels of aerobic endurance. Prolonged treatment with androgens seems to be required, however, before many anemic patients respond favorably (Gurney, 1976). The effect of supplementary androgens on erythropoiesis in normal adult men and women has not been adequately assessed, but the often inconsistent effects in anemic patients do not give one much reason to expect a significant effect of androgens on erythropoiesis in normal athletes. Therefore, one should also not expect to see a reproducible effect of supplementary steroid administration on maximal oxygen uptake and related variables.

Changes in Endogenous Androgens with Exercise

It has long been established that a large muscle can provide greater contractile force than a small one and that chronic overload of a muscle can, under the appropriate conditions, cause increased muscular growth (Goldberg, Etlinger, Goldspink, & Jablecki, 1975). If it could be demonstrated that exercise-induced muscular growth was associated with increased levels of natural androgenic hormones, this would suggest that steroid supplements might be useful for stimulating muscular growth.

Acute Exercise and Changes in Androgenic Hormones. The effects of a single bout of exercise on testosterone concentrations in blood plasma are quite variable. After a weight training session Fahey, Rolph, Dungmee, Nagel, and Mortara (1976) found increased testosterone levels in college-aged males but no change for college-aged females or for high-school-aged males. Skierska, Ustupska, Biczowa, and Lukaszewska (1976) studied the effects of 30 minutes of weight lifting in well trained male weight lifters and reported no change in testosterone concentrations.

Strenuous cycling or running for 10-30 minutes has been associated with substantial increases in plasma androgen concentrations in some studies (Brisson, Volle, Desharnais, Dion, & Tanaka, 1977; Gawel, Alaghband-Zadah, Park, & Rose, 1979; Sutton, Coleman, Casey, & Lazarus, 1973); increases of 20% or less, which might be explained by a loss of plasma volume during exercise (Galbo, Hummer, Petersen, Christensen, & Bie, 1977; Kuoppasalmi, Naveri, Rehunen, Harkonen, & Adlercreutz, 1976; Wilkerson, Horvath, & Gutin, 1980); and no significant change in androgens (Lamb, 1975).

Marathon running resulted in increased androgen levels in a study by Demers, Harrison, Halbert, and Santen (1981), but decreased androgen concentrations in other investigations (Dessypris, Kuoppasalmi, & Adlercreutz, 1976; Morville, Pesquies, Guezennec, Serrurier, & Guignard, 1979). In another study of long-duration exercise, Sutton et al. (1973) reported that both male and female Olympic-caliber rowers and swimmers exhibited increased concentrations of plasma androgens after maximal training sessions but not after an hour of submaximal work. Galbo et al. (1977) found increased testosterone concentrations during running exercise of 80 minutes duration, but de Lignieres, Plas, Commandre, Morville, Viani, and Plas (1976) observed decreased testosterone levels after prolonged cycling.

To summarize, it appears that strenuous, short-duration exercise usually results in a rather small increase in plasma concentrations of testosterone but that moderate, brief activity or prolonged work often is not associated with significant changes in testosterone levels. The data of Wilkerson et al. (1980) show that some of the observed increases in testosterone concentrations with exercise can be explained by hemoconcentration and that total circulating testosterone levels may be little changed by exercise. Sutton, Coleman, and Casey (1978), on the other hand, suggested that the increased androgen concentrations in plasma are caused by a *reduced degradation* of the hormones by the liver, which ordinarily is the principal site of destruction of anabolic hormones. Because blood flow to the liver is reduced as a function of the relative intensity of exercise (Rowell, 1974), it is logical to assume that part of the increase in testosterone concentration with heavy exercise is caused by reduced clearance of the hormone from the blood and not by increased secretion of testosterone from the testes.

Chronic Exercise and Changes in Androgenic Hormones. There is no evidence that physical training over a period of days or weeks is associated with increased plasma concentrations of testosterone. Hetrick and Wilmore (1979) measured testosterone levels at rest in men and women at the beginning, during, and at the end of an 8-week weight training program. They found no significant differences for control or training groups and no significant correlations between androgen levels and changes in strength. In another study, repeated cycling exercise over a period of 3 days did not cause any consistent change in testosterone levels at rest measured at four different times throughout the day (de Lignieres et al., 1976). Young, Ismail, Bradley, and Corrigan (1976) found no consistent association between testosterone concentrations and fitness training for 12 weeks in adult men. The fitness training emphasized calisthenics, jogging, and recreational sports activities. Since cycling and jogging are not associated with large increments in muscle growth or strength, one might not expect any consistent increase in testosterone with training that emphasizes such activities.

Chronic Exercise and Changes in Testosterone Uptake by Skeletal Muscle. If physical training caused testosterone to be taken up more readily by skeletal muscles, a growth-promoting effect on muscles could occur in the absence of an increased level of circulating hormone. McManus, Lamb, Judis, and Scala (1975) were unable to detect any effect of treadmill training on the uptake of radioactive testosterone into skeletal muscles of guinea pigs, but Rogozkin and Feldkoren (1979) found an increased testosterone-binding capacity in skeletal muscles of rats forced to swim 10-20 minutes daily with 6% of their body weights attached to their bodies. Neither running nor swimming would be expected to cause marked muscular growth. There have been no studies reported on the effects of weight training on testosterone uptake or binding.

Research Findings of Increased Performance

Evidence related to the effectiveness of anabolic steroid administration on body composition and athletic performance has come from both laboratory animal studies and studies on human beings.

Studies on Laboratory Animals

Only a few of the studies performed on laboratory animals have suggested that administration of supplementary anabolic steroids to sexually intact animals has positive effects on body composition or "athletic" performance. In intact female rats, Hervey and Hutchinson (1973) observed an increase in lean body mass without an increase in body weight when high doses of testosterone were injected. These high doses decreased lean body mass and body weight in male rats. Positive effects of intramuscular injections of anabolic steroids on force production by isolated muscle were shown in female rats by Exner, Staudte, and Pette (1973a).

Studies on Human Beings

Because natural androgens such as testosterone are quickly inactivated by the liver if they are consumed orally, pharmaceutical companies have developed synthetic anabolic steroids that can be taken in tablet form without rapid inactivation. There are a dozen or more such oral preparations available, but the most commonly abused steroid in athletics in methandrostenelone (Δ'-17 α-methyltestosterone), which is sold under the trade name Dianabol. The clinical dosage for methandrostenelone in therapy for hypogonadism is usually 10-30 mg/day, but testimonial evidence suggests that some athletes consume 100 mg or more daily.

Experimentation with androgenic-anabolic steroids in human beings is beset with difficulties. First, experiments should be done on a double-blind basis to avoid confounding the results by a placebo effect. Ariel and Saville (1972) showed that strength gains can occur in subjects treated with inert capsules if the subjects are told that the capsules contain steroids. Unfortunately, it appears that many subjects can distinguish between steroid and placebo; Freed et al. (1975) reported that all 13 of their subjects in a "double-blind" study correctly guessed when they were consuming the methandrostenolone capsules, presumably because of a mild euphoric effect of the drug. Second, it is unethical to treat human subjects over long periods with massive doses of steroids that may be harmful to their health; yet testimonial evidence indicates that many athletes believe such massive doses are the keys to improvements in athletic performance. Finally, athletic performance can fluctuate widely because of largely unknown psychological and physiological phenomena. Therefore, any reproducible positive effect of steroid administration must be substantial if that effect is to be detected in the face of the normal variation in measures of athletic performance. Because of these problems, it is perhaps too much to expect that experiments on human beings should have clearly answered the question of whether administration of anabolic steroids improves athletic performance.

Most of the studies of anabolic steroids and athletic performance in human beings have reported data on various measures of muscular strength and of tissue growth, for example, body weight, lean body mass, body density, and limb girth. A smaller number of papers include data on plasma hormone levels and on cardiovascular function, especially as reflected by maximal oxygen uptake. In this review, no human studies are included that did not meet two minimal criteria: (a) All groups must have consisted of at least five subjects for the duration of the study. (b) A control group must have been studied at the same time as the steroid group unless the study was based on a crossover design. Nineteen separate studies are reviewed, 13 of which were apparently conducted on a double-blind basis (Casner, Early, & Carlson, 1971; Fahey & Brown, 1973; Fowler, Gardner, & Egstrom, 1965; Golding et al., 1974; Hervey, 1975; Hervey, Hutchinson, Knibbs, Burkinshaw, Jones, Norgan, & Levell, 1976; Hervey, Knibbs, Burkinshaw, Morgan, Jones, Chettle, & Vartsky, 1981; Johnson, Fisher, Silvester, & Hofheins, 1972; Johnson, Roundy, Allsen, Fisher, & Silvester, 1975; Loughton & Ruhling, 1977; O'Shea, 1971; Steinbach, 1968; Stromme, Meen, & Aakvaag, 1974; Win-May & Mya-Tu, 1975). (Hervey [1975] and Hervey et al. [1976] reports result from the same experiment.) Four studies were conducted on a single-blind basis (Bowers & Reardon, 1972; Stamford & Moffatt, 1974; Ward, 1973; Weiss & Müller, 1968). In two studies the subjects were informed that they were or were not receiving the steroid (Johnson & O'Shea, 1969; Keul, Deus, & Kindermann, 1976). In all of the studies, subjects trained with weights during control and steroid treatment periods.

Increased Body Weight. In 12 of 18 studies reporting body weight changes, increase of body weight during the training period for steroid-treated subjects was significantly greater than for control subjects (Bowers & Reardon, 1972; Casner et al., 1971; Hervey et al., 1976; Hervey et al., 1981; Johnson et al., 1972; Johnson & O'Shea, 1969; Loughton & Ruhling, 1977; O'Shea, 1971; Stamford & Moffatt, 1974; Steinbach, 1968; Weiss & Müller, 1968; Win-May & Mya-Tu, 1975). The increases in body weight for the steroid-treated groups over the control groups ranged from 1.3 to 3.6 kg and averaged about 2.2 kg. There seems to be no common pattern of type of steroid used, method of drug administration, drug dosage, diet, training program, or type of subject that explains differences in the magnitude of steroid effects on body weight. The overall evidence suggests that the administration of Dianabol up to 100 mg/day (Hervey et al., 1976, 1981) to subjects undergoing weight training for periods of 3-12 weeks can be expected to improve body weight only slightly over that which would occur with training alone. The effect of longer periods of steroid use on body weight during training has not been adequately tested, but results from animal reseach suggest that the effect would be minimal.

Increased Limb Girth and Lean Body Mass. The rather small effects of anabolic steroid treatment on body weight show that large increases in limb girth and lean body mass should not be expected to follow steroid administration. Hervey et al. (1976, 1981) reported increases of 0.5-1.3 cm in calf, arm, and thigh girths and in muscle widths determined by x-ray following 6 weeks of weight training and Dianabol (100 mg/day). However, during the control period of weight training with placebo, these subjects exhibited decreased body weights and limb girths, findings totally unexpected after a rigorous weight training program. It is therefore difficult to interpret the significance of the reports of Hervey's group. Win-May and Mya-Tu (1975) also reported consistently greater effects of training on limb girths for steroids (5 mg Dianabol daily) over placebo.

In studies where changes in lean body mass were determined by hydrostatic weighing techniques (a more valid procedure than skin-fold measurements), Hervey et al. (1976, 1981) and Ward (1973) showed a significant advantage of steroid treatment over placebo. The differences between control and steroid groups were 2-3 kg of calculated lean body mass. It should again be pointed out that the placebo treatment in the reports by Hervey et al. resulted in a loss of lean body mass, a circumstance which probably exaggerated the steroid effect. Hervey et al. (1981) also reported a positive effect of steroids on whole-body nitrogen retention, but the gain in nitrogen appeared to be too large to be accounted for by the gains in body weight or lean body mass.

Increased Strength Performance. Nine of 19 studies reviewed described steroid-associated increases in most of the strength measures taken (Bowers & Reardon, 1972; Hervey et al., 1981; Johnson et al., 1972; Johnson & O'Shea, 1969; O'Shea, 1971; Stamford & Moffat, 1974; Steinbach, 1968; Ward, 1973; Win-May & Mya-Tu, 1975). When gains in strength with steroid use were described, the difference between steroid and control groups was about 8 kg for maximal lifts in the bench press and 11 kg in the squat; these were the two most widely reported strength measures. Differences in diet or steroid dose do not seem to explain why only about half the studies reviewed showed no consistent effect of steroid treatment on strength measurements. For example, subjects in both 1975 and 1981 studies by Hervey et al. used 100 mg of Dianabol daily for 6 weeks, but a significant effect of steroid use on strength was detected only in the most recent study. It has been suggested that the effectiveness of steroids on strength development is only likely to be detected in experienced lifters because strength gains due to training alone are so great for inexperienced trainees that the smaller effect of steroids is masked (Wright, 1980). This explanation could account for the significant effect of anabolic steroids on strength observed in the 1981 study of Hervey et al., in which the subjects were experienced lifters who were already in training, relative to their 1976 study, in which the subjects were relatively inexperienced physical education students.

Increased Maximal Oxygen Uptake. One study showed a beneficial effect on maximal oxygen uptake as predicted by heart rate response to submaximal work (Johnson & O'Shea, 1969).

Research Findings of Detrimental or Indefinite Effects

Studies on Laboratory Animals

The vast majority of animal studies show no significant effect of anabolic steroid treatment on body weight, body composition, or muscular performance relative to controls that participate in a training program.

Hickson, Heusner, Van Huss, Jackson, Anderson, Jones, and Psaledas (1976) found no effect of Dianabol on body weight, muscle weight, or lean body mass in rats trained by treadmill sprints for 8 weeks. A similar lack of Dianabol effects on muscle growth in trained rats was reported by Brown and Pilch (1972).

Nandrolone decanoate, another anabolic steroid, was ineffective in enhancing body weight and swim time to exhaustion more than swim training alone (Young, Crookshank, & Ponder, 1977), and did not cause substantial effects on body weight, muscle weight, muscle protein, or muscle contractile characteristics in male rats trained with static contractions (Exner, Staudte, & Pette, 1973b).

Rogozkin (1975) and Rogozkin and Feldkoren (1979) reported only a slight increase in body weight of rats treated with Dianabol or nandrolone decanoate and trained by brief swim periods, and Hervey and Hutchinson (1973) found no effect of testosterone injections on body weight and body composition in rats. Dianabol had no effect on body weight, specific gravity, lean body weight, or body fat in rats trained by running up steep grades with weights attached to their backs (Stone, Rush, & Lipner, 1978). This type of uphill treadmill training improved contractile characteristics in rat leg muscles, but Dianabol treatment did not enhance this training effect (Stone & Lipner, 1978).

One study has been described in which six monkeys were given daily oral doses of Dianabol (2.2 mg/kg) for 60 days (Richardson, 1977). These monkeys also received a high protein diet and were compared with control animals that received no steroid. The monkeys were trained with weight lifting exercises. The steroid group did not exhibit any significant differences from the controls in body weight gain and gained slightly less strength than the controls.

Studies on Human Beings

Indefinite Effects on Body Weight. Six of 18 studies reviewed showed no significant effect of anabolic steroid administration on body weight (Fahey & Brown, 1973; Fowler et al., 1965; Golding et al., 1974; Johnson et al., 1975; Stromme et al., 1974; Ward, 1973).

Indefinite Effects on Limb Girth and Lean Body Mass. In seven of ten studies where changes in limb girth were reported, no important or consistent effect on limb girth was found (Fahey & Brown, 1973; Golding et al., 1974; Johnson et al., 1972; Johnson & O'Shea, 1969; Stamford & Moffatt, 1974; Ward, 1973; Weiss & Müller, 1968).

Three of six studies on human beings could detect no significant effect of anabolic steroids on lean body mass as estimated by hydrostatic weighing (Casner et al., 1971; Fahey & Brown, 1973; Golding et al., 1974).

Indefinite Effects on Strength Performance. Of 19 studies reviewed, 10 showed indefinite effects of anabolic steroid treatment on measures of muscular strength (Casner et al., 1971; Fahey & Brown, 1973; Fowler et al., 1965; Golding et al., 1974; Hervey et al., 1976; Johnson et al., 1975; Keul et al., 1976; Loughton & Ruhling, 1977; Stromme et al., 1974; Weiss & Müller, 1968). Steroid dosages as high as 100 mg of Dianabol daily for 6 weeks were used in these studies (Hervey et al., 1976). Accordingly, it does not appear that large doses of steroids are necessarily the key to strength improvements. It is true that subjects in studies that showed indefinite effects of steroids on strength as a rule were less experienced in weight lifting than those who participated in experiments that resulted in significant strength improvements associated with drug use. However, speculation that subjects must be experienced with lifting to achieve positive effects of steroid use (Wright, 1980) should be accorded little more credence than speculation that experienced lifters may be better able to distinguish steroids from placebos and exert themselves acccordingly during testing of muscular strength.

Indefinite Effects on Maximal Oxygen Uptake. In seven of nine studies in which maximal oxygen uptake data were reported, no significant effect of anabolic steroid administration was detected (Bowers & Reardon, 1972; Fahey & Brown, 1973; Hervey et al., 1976; Johnson et al., 1972; Johnson et al., 1975; Keul et al., 1976; Win-May & Mya-Tu, 1975), and in one study a decrease in maximal oxygen uptake was observed in the steroid condition (Stromme et al., 1974).

Potentially Deleterious Side Effects of Steroid Administration. It is clear that long-term administration of anabolic steroids can result in harmful and potentially deadly side effects. Liver diseases, including liver cancer, have been associated with androgenic-anabolic steroid therapy (Farrell, Joshua, Uren, Baird, Perkins, & Kronenberg, 1975; Johnson, 1975; Stang-Voss & Appell, 1981; Westaby, Ogle, Paradinas, Randell, & Murray-Lyon, 1977; Wright, 1980). A case study has also been reported in which a fatal kidney tumor was associated with years of steroid abuse by a body builder (Prat, Gray, Stolley, & Coleman, 1977). There have been suggestions that prolonged use of anabolic steroids could lead to chronic elevation of blood cholesterol and triglycerides, which would increase the risk of early cardiovascular disease (Shephard, Killinger, & Fried, 1977; Wright, 1980).

A number of abnormal changes in the reproductive system are also associated with steroid administration (Wright, 1980). Endogenous testosterone levels usually are depressed when androgenic steroids are administered (Hervey et al., 1976; Shephard et al., 1977; Stromme et al., 1974; Thomson, Pearson, & Costill, 1981), but these reductions in testosterone may (Shephard et al., 1977; Wright, 1980) or may not (Hervey et al., 1976; Stromme et al., 1974; Fahey & Brown, 1973) be associated with reductions in follicle-stimulating hormone or interstitial-cell-stimulating hormone. Upon prolonged use of certain types of steroids, infertility, loss of sex drive, testicular atrophy, and abnormal structural changes may occur (Wright, 1980). Most of these changes are usually reversible after discontinuing use of the steroids (Wright, 1980).

Other side effects of steroid use include the development of male pattern baldness, acne, and increased facial and body hair (Wright, 1980). In women a deepening of the voice, increased facial and body hair, clitoral enlargement, and male pattern baldness may occur and be irreversible after cessation of drug use (Wright, 1980). Menstrual irregularities may also occur (Wright, 1980).

It is a fact that relatively few cases have been reported where steroid use by athletes has been associated with life-threatening disease. However, it may be that 20 years or more are required before some of the potential long-term effects of steroid abuse, such as liver cancer and early coronary heart disease, are observed.

Summary and Conclusions

Experimental and clinical evidence from studies of laboratory and domestic animals and human beings suggests that androgenic-anabolic steroid administration can be effective in increasing body weight, lean body mass, and red blood cell production in sexually immature or hypogonadal organisms. Only slight or insignificant effects should be expected from even large doses of steroids in normal, sexually mature animals, however. In human beings an increase of body weight over control groups usually amounts to about 2.2 kg, but the extent to which the weight gain is accounted for by increased muscle mass, by growth of nonmuscle tissue or by water retention is unclear.

The overwhelming majority of the evidence shows that no improvement in maximal oxygen uptake can be associated with the use of anabolic steroids.

There are contradictory reports on whether endogenous levels of plasma or muscular testosterone are altered with single or habitual bouts of exercise. At present there is no firm evidence that natural androgens are responsible for the increased muscle mass that accompanies overload training in sexually mature, well fed athletes.

With few exceptions, studies on laboratory rats and monkeys show that the administration of androgenic-anabolic steroids to normal animals has no reliable effect on the structure or performance of typical skeletal muscles. Studies on human beings are more evenly divided; about half of the experiments show small-to-moderate improvements in strength with steroid use and half show indefinite results. The lack of a placebo that is indistinguishable from the steroid in effects on mood makes it difficult to interpret performance improvements with steroids. It is clear, however, that many persons will not experience any beneficial effect of steroid use on muscular strength.

Information currently available is inadequate to assess the long-term effects of administration of massive doses of androgenic-anabolic steroids on human athletic performance, but the increasing risks of serious medical side effects with increasing doses and durations of steroid administration should dissuade any rational person from attempting to determine these effects.

References

ARIEL, G., & Saville, W. Anabolic steroids: The physiological effects of placebos. *Medicine and Science in Sports*, 1972, **4**, 124-126.

BOWERS, R., & Reardon, J. Effects of methandrostenolone (Dianabol) on strength development and aerobic capacity. *Medicine and Science in Sports*, 1972, **4**, 54. (Abstract)

BRISSON, G.R., Volle, M.A., Desharnais, M., Dion, M., & Tanaka, M. Pituitary-gonadal axis in exercising men. *Medicine and Science in Sports*, 1977, **9**, 47. (Abstract)

BROWN, B.S., & Pilch, A.H. The effects of exercise and Dianabol upon selected performances and physiological parameters in the male rat. *Medicine and Science in Sports*, 1972, **4**, 159-165.

CASNER, S., Early, R., & Carlson, B.R. Anabolic steroid effects on body composition in normal young men. *Journal of Sports Medicine and Physical Fitness*, 1971, **11**, 98-103.

DE LIGNIERES, B., Plas, J.N., Commandre, F., Morville, R., Viani, J.-L., & Plas, F. Secretion testiculaire d'androgenes apres effort physique prolonge chez l'homme. *La Nouvelle Presse Medicale*, 1976, **5**, 2060-2064.

DEMERS, L.M., Harrison, T.S., Halbert, D.R., & Santen, R.J. Effect of prolonged exercise on plasma prostaglandin levels. *Prostaglandins and Medicine*, 1981, **6**, 413-418.

DESSYPRIS, A., Kuoppasalmi, K., & Adlercreutz, H. Plasma cortisol, testosterone, androstenedione and luteinizing hormone (LH) in a noncompetitive marathon run. *Journal of Steroid Biochemistry*, 1976, **7**, 33-37.

DOHM, G.L., Tapscott, E.B., & Louis, T.M. Skeletal muscle protein turnover after testosterone administration in the castrated male rat. *IRCS Medical Science: Physiology*, 1979, **7**, 40.

EXNER, G.U., Staudte, H.W., & Pette, D. Isometric training of rats—Effects upon fast and slow muscle and modification by an anabolic hormone (nondrolone decanoate) I. Female rats. *Pflügers Archiv*, 1973, **345**, 1-14. (a)

EXNER, G.U., Staudte, H.W., & Pette, D. Isometric training of rats—effects upon fast and slow muscle and modification by an anabolic hormone (nondrolone decanoate) II. Male rats. *Pflügers Archiv*, 1973, **345**, 15-22. (b)

FAHEY, T.D., & Brown, C.H. The effects of an anabolic steroid on the strength, body composition, and endurance of college males when accompanied by a weight training program. *Medicine and Science in Sports*, 1973, **5**, 272-276.

FAHEY, T.D., Rolph, R., Dungmee, P.M., Nagel, J., & Mortara, S. Serum testosterone, body composition and strength of young adults. *Medicine and Science in Sports*, 1976, **8**, 31-34.

FARRELL, G.C., Joshua, D.E., Uren, R.F., Baird, P.J., Perkins, K.W., & Kronenberg, H. Androgen-induced hepatoma. *Lancet*, 1975, **i**, 430-431.

FOWLER, V.R. Some aspects of the use of anabolic steroids in pigs. In F.C. Lu & J. Rendel (Eds.), *Anabolic agents in animal production*. Stuttgart: Georg Thieme, 1976.

FOWLER, W.M., Jr., Gardner, G.W., & Egstrom, G.H. Effect of an anabolic steroid on the physical performance of young men. *Journal of Applied Physiology*, 1965, **20**, 1038-1040.

FREED, D.L.J., Banks, A.J., Longson, D., & Burley, D.M. Anabolic steroids in athletics: Crossover double-blind trial on weightlifters. *British Medical Journal*, 1975, **2**, 471-473.

GALBO, H., Hummer, L., Petersen, J.B., Christensen, N.J., & Bie, N. Thyroid and testicular hormone responses to graded and prolonged exercise in man. *European Journal of Applied Physiology*, 1977, **36**, 101-106.

GAWEL, M.J., Alaghband-Zadah, J., Park, D.M., & Rose, F.C. Exercise and hormonal secretion. *Postgraduate Medical Journal*, 1979, **55**, 373-376.

GOLDBERG, A.L., Etlinger, J.D., Goldspink, D., & Jablecki, C. Mechanism of work-induced hypertrophy of skeletal muscle. *Medicine and Science in Sports*, 1975, **7**, 248-261.

GOLDING, L.A., Freydinger, J.E., & Fishel, S.S. Weight, size and strength—unchanged by steroids. *Physician and Sportsmedicine*, 1974, **2**, 39-45.

GURNEY, C.W. The hematologic effects of androgens. In C.D. Kochakian (Ed.), *Anabolic-androgenic steroids*. Berlin: Springer-Verlag, 1976.

HEITZMAN, R.J. The effectiveness of anabolic agents in increasing rate of growth in farm animals: Report on experiments in cattle. In F.C. Lu & F. Rendel (Eds.), *Anabolic agents in animal production*. Stuttgart: Georg Thieme, 1976.

HERVEY, G.R. Are athletes wrong about anabolic steroids? *British Journal of Sports Medicine*, 1975, **9**, 74-77.

HERVEY, G.R., & Hutchinson, I. The effects of testosterone on body weight and composition in the rat. *Journal of Endocrinology*, 1973, **57**, xxiv-xxv.

HERVEY, G.R., Hutchinson, I., Knibbs, A.V., Burkinshaw, L., Jones, P.R.M., Norgan, N.G., & Levell, M.J. "Anabolic" effects of methandieone in men undergoing athletic training. *Lancet*, 1976, **ii**, 699-702.

HERVEY, G.R., Knibbs, A.V., Burkinshaw, L., Morgan, D.B., Jones, P.R.M., Chettle, D.R., & Vartsky, D. Effects of methandienone on the performance and body composition of men undergoing athletic training. *Clinical Science*, 1981, **60**, 457-461.

HETRICK, G.A., & Wilmore, J.H. Androgen levels and muscle hypertrophy during an eight week weight training program for men/women. *Medicine and Science in Sports*, 1979, **11**, 102. (Abstract)

HETTINGER, T. *Physiology of strength*. Springfield, IL: Charles C. Thomas, 1961.

HICKSON, R.C., Heusner, W.W., Van Huss, W.D., Jackson, D.E., Anderson, D.A., Jones, D.A., & Psaledas, A.T. Effects of Dianabol and high-intensity sprint training on body composition of rats. *Medicine and Science in Sports*, 1976, **8**, 191-195.

JOHNSON, F.L. The association of oral androgenic-anabolic steroids and life threatening disease. *Medicine and Science in Sports*, 1975, **7**, 284-286.

JOHNSON, L.C., Fisher, G., Silvester, L.J., & Hofheins, C.C. Anabolic steroid: Effects on strength, body weight, oxygen uptake and spermatogenesis upon mature males. *Medicine and Science in Sports*, 1972, **4**, 43-45.

JOHNSON, L.C., & O'Shea, J.P. Anabolic steroid: Effects on strength development. *Science*, 1969, **164**, 957-959.

JOHNSON, L.C., Roundy, E.S., Allsen, P.E., Fisher, A.G., & Silvester, L.J. Effect of anabolic steroid treatment on endurance. *Medicine and Science in Sports*, 1975, **7**, 287-289.

KEUL, J., Deus, B., & Kindermann, W. Anabole hormone: Schädigung, Leistungsfähigkeit und Stoffwechsel. *Medizinische Klinik*, 1976, **71**, 497-503.

KOCHAKIAN, C.D. Body and organ weights and composition. In C.D. Kochakian (Ed.), *Anabolic-androgenic steroids*. Berlin: Springer-Verlag, 1976.

KOCHAKIAN, C.D., & Endahl, B.R. Changes in body weight of normal and casterated rats by different doses of testosterone propionate. *Proceedings of the Society for Experimental Biology and Medicine*, 1959, **100**, 520-522.

KROTKIEWSKI, M., Kral, J.G., & Karlsson, J. Effects of castration and testosterone substitution on body composition and muscle metabolism in rats. *Acta Physiologica Scandinavica*, 1980, **109**, 233-237.

KUOPPASALMI, K., Naveri, H., Rehunen, S., Harkonen, M., & Adlercreutz, H. Effect of strenuous anaerobic running exercise on plasma growth hormone, cortisol, luteinizing hormone, testosterone, androstenedione, estrone and estradiol. *Journal of Steroid Biochemistry*, 1976, **7**, 823-829.

LAMB, D.R. Androgens and exercise. *Medicine and Science in Sports*, 1975, **7**, 1-5.

LANDAU, R.L. The metabolic effects of anabolic steroids in man. In C.D. Kochakian (Ed.), *Anabolic-androgenic steroids*. Berlin: Springer-Verlag, 1976.

LOUGHTON, S.J., & Ruhling, R.O. Human strength and endurance responses to anabolic steroid and training. *Journal of Sports Medicine and Physical Fitness*, 1977, **17**, 285-296.

MCMANUS, B.M., Lamb, D.R., Judis, J.J., & Scala, J. Skeletal muscle leucine incorporation and testosterone uptake in exercised guinea pigs. *European Journal of Applied Physiology*, 1975, **34**, 149-156.

MICHEL, G., & Baulieu, E-E. Androgen receptor in rat skeletal muscle: Characterization and physiological variations. *Endocrinology*, 1980, **107**, 2088-2098.

MORVILLE, R., Pesquies, P.C., Guezennec, C.Y., Serrurier, B.D., & Guignard, M. Plasma variations in testicular and adrenal androgens during prolonged physical exercise in man. *Annals of Endocrinology*, 1979, **40**, 501-510.

NESHEIM, M.C. Some observations on the effectiveness of anabolic agents in increasing the growth rate of poultry. In F.C. Lu & J. Rendel (Eds.), *Anabolic agents in animal production*. Stuttgart: Georg Thieme, 1976.

O'SHEA, J.P. The effects of an anabolic steroid on dynamic strength levels of weight lifters. *Nutrition Reports International*, 1971, **4**, 363-370.

PRAT, J., Gray, G.F., Stolley, P.D., & Coleman, J.W. Wilm's tumor in an adult associated with androgen abuse. *Journal of the American Medical Association*, 1977, **21**, 2322-2323.

RICHARDSON, J.H. A comparison of two drugs on strength increase in monkeys. *Journal of Sports Medicine and Physical Fitness*, 1977, **17**, 251-254.

ROGOZKIN, V. Anabolic and androgenic effects of methandrostenolone ("Nerobol") during systematic physical activity in rats. *British Journal of Sports Medicine*, 1975, **9**, 65-69.

ROGOZKIN, V. Metabolic effects of anabolic steroid on skeletal muscle. *Medicine and Science in Sports*, 1979, **11**, 160-163.

ROGOZKIN, V., & Feldkoren, B. The effects of retabolil and training on activity of RNA-polymerase in skeletal muscles. *Medicine and Science in Sports*, 1979, **11**, 345-347.

ROWELL, L.B. Human cardiovascular adjustments to exercise and thermal stress. *Physiological Reviews*, 1974, **51**, 75-159.

RYAN, A.J. Athletics. In C.D. Kochakian (Ed.), *Anabolic-androgenic steroids*. Berlin: Springer-Verlag, 1976.

SHEPHARD, R.J., Killinger, D., & Fried, T. Responses to sustained use of anabolic steroid. *British Journal of Sports Medicine*, 1977, **11**, 170-173.

SKIERSKA, E., Ustupska, J., Biczowa, B., & Lukaszewska, J. Effect of physical exercise on plasma cortisol, testosterone, and growth hormone levels in weight lifters. *Endokrynologia Polska*, 1976, **27**, 159-165.

STAMFORD, B.A., & Moffatt, R. Anabolic steroid: Effectiveness as an ergogenic aid to experienced weight trainers. *Journal of Sports Medicine and Physical Fitness*, 1974, **14**, 191-197.

STANG-VOSS, C., & Appell, H.-J. Structural alterations of liver parenchyma induced by anabolic steroids. *International Journal of Sports Medicine*, 1981, **2**, 101-105.

STEINBACH, M. Über den Einfluss anaboler Wirkstoffe auf Körpergewicht, Muskelkraft und Muskeltraining. *Sportarzt und Sportmedizin*, 1968, **11**, 485-492.

STEROID bust. *Time*, July 27, 1981, p. 61.

STONE, M.H., & Lipner, H. Responses to intensive training and methandrostenelone administration: I. Contractile and performance variables. *Pflügers Archiv*, 1978, **375**, 141-146.

STONE, M.H., Rush, M.E., & Lipner, H. Responses to intensive training and methandrostenelone administration: II. Hormonal, organ weights, muscle weights, and body composition. *Pflügers Archiv*, 1978, **375**, 147-151.

STROMME, S.B., Meen, H.D., & Aakvaag, A. Effects of an androgenic-anabolic steroid on strength development and plasma testosterone levels in normal males. *Medicine and Science in Sports*, 1974, **6**, 203-208.

SUTTON, J.R., Coleman, M.J., & Casey, J.H. Testosterone production rate during exercise. In F. Landry & W.A.R. Orban (Eds.), *Third international symposium on biochemistry of exercise, Book 3*. Miami: Symposia Specialists, 1978.

SUTTON, J.R., Coleman, M.J., Casey, J., & Lazarus, L. Androgen responses during physical exercise. *British Medical Journal*, 1973, **163**, 520-522.

THOMSON, D.P., Pearson, D.R., & Costill, D.L. Use of anabolic steroids by national level athletes. *Medicine and Science in Sports and Exercise*, 1981, **13**, 11. (Abstract)

TRENKLE, A. The anabolic effect of estrogens on nitrogen metabolism of growing and finishing cattle and sheep. In F.C. Lu & J. Rendel (Eds.), *Anabolic agents in animal production*. Stuttgart: Georg Thieme, 1976.

VANDERWAL, P. General aspects of the effectiveness of anabolic agents in increasing protein production in farm animals, in particular bull calves. In F.C. Lu & J. Rendel (Eds.), *Anabolic agents in animal production*. Stuttgart: Georg Thieme, 1976.

VERMEULEN, A. Plasma levels and secretion rate of steroids with anabolic activity. In F.C. Lu & J. Rendel (Eds.), *Anabolic agents in animal production*. Stuttgart: Georg Thieme, 1976.

WARD, P. The effect of an anabolic steroid on strength and lean body mass. *Medicine and Science in Sports*, 1973, **5**, 277-282.

WEISS, V., & Müller, H. Zur Frage der Beeinflussung des Krafttrainings durch anabole Hormone. *Schweizerische Zeitschrift für Sportmedizin*, 1968, **16**, 79-89.

WESTABY, D., Ogle, S.J., Paradinas, F.J., Randell, J.B., & Murray-Lyon, I.M. Liver damage from long-term methyltestosterone. *Lancet*, 1977, **ii**, 261-263.

WILKERSON, J.E., Horvath, S.M., & Gutin, B. Plasma testosterone during treadmill exercise. *Journal of Applied Physiology*, 1980, **49**, 249-253.

WIN-MAY, M., & Mya-Tu, M. The effect of anabolic steroids on physical fitness. *Journal of Sports Medicine and Physical Fitness*, 1975, **15**, 266-271.

WRIGHT, J.E. Anabolic steroids and athletics. *Exercise and Sport Sciences Reviews*, 1980, **8**, 149-202.

YOUNG, M., Crookshank, H.R., & Ponder, L. Effects of an anabolic steroid on selected parameters in male albino rats. *Research Quarterly of the American Alliance for Health, Physical Education and Recreation*, 1977, **48**, 653-656.

YOUNG, R.J., Ismail, A.H., Bradley, A., & Corrigan, D.L. Effect of prolonged exercise on serum testosterone levels in adult men. *British Journal of Sports Medicine*, 1976, **10**, 230-235.

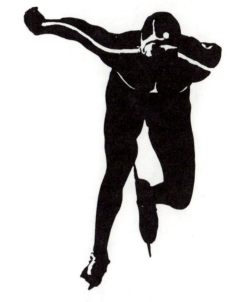

Part 3
Physiological
Ergogenic Aids

7

Oxygen

Alfred F. Morris

A basic unresolved problem in exercise physiology is to identify
the factor(s) primarily responsible for the limiting of human physical performance of a total body nature (Keul, 1973). Whenever exercise scientists discuss this critical problem, at least two major
categorical viewpoints are proposed. Either delivery of O_2 to the
working muscle by the cardiovascular system (central mechanisms) or metabolic capacity of the working muscle to utilize O_2
(peripheral mechanisms) is viewed as a possible limiting factor
(Keul, 1973). It is the purpose of this review to examine the effects
of supplemental O_2 as an ergogenic (work-enhancing) agent
within the scope of these proposed factors limiting human performance.

Methodological Problems with the Use
of Supplemental Oxygen

Many confounding factors must of necessity enter into any discus-

Alfred F. Morris, Ph.D., F.A.C.S.M., is with the Division of Rehabilitation Education at the University of Illinois in Urbana-Champaign.

sion of the role of supplementary O_2 as an ergogenic aid. One consideration is how the extra O_2 is administered to the subject. First, does the subject receive hyperoxygenated air or pure O_2 at normal atmospheric pressure, or, secondly, does the subject inhale compressed air or use compressed hyperoxygenated air or pure O_2? In the first case it is possible to increase the O_2 tension up to one atmosphere (1 atm) or 760 mm, while in the second instance, increases of O_2 could be inhaled at tensions above 1 atm.

A second major consideration of using supplemental O_2 in an attempt to improve human performance revolves around when to administer the supplemental O_2. Various experimenters have administered oxygen before, during, or after a particular work task. In relation to this point, the time frame of the supplemental O_2 administration, that is, the elapsed time between inhalation and performance, the elapsed time during the work task, or the timing of O_2 administration after the work task, may be crucial.

There are still other important methodological considerations when examining this area of ergogenics. A part of the problem in determining the benefits of supplemental O_2 lies with possible errors of measurement in estimating O_2 consumption ($\dot{V}O_2$) when breathing high concentrations of O_2 (Hill, Long, & Lupton, 1924; Welch, Mulin, Wilson, & Lewis, 1974; Wilmore, 1972). As the O_2 content in inspired air is increased over 21% up to 80, 90, or 100%, the nitrogen (N_2) fraction must decrease, and the error of estimation of maximal oxygen uptake ($\dot{V}O_2$ max) increases (Hill et al., 1924). For a more indepth explanation of this measurement procedure, see Welch et al. (1974) for two suggested methods to calculate $\dot{V}O_2$ max when mixtures of 80% (or greater) of O_2 are inhaled.

In addition, the loss of N_2 from body water must be considered (Wilmore, 1972). By directly measuring carbon dioxide (CO_2) production, the problem of N_2 loss and changes in pressure of O_2 can be partially corrected. If one measures ventilation, O_2, and CO_2 production and from these estimates the respiratory exchange ratio (R), the resulting corrected O_2 uptake values may be more accurate.

Finally, what parameters are to be measured when the subject inhales the extra oxygen? Should the experimenters examine human performance in terms of regular, established work tasks like increased pedaling, running, or lifting performance? Are anaerobic or aerobic tasks to be evaluated? Or should investigators examine various physiological parameters such as $\dot{V}O_2$ max, heart rate, cardiac output, stroke volume, and ventilation? Or should lactic acid production and the response of the skeletal muscle cells be monitored? All these factors (and others such as age, sex, and level of training) might serve to complicate any discussion of the possible role of supplemental O_2 and human performance.

Methodological Approaches to the Study of Supplemental Oxygen as an Aid to Human Performance

There are several different approaches to the study of supplemental O_2 and human performance. The work of two outstanding researchers representing two different laboratories and approaches to this topic are reviewed below.

Kaijser (1973) studied O_2 as a limiting factor in all-out physical performance. He noted that if one wishes to determine whether supplemental O_2 may enhance muscular aerobic performance by facilitating either central or peripheral mechanisms, the following four experimental models may be used: (a) The blood O_2 content can be increased and performance studied. (b) An experimental model that would heat or cool the exercising muscle should predict an increase or decrease in the maximal metabolic rate of the working muscle. Kaijser (1973) reported that cooling a muscle inhibits its performance, indicating that metabolic factors are crucial to muscle performance. (c) Increase the exercising muscle mass; that is, add arm work to the already exercising leg muscle mass. If O_2 uptake is increased, then metabolic and not circulatory factors may be rate limiting. (d) Maximum cardiac output could be manipulated to see if it affects performance, thus testing central mechanisms. On the basis of his work involving supplemental O_2 and performance, Kaijser (1969, 1970, 1973) concluded that the central mechanism is not the main limiting factor for performance for the average subject.

Another experimental strategy was employed by Welch, Bonde-Petersen, Graham, Klausen, and Secher (1977). They attempted to corroborate Kaijser's findings to see if the limiting factor to human performance resided in the periphery, that is, in the working skeletal muscle. However, in an attempt to improve on earlier studies, they decided to monitor leg blood flow and metabolism of six active young males during bicycle ergometer exercise. They administered supplemental O_2 at 60% or 100% while working their subjects at about 55% to 70% of each subject's maximal aerobic capacity. Their findings are contradictory to those previously reporting increases in peripheral O_2 uptake during exercise under hyperoxic conditions and do not support the thesis held by Kaijser (1973).

From these two examples (Kaijser, 1973; Welch et al., 1977) several approaches to the question of the effect of supplemental O_2

on performance may be seen. Both investigations attempted to evaluate the effect of supplemental O_2 on peripheral muscle metabolic function and, using different strategies, came to different conclusions.

Format for Review

This review will have as its major format a discussion of the effect of supplemental O_2 on various physiological parameters and performance. For discussion purposes stated in the initial paragraph, the relationship of supplemental O_2 and limits to human performance will be discussed. The first area of discussion will focus on the delivery of O_2 to the working muscles by the cardiovascular system. This will essentially involve central mechanisms of heart rate, cardiac output, and stroke volume. It will also include ventilation and respiratory aspects.

A second area for discussion will review studies to see how O_2 may limit local muscular metabolism, or peripheral mechanisms. That is, how is supplemental O_2 related to the inner workings of the skeletal muscle cell in the periphery? Included in this discussion will be topics of lactic acid production, oxygen debt, and aerobic versus anaerobic metabolism. Some factors overlap both areas. For example, should $\dot{V}O_2$ max be considered a central or peripheral factor? Obviously, it is affected by both central and peripheral factors. Within the constraints imposed here, the purpose of this chapter is to examine studies in which supplemental O_2 was used to aid human performance or individual parameters of human performance. The first section is an evaluation of O_2 as an ergogenic aid for central mechanisms. The second section deals with O_2 as an aid to peripheral factors. The last section examines O_2 as an aid to actual performance (including psychomotor performance).

Theoretical Considerations

O_2 administration could aid human performance by improving O_2 transport by the cardiovascular-respiratory complex. In essense, $\dot{V}O_2$ max represents the interaction of the cardiac output and the arterio-venous O_2 difference. To improve O_2 transport, either the cardiac output or the arterial saturation could be increased. An increased O_2 pressure (PO_2) in the lungs could increase the alveolar PO_2 and the pressure gradient to the arterial blood. In fact, Wilmore (1972) suggests that this increased pulmonary diffusion capacity may be the most significant factor relating increased performance with O_2 supplementation.

Mathews & Fox (1976) list four factors that affect pulmonary diffusion and uptake of O_2 by the blood: (a) the PO_2 in the blood, (b) the temperature of the blood, (c) the acidity of the blood, and (d) the amount of CO_2 in the blood. The pressure gradient for a gas determines the speed and amount of diffusion. If additional O_2 is to be delivered to the blood from the alveoli, the pressure gradient has to be sufficient. Let us assume that the PO_2 in the venous blood fell to 20 mmHg and the PO_2 of alveoli is 120 mmHg. The pressure gradient would be 100 mmHg. If 100% O_2 were being breathed, the alveolar PO_2 might rise to 700 mmHg and the pressure gradient to about 600 mmHg. This would create a great driving force for O_2 diffusion.

Buskirk, Kollias, Piconreatigue, Akers, Prokop, & Baker (1967) have reported a linear decrease in PO_2 with high altitudes. Greater concentrations of supplemental O_2 at sea level should result, theoretically, in linear increases of PO_2. However, the O_2 uptake by the blood is not linear, due to the phenomenon of hemoglobin saturation of O_2 in arterial blood as demonstrated by the classic elongated s-shape of the oxyhemoglobin dissociation curve. A drop of pH (or greater acidity of the blood) and a blood temperature rise (as in prolonged intense exercise) displace the dissociation curve to the right, which could reduce arterial saturation at the lung level. At the muscular level, this lower pH and higher temperature could foster greater O_2 dissociation from the blood to the muscle tissues.

During exercise, studies at normal O_2 pressure have revealed that arterial PO_2 is typically maintained near optimal levels, that is, 95% or greater saturation. (Wilson, Welch, & Liles, 1975). With increased alveolar PO_2 from O_2 supplementation, however, the O_2 capacity of the blood could be increased to 100% saturation. Although this is not a great increase in O_2 saturation, it is nevertheless an increase of about 5%. Moreover, arterial saturation may decrease during severe exercise as low as 85% (deVries, 1980). With this lower saturation, supplemental O_2 administered during maximal exercise might be expected to improve performance.

Beneficial Effects on Central Mechanisms of Oxygen Administered During Exercise

Although this section is devoted primarily to central mechanisms, a number of the studies reviewed also reported data on lactic acid levels. Production of lactic acid would represent anaerobic work and hence decreased aerobic efficiency. Thus, if lactic acid levels are lowered by O_2 supplementation, the muscle tissues may be more aerobic. This could be due to either increased O_2 supply or increased O_2 uptake by the muscle. Although apparently more related to peripheral factors, some lactic acid data will be presented in this section when they were an integral part of the study.

In one early study Nielsen and Hansen (1937) found reductions in ventilation when supplemental O_2 was consumed during heavy work. This was not the case for mild exercise. In a later study Asmussen and Nielsen (1946) noted that ventilation volumes were lower during O_2 inhalation. When subjects worked near their $\dot{V}O_2$ max, supplemental O_2 was effective in reducing ventilation by 21%. Measurements of blood lactate, in response to ambient air or O_2 enriched air, revealed that supplemental O_2 lowered blood lactate levels. These experiments revealed that as O_2 content of gas mixtures rose from 21 to 30, 60, and 100%, subjects exercising on a bicycle ergometer demonstrated a stepwise lowering of blood lactate with increased O_2 content. Also noted was a decrease in ventilation as supplemental O_2 was added to the inspired gas. These scientists speculated that O_2 inhalation acts on peripheral chemoreceptors as well as on the respiratory center.

Miller, Perdue, Teague, and Fereber (1952) studied O_2 supplementation during treadmill work. Heart rate and blood pressure values were not changed due to the supplemental O_2 breathing; however, as in earlier studies, blood lactate levels were lowered when subjects breathed additional O_2. In addition, in exhaustive runs, the time for these runs lengthened (time to exhaustion) 7.3-8.9 minutes as a result of supplemental O_2.

One of the more thorough studies done on supplemental O_2 breathing and performance was done by Bannister and Cunningham (1954). These British workers had trained runners exercise to exhaustion on a treadmill while breathing gas mixtures with O_2 content of 33%, 66%, or 100%. However, one major deficiency of this and other earlier studies was the fact that the subjects knew which mixture they were inhaling; therefore, the psychological or placebo effect was not accounted for. Results indicated that performances were generally better when the subjects inhaled 66% O_2 compared to ambient air or mixtures of 33% or 100% O_2. Pulmonary ventilation as well as blood lactate levels were decreased. In addition to these physiological measurements, Bannister and Cunningham reported that their subjects felt that the exhaustive runs were easier when inhaling supplemental O_2.

Cunningham (1966) studied the effects of breathing high concentrations of O_2 on treadmill performance time, lactic acid concentrations, and O_2 debt. He had seven active subjects run several tests to exhaustion while breathing 70% O_2 or ambient air. Results indicated that subjects performed significantly longer while breathing supplemental O_2. In addition, maximal heart rate was not affected by inspiring the additional oxygen, although he reported longer steady-state levels for the supplemental O_2 subjects. Finally, Cunningham noted a lower O_2 debt in the first minute of recovery after breathing O_2.

Hughes, Clode, Edwards, Goodwin, and Jones (1968) had subjects breathe 11, 16, 21, and 33% O_2 during bicycle ergometer work tasks. They found lower ventilation volumes, heart rates, cardiac output, and peak lactate values at submaximal loads when 33% O_2 was inhaled. Also, blood pH was lower when O_2 at 33% was breathed.

Taunton, Banister, Patrick, Oforsagd, and Duncan (1970) studied the exercise capacity of two subjects who performed on a bicycle ergometer at four different work rates while breathing air at 1 and 2 atm and while breathing O_2 at 2 atm. Results indicated that $\dot{V}O_2$ max was greater when subjects breathed air at 2 atm and still higher when they breathed O_2 at 2 atm. O_2 production exhibited the opposite response. The ventilation equivalent was highest for work with ambient air (1 atm) and lowest with supplemental O_2 inhalation at 2 atm.

In a second report, the same investigators (Banister, Taunton, Patrick, Oforsagd, & Duncan, 1970) compared the effects of supplemental O_2 at 2 atm and normal air breathing on heavy bicycle work (1,500 kpm/min for 5 min). Results indicated that peak heart rates decreased from 173 to 159 beats/min for the hyperoxic and hyperbaric O_2 mixture; pulmonary ventilation dropped from 138 to 95 l/min; CO_2 was decreased and O_2 uptake was increased; and lactic acid levels were lower and a higher blood pH resulted from O_2 inhalation. The authors attributed these changes to high arterial and tissue O_2 tension and to a diminution of possible adverse affects of O_2 on enzyme systems in glycolysis.

Wyndham, Strydom, Van Rensburg, and Rogers (1970) devised a unique experiment to observe the effects of exercising underground (in a mine at a depth of 1,828 m) and at altitude (1,763 m) on O_2 consumption and running performance. $\dot{V}O_2$ max values were recorded at altitude and then immediately after descent into the mine. (This actually mimicked a return to sea level because ground level was at 1,763 m above sea level). A second experimental group was studied with the same baseline tests (at altitude, 1,763 m) and then at a depth of 3,033 m, or about 1,270 m, below sea level. The recorded barometric pressures at these sites were 630 mmHg at ground level (1,763 m), 765 mmHg at 1,825-m depth (approximately sea level), and 865 mmHg at 3,033-m depth (1,270 below sea level). Thus, exercising at the greatest depth would be approximately equal to exercising while consuming an O_2 mixture of about 24%. The researchers reported that the subjects were able to perform better at the deep mine level. Also, $\dot{V}_2$ max levels were greater at the depth of 3,033 m. Finally, maximum heart rate levels and maximum pulmonary ventilation volumes were greater at the lower depths. This indicated a greater efficiency while working at moderate depths.

In the middle and late 1970s, researchers became much more sophisticated in their research designs and began to explore in more detail possible factors accounting for the increased performance with supplemental O_2 breathing. Several investigators began to measure CO_2 production and tissue blood flow and also began attempts to mask the cues as to which gaseous mixtures the subjects were breathing in an attempt to control the placebo effect in supplemental oxygen studies. Some of these studies are reviewed below.

Wilson and Welch (1975) tried to assess the effect of various enriched O_2 mixtures on treadmill running of nine active males while measuring $\dot{V}O_2$ max. The gas mixtures used were 20%, 40%, 60%, 80%, or 100% O_2. All subjects worked to exhaustion and were blind as to which O_2 mixture they were inhaling. The results indicated that running times increased as the percentage of O_2 increased. This was in contradiction to other studies (Bannister & Cunningham, 1954; Briggs, 1920) that had indicated breathing a mixture of about 60 to 66% supplemental O_2 appeared to be the best percentage for optimal performance. Wilson and Welch (1975) also noted that ventilation decreased when subjects breathed the hyperoxic mixtures but that maximal heart rates were not significantly different regardless of the O_2 fraction of the inspired gas.

Swedish researchers (Ekblom, Huot, Stein, & Thorstenson, 1975) have studied the effects of changes in arterial O_2 content on circulation and physical performance during both treadmill and bicycle ergometer work. The treadmill runs were to exhaustion while the bicycle ergometer exercises were submaximal. The nine subjects were moderately active and were tested under three experimental conditions: first, while the subjects inhaled ambient air (control), second, while the subjects inhaled a 50% O_2 mixture, and third, while subjects rebreathed a CO_2 mixture to simulate a hypoxic condition. Results showed that $\dot{V}O_2$ max was significantly higher in hyperoxia (4.99 l/min) and significantly lower in hypoxia (3.80 l/min) than in the control condition (4.43 l/min). Also, physical performance was congruent with the $\dot{V}O_2$ changes. Finally, measurement of cardiac output was similar in hyperoxia as in the control condition, but was significantly lower in hypoxia. This was mainly due to a lower stroke volume. Because a correlation between $\dot{V}O_2$ and transported O_2, that is, O_2 content of arterial blood × maximal cardiac output, was found, the investigators suggested that central circulation might be an important limiting factor for human maximal aerobic power.

Dressendorfer, Wade, and Bernauer (1977) investigated the relationship of increased airway resistance and hyperoxia on aerobic work tolerance. Seven men, four of whom were trained endurance athletes, were given cycling tests to exhaustion while being artificially submitted to three inspiratory resistance levels. Submaximal $\dot{V}O_2$ was not affected by increased resistance to breathing; however, the increased resistance did decrease $\dot{V}O_2$ and pulmonary ventilation at maximal exercise levels. During the trial with the highest airway resistance, heart rate and endurance time on the bicycle ergometer were reduced. Breathing O_2-enriched air (35% O_2) increased $\dot{V}O_2$ max and peak heart rate as well as endurance time, suggesting that aerobic work tolerance under added stress (artificially imposed airway resistance) was affected by the increased work of breathing and reduced ventilatory capacity and was partially improved by moderate hyperoxia, apparently because the ventilatory limit may have been partially compensated.

In another report, Wilson and Welch (1980) hypothesized that improvement in exercise tolerance due to O_2 supplementation may be attributed to (a) a decreased anaerobiosis in the working muscle cell, (b) a decreased cost of breathing, or (c) the reduction of a possible metabolic depressant, (N_2 acting as a metabolic depressant). To test these hypotheses, 10 subjects ran to exhaustion on a treadmill breathing one of four mixtures of O_2, N_2, or helium (He): 20% O_2/80% N_2, 20% O_2/80% He, 80% O_2/20% N_2, or 80% O_2/20% He. Results indicated that running time to exhaustion increased significantly on both hyperoxic mixtures and on both He/O_2 mixtures. The authors speculated that although the peak ventilatory volumes were higher with the He/O_2 mixtures, the mass of the ventilatory gasses was significantly less (a 20% O_2/80% He mixture is only about a third as dense as room air), which might result in a reduction in the cost of breathing. Wilson and Welch (1980) concluded that their data favor the second hypothesis that supplementary O_2 or O_2 in combination with He seemed to decrease the cost of breathing and result in increased tolerance to exhaustive exercise.

The above studies have in the main indicated increased cardiovascular, respiratory, and ventilatory functions with increased O_2 supplementation. Many of these studies mentioned increased metabolic function as well. The following section reviews studies suggesting that increased human performance via O_2 supplementation is governed primarily by the peripheral metabolic capacity of the working muscles.

Beneficial Effects on Peripheral Mechanisms of Oxygen Administered During Exercise

In most of the studies involving supplemental O_2, subjects exercised while actually breathing a mixture high in O_2 content. In one such early study (Feldman & Hill, 1911) subjects inhaled either concentrated O_2 solutions or ambient air at sea level conditions to see how their performance was affected. Supplemental O_2 seemed to lower lactic acid production resulting from exercise. The authors concluded that the increased lactic acid produced during exercise might be due to a need for more O_2.

Fragraeus (1974) examined the effects of acute exposure to the hyperbaric environment on physiological functions in submaximal and maximal exercise. Hyperbaric conditions ranged up to 6.0 atm. In addition, He-O_2 mixtures were inhaled at hyperbaric pressures. Results generally indicated that exercise at 1.4 atm produced the most favorable performances. With higher pressures at 4.5-6.0 atm, it was theorized that the higher gas density may have caused an increase in airway resistance and hence an increase in the work of breathing. Dressendorfer, Wade, and Bernauer (1977) later came to a similar conclusion. However, another interesting finding by Fagraeus (1974) was that muscle metabolite levels (ATP, CP, lactate, pyruvate, and glucose), glycogen depletion, and O_2 deficit at end points of exhaustion were not significantly changed as air pressure was raised in the hyperbaric conditions. This was observed in spite of significant increases in $\dot{V}O_2$ max. Also, peak blood lactate was not changed as subjects received the hyperbaric mixtures. The later findings might suggest that although performance times were better and $\dot{V}O_2$ max was higher, the muscle metabolism could not keep pace with the increasing demands of the exercise task.

As previously mentioned, Welch et al. (1974) noted possible errors in $\dot{V}O_2$ measurements when high concentrations of supplemental O_2 were inhaled during heavy exercise. In an attempt to correlate findings observed in human subjects with events occurring in the muscle, they used an *in situ* muscle preparation in dogs to evaluate local arterial and venous flow, periodically taking blood samples for measurements of O_2 consumed and CO_2 produced. The results indicated a 20% higher $\dot{V}O_2$ max when their six human subjects breathed a mixture of 80% O_2. This was accompanied by a 30-35% decrease in ventilation and a slight decrease in CO_2 production. In the *in situ* dog muscle preparation, neither $\dot{V}O_2$ nor $\dot{V}CO_2$ changed during contractions whether the animal was breathing air or 100% O_2. Welch et al. suggested that since increased metabolic rates in humans cause increases in $\dot{V}CO_2$, it might be possible that the apparent increased $\dot{V}O_2$ observed with supplemental O_2 may be due to something other than increased O_2 utilization in the mitochondria. Stainsby (1973), working on *in situ* dog calf muscles, reached a similar conclusion, noting that the rate-limiting metabolite is probably not O_2. Stainsby further speculated that the rate-limiting process seems to be the excitation-contraction coupling system in the contraction apparatus itself. This explanation also hints of a metabolic failure.

In a related study, the same workers (Wilson et al., 1975) examined the effects of supplemental O_2 inhalation during bicycle ergometer work of submaximal intensity. Four men who were physically active and moderately trained as cyclists rode at either 40% or 80% of their maximal aerobic capacity for 30 minutes while breathing either a 21% or 60% O_2 mixture. The $\dot{V}CO_2$ showed no significant change during the 40% exercise tests, but was significantly decreased during the 80% intensity rides. Furthermore, the respiratory quotient decreased during the hyperoxic tests which would suggest a slight shift from carbohydrate metabolism to fatty acid metabolism.

In an attempt to improve on earlier studies, Welch and co-workers (1977) decided to monitor leg blood flow and metabolism of six young males during bicycle ergometer exercise. They administered supplemental O_2 at 60% or 100% while working their subjects at about 55% to 70% of each subject's maximal aerobic capacity. The major findings of this study were: (a) that leg blood flow is reduced with supplemental O_2, (b) that the $\dot{V}O_2$ of the exercising limb is not changed during hyperoxia, (c) that O_2 delivery (the product of blood flow × arterio-venous O_2 difference) is not significantly different with supplemental oxygen, and (d) the blood pressure is not greatly affected by hyperoxia. The authors concluded that, because blood pressure was not different during hyperoxia and leg blood flow was reduced by 11%, this may indicate an increased resistance to blood flow in the exercising limb. These findings are contradictory to other studies reporting increases in oxygen uptake during exercise under hyperoxic conditions.

Effects of Oxygen Administered Before Exercise

Should supplemental O_2 given prior to exercise affect subsequent performance? McArdle, Katch, and Katch (1981) explained that a 70-kg person may have about 5,000 ml of blood. If such persons breathed a hyperoxic mixture prior to exercise, they may potentially "store" about 70 ml of O_2 in the total blood volume (5,000 ml of blood $\times$ 1.4 ml "extra" O_2 per 100 ml of blood, or 1.4 ml $O_2 \times 50$ = 70 ml). Therefore, the pre-exercise O_2 breathing may help only if the performance took place immediately after the supplemental O_2 inhalation and only if the exercise duration were about 2 minutes or less in duration (e.g., an 800-meter foot race). Furthermore, if ambient air were breathed in the interval (between supplemental O_2 breathing and the beginning of the exercise effort), the "extra" oxygen "stored" might be dissipated.

One of the earliest reported studies was done by Hill and McKenzie (1909), who recorded the effects of O_2 supplementation for 3 minutes on the subsequent performance of running distance of 250 and 880 yards. They noted that following O_2 breathing, running performances improved. In addition, the subjects noted a two-fold increase in breath-holding time after O_2 inhalation. On a weight lifting task that involved weight lifting while holding one's breath, individuals who followed forced breathing of O_2 were able to do more work.

Douglas and Haldane (1909) studied oxygen inhalation or quite forced breathing for 3 minutes on subjects' abilities to run up and down a 40-foot stairway two times. Results indicated only a slight effect on postexercise heart rate and no significant increase in performance. Hill and Flack (1909) reported heart rate, respiration, and blood pressure in subjects who ran a flight of stairs (26 steps) as fast as possible eight or nine times. Certain subjects who breathed O_2 prior to this exercise had better running times than others who breathed normal air. One year later, Hill and Flack (1910) again observed increases on a running, stepping task and weight lifting after subjects breathed supplemental O_2. Their overall conclusions were that subjects could perform better in the initial aspects of a race if the race were shorter than a half mile. Hill and Flack (1910) attributed increases in performance to an increased storage of O_2 or to an increased tolerance of CO_2 accumulation in the individual.

Karpovich (1934), after observing that certain Japanese Olympic swimmers had used O_2 prior to competing in 1932, studied the effect of O_2 supplementation on swimming performance. He found that several athletes increased their swimming performance in

100-to 200-yard swims when they had supplemental O_2 prior to the event. Neither the 50-yard swim times nor the 440-yard swim times were significantly altered. Morris (1978) has noted that swim distances of 100-200 yards are about equal to running distance of 400-800 yards in terms of energy source utilization (about half anaerobic and half aerobic), so the findings of Karpovich (1934) seem to concur with those of Hill and Flack (1909, 1910).

Miller et al. (1952) introduced supplemental O_2 in a blind procedure to several subjects and noted no significant improvement in exercise or recovery. There were no changes in heart rate, blood pressure, blood lactate, endurance, or subjective impressions of his subjects.

Elbel, Ormond, and Close (1961) used trained individuals in treadmill tests to determine the effects of supplemental O_2 prior to 5 minutes of running. They reported that O_2 breathing prior to the treadmill run resulted in a lower pulse rate at rest and during the first 2 minutes of the treadmill run.

Effects of Oxygen Administered in the Post-Exercise Period

Some early studies alluded to beneficial effects of supplemental O_2 during recovery from exercise (Hill & Flack, 1909, 1910) and on succeeding efforts. There were certain deficiencies in these studies, however. Very often the experimenters served as subjects and knew which gas mixtures they were inhaling, thereby introducing a bias. Other evidence that breathing O_2-enriched air in the recovery period following exercise aids recovery is not without controversy. Elbel et al. (1961) found post-exercise recovery heart rates were consistently lower when subjects breathed O_2 in the recovery period. However, respiration rates were surprisingly elevated. Hagerman, Bowers, Fox, and Ersing (1968) observed a trend toward quicker recovery with supplemental O_2, although no significant differences were reported on recovery pulse rates. They studied bicycle ergometer work.

Weltman and colleagues (Weltman, Stamford, Moffatt, & Katch, 1977; Weltman, Katch, & Sady, 1978), in an extensive study of the effects of supplemental O_2 on recovery and subsequent work tasks on a bicycle ergometer, found no significant increase in the number of pedal revolutions for a 60-second interval and in total work output of a 60-second all-out ride. Subjects were allowed to breathe room air or 100% O_2 for either 10 or 20 minutes; then they repeated the 60-second all-out bike ride. Riding performance and blood lactic acid levels showed no difference between both conditions. The investigators suggested that hyperoxic inhalation did not alter lactate production and removal.

Supplemental Oxygen and Psychomotor Speed

Psychomotor speed performances are tested with small motor tasks, e.g., finger tapping, reaction times with hand or arm movements, and crossing out symbols with a pen or pencil. These psychomotor performances, which are nonexhaustive, are contrasted with gross motor activities, which have been reported earlier, for example, exhaustive running, cycling, or stair climbing.

In an excellent recent review of psychomotor speed and aging, Spirduso (1980) stated that supplemental O_2 treatments often significantly improved perceptual and psychomotor functioning in patients as well as aged healthy subjects. The mechanisms suggested were that hyperbaric O_2 might affect autoregulatory mechanisms, which might in turn improve cerebral blood flow. It is known that adequate cerebral blood flow is critical to normal mental functioning and psychomotor performance.

General Summary and Conclusions

The use of supplemental O_2 breathing mixtures prior to, during, and following strenuous exercise has been theorized to be an ergogenic aid to muscular performance. This review reveals that there is little or no effect (other than perhaps psychologically) in inhaling oxygen-enriched air prior to or following exhaustive exercise. However, breathing supplemental oxygen during exercise seems to facilitate maximum human performance and improve endurance, but the exact mechanism(s) remains unclear. Many investigators have reported increases in $\dot{V}O_2$ max, reductions in blood lactic acid, and lowering of the ventilatory rate in subjects breathing supplemental oxygen during work bouts. Most experimenters also report some increases in human physical performance.

For military operations or in a clinical setting, supplemental oxygen may have a purpose, but for the athlete it is impractical. Even if athletes could somehow strap an oxygen breathing apparatus to their bodies during exercise, it would probably impede their performance more than it could possibly aid it. And, finally, according to the present international rules, such artificial aids would be illegal.

References

ASMUSSEN, E., & Nielsen, M. The cardiac output in rest and work at low and high oxygen pressure. *Acta Physiologicia Scandinavica*, 1946, **35**, 73-83.

BANISTER, E.W., Taunton, J.E., Patrick, T., Oforsagd, P., & Duncan, W.R. Effect of oxygen at high pressure, at rest and during severe exercise. *Respiration Physiology*, 1970, **10**, 74-84.

BANNISTER, R.G., & Cunningham, D.J.C. The effects on the respiration and performance during exercise of adding oxygen to the inspired air. *Journal of Physiology*, 1954, **125**, 118-137.

BRIGGS, H. Physical exertion, fitness, and breathing. *Journal of Physiology*, 1920, **54**, 292-318.

BUSKIRK, E.R., Kollias, J., Piconreatigue, E., Akers, R., Prokop, E., & Baker, P. Physiology and performance of track athletes at various altitudes in the United States and Peru. In R. Goddard (Ed.), *The effects of altitude on physical performance*. Chicago: The Athletic Institute, 1967.

CUNNINGHAM, D.A. Effects of breathing high concentrations of oxygen on treadmill performance. *Research Quarterly*, 1966, **37**, 491-494.

deVRIES, H.A. *Physiology of exercise*. Dubuque, IA: Wm. C. Brown, 1980.

DOUGLAS C.E., & Haldane, J.S. The effects of previous forced breathing and oxygen inhalation on the distress caused by muscular work. *Journal of Physiology*, 1909, **39**, 1-4.

DRESSENDORFER, R.H., Wade, C.E., & Bernauer, E.M. Combined effects of breathing resistance and hyperoxia on aerobic work tolerance. *Journal of Applied Physiology*, 1977, **42**, 444-448.

EKBLOM, B., Huot, R., Stein, E.M., & Thorstenson, A.T. Effect of changes in arterial oxygen content on circulation and physical performance. *Journal of Applied Physiology*, 1975, **39**, 71-75.

ELBEL, E.R., Ormond, D., & Close, D. Some effects of breathing oxygen before and after exercise. *Journal of Applied Physiology*, 1961, **16**, 48-52.

FAGRAEUS, L. Cardiorespiratory and metabolic functions during exercise in the hyperbaric environment. *Acta Physiologicia Scandinavica*, 1974, **92**, 1-40. (Supplement 414)

FELDMAN, I., & Hill, L. The influence of oxygen inhalation on the lactic acid produced during hard work. *Journal of Physiology*, 1911, **42**, 439-443.

HAGERMAN, F.C., Bowers, R.W., Fox, E.L., & Ersing, W.W. The effects of breathing 100 percent oxygen, during rest, heavy work, and recovery. *Research Quarterly*, 1968, **39**, 965-975.

HILL, A.V., Long, C.N.H., & Lupton, H. Muscular exercise, lactic acid and the supply and utilization of oxygen. *Proceedings of the Royal Society*, 1924, **97**, 155-167.

HILL, L., & Flack, M. The influence of oxygen on athletes. *Journal of Physiology*, 1909, **38**, 28-36.

HILL, L., & Flack, M. The influence of oxygen inhalations on muscular work. *Journal of Physiology*, 1910, **40**, 347-372.

HILL, L., & McKenzie, J. The effect of oxygen inhalation on muscular exertion. *Journal of Physiology*, 1909, **39**, 33-38.

HUGHES, R.L., Clode, M., Edwards, R.H.T., Goodwin, T.S., & Jones, N.L. Effect of inspired O_2 on cardiopulmonary and metabolic responses to exercise in man. *Journal of Applied Physiology*, 1968, **24**, 336-347.

KAIJSER, L. Physical exercise under hyperbaric oxygen pressure. *Life Sciences*, 1969, **8**, 929-932.

KAIJSER, L. Limiting factors for aerobic muscle performance: The influence of varying oxygen pressure and temperature. *Acta Physiologicia Scandinavica*, 1970, **79**, 1-96. (Supplement 346)

KAIJSER, L. Oxygen supply as a limiting factor in physical performance. In J. Keul (Ed.), *Limiting factors of physical performance*. Stuttgart: Georg Thieme, 1973.

KARPOVICH, P.V. Effects of oxygen inhalation on swimming performance. *Research Quarterly*, 1934, **5**, 24-28.

KEUL, J. (Ed.). *Limiting factors of physical performance*. Stuttgart: Georg Thieme, 1973.

MATHEWS, D.K., & Fox, E.L. *The physiological basis of physical education and athletics*. Philadelphia: W.B. Saunders, 1976.

MCARDLE, W.D., Katch, F.I., & Katch, V.L. *Exercise physiology: Energy, nutrition, and human performance*. Philadelphia: Lea & Febiger, 1981.

MILLER, A.T., Jr., Perdue, H.L., Teague, E.L., Jr., & Fereber, J.A. Influence of oxygen administration on cardiovascular function during exercise and recovery. *Journal of Applied Physiology*, 1952, **5**, 165-168.

MORRIS, A.F. Comparing and contrasting two similar sports: Swimming and track. *Journal of Sports Medicine and Physical Fitness*, 1978, **18**, 409-415.

NIELSEN, M., & Hansen, O. Maximale Körperliche Arbeit bei Atmung O_2-reicher Luft. *Scandinavia Archives of Physiology*, 1937, **76**, 37-59.

SPIRDUSO, W.W. Physical fitness, aging, and psychomotor speed: A review. *Journal of Gerontology*, 1980, **35**, 850-865.

STAINSBY, W.N. Critical oxygen tensions in muscle. In J. Keul (Ed.), *Limiting factors of physical performance*. Stuttgart: George Thieme, 1973.

TAUNTON, J.E., Banister, E.W., Patrick, T.R., Oforsagd, P., & Duncan, W.R. Physical work capacity in hyperbaric environments and conditions of hyperoxia. *Journal of Applied Physiology*, 1970, **28**, 421-427.

WELCH, H.G., Bonde-Petersen, F., Graham, T., Klausen, K., & Secher,

N. Effects of hyperoxia on leg blood flow and metabolism during exercise. *Journal of Applied Physiology*, 1977, **42**, 385-390.

WELCH, H.G., Mulin, J.P., Wilson, G.D., & Lewis, J. Effects of breathing O_2-enriched gas mixtures on metabolic rate during exercise. *Medicine and Science in Sports*, 1974, **6**, 26-32.

WELTMAN, A., Katch, V., & Sady, S. Effects of increasing oxygen availability on bicycle ergometer endurance performance. *Ergonomics*, 1978, **21**, 427-432.

WELTMAN, A.L., Stamford, B.A., Moffatt, R.J., & Katch, V.L. Exercise recovery, lactate removal, and subsequent high intensity exercise performance. *Research Quarterly*, 1977, **48**, 786-796.

WILMORE, J.H. Oxygen. In W.P. Morgan (Ed.), *Ergogenic aids and muscular performance*. New York: Academic Press, 1972.

WILSON, B.A., Welch, H.G., & Liles, J.N. Effects of hyperoxic gas mixtures on energy metabolism during prolonged work. *Journal of Applied Physiology*, 1975, **39**, 267-271.

WILSON, G.D., & Welch, H.G. Effects of hyperoxic gas mixtures on exercise tolerance in man. *Medicine and Science in Sports*, 1975, **7**, 48-52.

WILSON, G.D., & Welch, H.G. Effects of varying concentrations of N_2/O_2 and He/O_2 on exercise tolerance in man. *Medicine and Science in Sports and Exercise*, 1980, **12**, 380-384.

WYNDHAM, C.H., Strydom, N.B., Van Rensburg, A.J., & Rogers, G.G. Effects on maximal intake of acute changes in altitude in a deep mine. *Journal of Applied Physiology*, 1970, **29**, 552-555.

8

Blood Doping

Melvin H. Williams

Certain athletes, such as distance runners, swimmers, or cyclists, have always been interested in various techniques or agents to help improve their endurance capacity. Hence, altitude training and such diverse compounds as alkaline salts, amphetamines, caffeine, iron supplements, vasodilators, vitamins B_{12} and E, among others, have been utilized in attempts to increase maximal oxygen uptake ($\dot{V}O_2$ max) and help prevent the physiological or psychological fatigue associated with prolonged aerobic exercise.

The role of blood is one of the prime determinants of $\dot{V}O_2$ max. The removal of 500 to 1,000 ml of blood, with concomitant loss of hemoglobin (Hb), has been shown to significantly reduce working capacity and $\dot{V}O_2$ max (Balke, Grillo, Konecci, & Luft, 1954; Ekblom, Goldbarg, & Gullbring, 1972; Howell & Coupe, 1964; Karpovich & Millman, 1942). On the other hand, athletic training at altitude has been theorized to enhance endurance performance upon subsequent return to sea level due to increased red blood cells (RBC) and Hb. Moreover, Oscai, Williams, and Hertig (1968)

Melvin H. Williams, Ph.D., F.A.C.S.M., is with the Human Performance Laboratory at Old Dominion University in Norfolk, Virginia.

suggested that increases in $\dot{V}O_2$ max through training are associated with increases in total blood volume and total Hb. Thus, it is theorized that increased blood volume and/or Hb may contribute to greater levels of $\dot{V}O_2$ max and performance in prolonged aerobic activity.

Training at altitude will elicit significant alterations in blood parameters that are theorized to increase aerobic work capacity. However, in recent years the technique of blood doping has been advocated as a method to mimic the effects of altitude training. In essence, blood doping is the infusion of blood into an athlete. It may be his own blood, which has been withdrawn 5-6 weeks earlier, or other cross-matched blood. The recommended technique is to use autologous blood. Following blood withdrawal, the athlete waits 5-6 weeks for his RBC to regenerate. During this time, his blood has been stored in a frozen state. The blood is then infused into the athlete from 1-7 days prior to the scheduled athletic event.

Blood doping has been purported to be an ergogenic aid on the European sports scene since 1971. It did not receive great public attention, however, until the 1976 Montreal Olympics, when several television sports commentators suggested the technique was being used by an Olympic champion. Following the 1976 Olympic Games, the United States Olympic Committee quietly approved the formation of a panel of experts to study the scientific and medical aspects of sports and their effects on the performance of world class athletes. Blood doping was earmarked as an important research area in attempts to help maximize American athletic potential (Amdur, 1976). Similar emphasis on blood doping research has also been encouraged by other countries.

Theoretical Benefits

The theory underlying blood doping is based upon possible increases in the O_2-carrying capacity of the blood. Endurance athletes usually have well developed cardiovascular systems and are able to produce more energy over prolonged periods, mainly as a result of a high $\dot{V}O_2$ max. Of the various physiological factors that govern $\dot{V}O_2$ max, the available evidence suggests gas transport is the limiting factor. Shephard (1971) indicated that $\dot{V}O_2$ max is normally limited by physiological rather than biochemical processes and concluded that overall conductance of O_2 can be augmented by an increase in blood Hb concentration or increased cardiac output. Thus, as the theory goes, by increasing either the blood volume or the RBC and Hb concentration, or both, the athlete may possess greater O_2-carrying capacity, a potentially desirable physiological state in aerobic endurance events.

Oxygen unloading to the tissues is governed by several independent variables expressed in the formula $\dot{V}O_2 = \dot{Q} \cdot (Sa_{O_2} - S\bar{v}_{O_2})$, where $\dot{V}O_2$ equals liters O_2, $\dot{Q}$ is cardiac output or blood flow, and $Sa_{O_2} - S\bar{v}_{O_2}$ represents the difference in arterial and mixed venous blood saturation with O_2. $Sa_{O_2} = 1.34 \cdot Hb$, where 1.34 equals ml of O_2 bound by 1 g Hb fully saturated, and Hb is hemoglobin concentration in grams. Therefore, to increase O_2 transport one can attempt to increase $\dot{Q}$, Hb, or Sa_{O_2}. O_2 utilization by the tissues is represented by $Sa_{O_2} - S\bar{v}_{O_2}$. The theoretical beneficial effects of blood doping have been attributed to its ability to increase blood volume (hypervolemia) and/or RBC and Hb concentration (polycythemia).

Theoretically, induced hypervolemia through blood doping could prove to be beneficial during an aerobic work task, as the increased total blood volume could increase the capacity for greater cardiac output. According to Gregersen and Chien (1968), the plasma volume is subordinate to the regulation of blood volume; the latter is held relatively constant at the expense of the former. Any attempt to increase blood volume forcibly by infusion of fluids, plasma, or RBC is promptly countered by restoration of blood volume to its previous level. The rate of change of fluid across the capillary wall is high, the plasma volume undergoing rapid changes in comparison to cell volume. Guyton (1981) stated that the increased cardiac output caused by an acute increase in blood volume, as through transfusion, lasts only a few minutes because the increased cardiac output increases the capillary pressure so that the fluid begins to transude out of the capillaries into the tissues, thereby returning blood volume to normal. He indicated the cardiac output would gradually return to normal in about 40 minutes. Calculations by Williams, Bocrie, Goodwin, and Perkins (1973), extrapolating data from Berne and Levy (1967), have indicated that a 500-ml blood transfusion would result in an efflux of approximately 250 ml of the plasma within 1 hour of transfusion. Thus, infusion of 500 ml whole blood, or packed RBC in normal saline to an equivalent 500 ml, would result primarily in an elevated Hb concentration, RBC count, and hematocrit (Hct) with little change in total blood volume.

As mentioned previously, the increased Hb concentration resulting from RBC infusion may be theorized to increase endurance capacity. Exercise, in and by itself, may elicit a reflex hemoconcentration with elevated Hb levels. Fahey and Rolph (1975) noted an increase in Hct during exercise that is apparently due to a shift of plasma to the extracellular space. Gregersen and Chien (1968) reported that 1 minute of violent exercise will reduce plasma volume by several hundred ml. In a recent study with 20 subjects, Williams and Ward (1977) noted a 4% and 9% increase in Hb and Hct, respectively, following a 1 mile run. Thus, it appears that nature attempts to increase the O_2 transport capacity during exercise via an increased Hb concentration and Hct. A number of reports (Ekblom et al., 1972; Ekblom, Wilson, & Astrand, 1976; Leavell & Thorup, 1976; Mollison, 1972; Williams, Lindhjem, & Schuster, 1978; Williams, Wesseldine, Somma, & Schuster, 1981) have shown increased resting Hb and Hct levels following the infusion of either whole blood or packed RBC. If this resting hemoconcentration could be augmented by the exercise-induced hemoconcentration, then the O_2-carrying capacity of the blood would be even further increased.

Blood doping may have another theoretical benefit. If a decreasing blood pH is a causative factor in the development of fatigue, then infusion of RBC may be useful in events where blood pH may decrease, such as the anaerobic stages near the climax of high-intensity aerobic work tasks. The Hb of the RBC is an excellent acid-base buffer; Guyton (1981) reported that the RBC are responsible for approximately 70% of all the buffering power of the whole blood. Recent research has noted a decreased lactate acidosis following exercise at 85 and 100% $\dot{V}O_2$ max when blood doping was used (Gledhill, Spriet, Froese, Wilkes, & Meyers, 1980).

On the other hand, RBC infusion could be a possible disadvantage to increasing physical performance if a marked polycythemia occurs. The RBC concentration is the prime determinant of blood viscosity, and the viscosity will rise with increasing Hct. Blood flow velocity has been reported to be inversely related to Hct level (Itzchak, Silverberger, Modan, Adar, & Deutsch, 1977). According to Williams, Beutler, Ersley, and Rundles (1972), at Hct readings higher than 50%, the viscosity of the blood increases exponentially, decreasing the transport of O_2 to the tissues. Following blood infusion in animals Replogle and Merrill (1970) noted a reduced peripheral O_2 content, inferring that the increased O_2-carrying capacity of the blood due to hemoconcentration was not sufficient to counterbalance the effect of reduced cardiac output. Guyton and Richardson (1961) indicated that polycythemia reduced the minute RBC flow to the tissues due to decreased venous return. Weisse, Calton, Kuida, and Hecht (1964), studying normovolemic polycythemia, noted a decreased cardiac output and O_2 transport during rest. Although they also noted a rise in O_2 transport with exercise in polycythemic animals, in only one case was the value greater than when the animals were normocythemic. It should be noted, however, that in these studies a high degree of polycythemia was created, well above a Hct of 50%. In most studies investigating the effect of blood infusion upon physical performance in humans, the Hct has not exceeded 50%, although Pace, Lozner, Consolazio, Pitts, and Pecora (1947) reported a 58.3% after the infusion of 2,000 ml of a 50% suspension of compatible RBC. Hence, the polycythemia created by infusion of 500-1,000 ml of blood may not increase the blood viscosity significantly enough to retard O_2 transport.

An important factor that may influence the theoretical efficacy of blood doping is the technique of storing the blood, as it may affect the oxygen-carrying capacity of the blood, particularly if the individual is to exercise within several hours after the infusion. The concentration of 2,3-diphosphoglycerate (2,3-DPG) in the RBC is important relative to the affinity of oxygen to Hb. Increased 2,3-DPG is associated with a reduced affinity of O_2 to Hb, therefore facilitating the release of O_2 from Hb when the blood reaches the muscles (Edington & Edgerton, 1976). Conversely, Hb affinity for O_2 is increased, with resultant tissue hypoxia, when intracellular 2,3-DPG concentration is diminished (Klein, 1973). Mollison (1972) has indicated that blood stored in acid-citrate-dextrose (ACD) will lose 60% of its 2,3-DPG in 1 week and 90% in 2 weeks. Bunn, Forget, and Ranney (1977), summarizing their own and other studies, indicated that during the first week of storage of blood with ACD, RBC become depleted of 2,3-DPG and, as a result, have increased O_2 affinity. However, they do note that following infusion of such donor cells into normal subjects, their content of 2,3-DPG returns to normal in 6-24 hours. This finding has been confirmed in three blood doping studies (Buick, Gledhill, Froese, Spriet, & Meyers, 1980; Ekblom et al., 1976; Williams et al., 1981) that evaluated 2,3-DPG levels before and after infusion, although the blood was frozen in two of the studies. Thus, in order to achieve the full O_2 transport capacity of RBC, physical performance should be undertaken after 6-24 hours postinfusion if the blood was stored in ACD. With frozen blood, performance may be undertaken shortly after infusion. It should be noted that another anticoagulant, citrate-phosphate-dextrose (CPD), has been reported to be a better preservative than ACD (Bunn et al., 1977; Huestis, Bove, & Busch, 1976).

The reported research relative to the effects of blood doping upon physical performance and associated parameters reveals conflicting results, perhaps because previous research may have been confounded by one of several factors, including the nature of the criterion workload task, a training effect on untrained subjects, absence of a control or placebo group, failure to measure selected blood variables such as Hb, absence of a double-blind protocol, differences in elapsed time between withdrawal and infusion, blood storage techniques, and volume of blood infused, These limitations should be kept in mind when interpreting the literature.

Supportive Research Findings

Two early studies investigated the effect of blood infusion upon submaximal work. Pace and others (1947) induced a polycythemia in five normal men by the infusion of 2,000 ml of 50% suspension of compatible erythrocytes at a rate of 500 ml/day for 4 days. The Hct value rose from 46.2 to 58.3%, and the polycythemia lasted 50 days. The O_2-carrying capacity of the arterial blood was increased 23%. Using the pulse rate during submaximal work as the criterion measure for adjustments to simulated hypoxic levels, the authors concluded that the transfusion conferred an advantage to the subjects when exposed to a simulated altitude. Gullbring, Holmgren, Sjostrand, and Strandell (1960) used the PWC (physical working capacity) PWC_{170}, a submaximal test monitoring heart rate (HR), to investigate the withdrawal and reinfusion effect of approximately 10% of the blood volume in six physicians. Performance was adversely affected on tests the day following withdrawal. The blood was reinfused 7 days after withdrawal, and a marked improvement in PWC_{170} was noted 1 hour postinfusion. Both of these studies are limited by the fact that submaximal exercise tasks may not accurately reflect maximal performance. Moreover, neither study involved control groups or double-blind protocol, and a training effect may also have confounded the results.

Ekblom and his associates (1972) studied the effects of blood loss and subsequent reinfusion on the PWC of seven nonathletic subjects. Three subjects, Group I, underwent a single venesection of 800 ml blood, while four subjects, Group II, lost 1,200 ml during three withdrawals of 400 ml each. Baseline values for HR, O_2 uptake, and submaximal and maximal work parameters were determined prior to the blood loss. PWC and $\dot{V}O_2$ max decreased substantially following withdrawal. Approximately 4 weeks later, the blood was reinfused. In Group I, the increased blood volume caused a significant increase in $\dot{V}O_2$ max, Hb, and maximal work time. The same increase in $\dot{V}O_2$ max was not noted in Group II because no preinfusion data was available from the preceding day. However, they did experience substantial increases in maximal work time and Hb when compared to base-line values. Although it was a highly sophisticated study, the data may have been confounded by a training effect and lack of a control group; in addition, no indication of a double-blind design was noted.

Von Rost, Hollman, Liesen, and Schulten (1975) infused the packed RBC from 900 ml blood into 17 athletic subjects, placed in three groups, in order to investigate the effect upon various performance parameters. Six of the subjects undertook treadmill tests for $\dot{V}O_2$ max and endurance time, and four of those six also had cardiac output determinations; five subjects did $\dot{V}O_2$ max tests on a bicycle ergometer; and six subjects undertook swimming performance tests ranging in duration from 1 to 16 minutes. The blood was infused into the subjects 3-4 weeks postwithdrawal. The tests, with some exceptions, appear to have been administered before and after both withdrawal and infusion. A fourth group of six subjects received infusions of either 500 ml normal saline, 500 ml of a collodial solution, or 250 ml of a protein solution. $\dot{V}O_2$ max and treadmill endurance time were studied; no blood was withdrawn from this group, and only a preinfusion and postinfusion test was administered. The authors reported a 9% increase in $\dot{V}O_2$ max and a 37% increase in treadmill endurance time following the RBC infusion, even though the Hb rise was very small; however, the results were not statistically significant due to large individual variability. The competitive swimmers improved their performance times, four of the six attaining personal bests; however, the authors noted that a placebo effect could not be discounted. Submaximal HR and $\dot{V}O_2$ were unchanged following RBC infusion. Maximal cardiac output did not appear to change. The saline solution prolonged treadmill endurance time but did not increase $\dot{V}O_2$ max. The authors concluded that the increased performances could be attributed to increased blood volume rather than to increased Hb levels. Although this report contained some useful information relative to the effect of blood doping, the lack of a sound control-group double-blind protocol clouds the results. The authors even noted that methodological difficulties and wide individual variation may create problems with interpretation of the data.

Ekblom and others (1976) studied five well trained subjects under three conditions: control, after venesection of 800 ml whole blood, and after reinfusion of 360 ml packed RBC (110 g Hb) about 30-35 days after venesection. Actually, the subjects were tested four times; basic data on $\dot{V}O_2$ max was collected before the experiment started. The preinfusion control trial was given 30 days postvenesection, and the results from this trial were not significantly different from the prevenesection data, even though the Hb and Hct were lower at the preinfusion trial compared to the prevenesection trial. Within 2-5 days after the control trial, the packed RBC were infused and the performance tests were conducted 1 day later. Both maximal and submaximal tests were administered to the subjects. A number of physiological measures were recorded throughout the investigation, including $\dot{V}O_2$ max, HR, SV, $\dot{Q}$, $C\bar{v}_{O_2}$, Ca_{O_2}, Sa_{O_2}, Pa_{O_2}, Pa_{CO_2}, and pH. Comparing the control and postinfusion trials, there was a 4.5% increase in Hb during the maximal exercise period, which was only about a third of that expected theoretically. There was a significant increase in $\dot{V}O_2$ max during the postinfusion trial, which the authors attributed to an increase in Ca_{O_2} (Hb concentration) and a lowering of $C\bar{v}_{O_2}$. There were no changes in maximal values for HR, SV, and $\dot{Q}$. It should be noted, however, that the report did not indicate whether there was an increase in physical performance capacity, even though the $\dot{V}O_2$ max increased by approximately 6%. In addition, there was no mention of a control group or double-blind procedure.

In a related study, Horstman, Weiskopf, Jackson, and Severinghaus (1976) studied the effect of an extended sojourn at high altitude (HA) and the specific role of HA-induced polycythemia upon sea-level work capacity. Nine subjects were divided into two groups and underwent $\dot{V}O_2$ max and endurance time to exhaustion tests prior to 4 weeks at altitude without physical training. One week prior to return to sea level, five subjects had 450 ml blood withdrawn, while the other four subjects were exposed to a sham withdrawal. Upon return to sea level, the performance tests were retaken. There was no significant difference in $\dot{V}O_2$ max and endurance time for the blood donor group, but the sham group increased significantly in both. Because the Hct of the sham group was significantly higher during the second trial as compared to the first and the blood donor group experienced no significant difference, the authors postulated that the increased work capacity was a function of the increased O_2 transport afforded by the HA-induced polycythemia.

Robertson, Gilcher, Metz, Bahnson, Allison, Skriner, Abbott, and Becker (1978) studied the effect of RBC reinfusion on metabolic and perceptual responses during exercise for five male mountain climbers. Separate treadmill tests were performed under four conditions: (a) preinfusion, normoxia (N_1); (b) postinfusion, normoxia (N_2); (c) preinfusion, hypoxia (H_1); and (d) postinfusion, hypoxia (H_2). Testing occurred immediately before and within 24 hours after reinfusion of four units of packed RBC. $\dot{V}O_2$, ventilation ($\dot{V}_E$), HR, respiratory rate/min (RR) and ratings of perceived exertion overall, chest and legs (RPE_o, RPE_c, RPE_L) were measured from the fifth to sixth minutes of submaximal exercise and at maximal work. Submaximal HR was lower at N_2 than N_1 and at H_2 than H_1. Maximal $\dot{V}O_2$, $\dot{V}_E$, RR, and performance time were higher at N_2 than N_1. $\dot{V}O_2$ and performance time were higher at H_2 than H_1.

RBC reinfusion decreased submaximal cardiac work and increased maximal aerobic capacity and performance time under normoxic and hypoxic conditions. RPE was not affected. However, no control group was utilized in this study.

In a subsequent study, Robertson, Gilcher, Metz, Casperson, Abbott, Allison, Skriner, Werner, Zelicoff, and Krause (1979) tested seven females on separate submaximal and maximal cycle ergometer tests in the following sequence: I—control tests; II—placebo test 48 hours after reinfusion of 350 ml of Plasmalyte; and III—reinfusion test 48 hours after reinfusion of 350 ml of packed red blood cells. $\dot{V}O_2$, $\dot{V}_E$, HR, $\dot{Q}$, a-v O_2 difference, and submaximal lactic acid were determined under normoxic and hypoxic conditions. Hct and Hb increased significantly following reinfusion. Significant differences were not found between the control and placebo tests. Submaximal HR decreased following reinfusion under normoxia and hypoxia. Lactic acid was similar between control and reinfusion tests. Under both normoxia and hypoxia maximal $\dot{V}O_2$ and performance time and a-v O_2 difference increased significantly following reinfusion. Maximal $\dot{Q}$ was unaffected by reinfusion. The investigators concluded that expansion of the Hb concentration improved physical work capacity via central circulatory adjustments under normoxia and hypoxia. However, there is no mention of a control group and it appears that the order of administration of the three tests was not counterbalanced and hence may have elicited a training effect.

Cottrell (1979) reported a study conducted by Moore and Parry with members of the British Army. Eight men had 405 ml of their blood frozen for 63 days. Six of the subjects then were infused with their own packed cells while two subjects served as controls. Performance was measured via a 6-minute ride on a bicycle ergometer designed to simulate uphill pedaling. HR was monitored continuously. On the basis of individual improvements in performance ranging from 1-5%, the authors concluded that this is further evidence that blood doping improves athletic performance. No statistical comparisons were made in this brief report, however, and no evidence of a double-blind protocol was presented. In addition, it appears that only HR data was measured, and a possible training effect could have influenced the reported results.

Using a double-blind design, Buick and others (1980) studied the effect of experimental polycythemia on maximal treadmill exercise in highly trained endurance runners. Blood was stored by freezing for autologous reinfusion after restoration of normocythemia. Hb, $\dot{V}O_2$ max, and endurance performance were assessed following sham reinfusion (50 ml saline) and reinfusion (900 ml whole blood) in random order. Control measurements were made prior to blood removal (C1), prior to reinfusion (C2), and at the termination of polycythemia (C3). No differences were observed in Hb and $\dot{V}O_2$ max among the C1, C2, C3, and post-sham-reinfusion tests. At 24 hours postreinfusion, there were significant increases in Hb, $\dot{V}O_2$ max, and running time to exhaustion. At 1 week postreinfusion, the increases were still present. The authors concluded that blood boosting increases $\dot{V}O_2$ max and also prolongs endurance time in highly trained runners and that these advantages persist for at least 1 week. However, the authors related the performance changes to Hb levels; although the Hb levels were down to normal at the termination of polycythemia (C3), performance time was significantly better than the control and sham trials. This finding was attributed to a "super-training effect", that is, the blood infusion allowed the athletes to train at a higher level during this period, and hence performance ability remained elevated. Another interesting finding was a lower blood lactate following the reinfusion trial, suggesting that the increased RBC may augment the buffering capacity of the blood.

Spriet, Gledhill, Froese, Wilkes, and Meyers (1980) investigated the effect of an elevated Hct upon central circulation and O_2 transport during maximal exercise. Four highly trained runners performed a maximal treadmill test at three Hct levels: 45.6, control; 49.2, following the infusion of approximately 800 ml autologous blood; and 50.5, following the infusion of an additional 400 ml blood. The values recorded for each of the three trials, in respective order as above, were as follows: $\dot{V}O_2$ max (ml/kg/min)—77.3, 80.3, 82.4; $\dot{Q}$ (liters/min)—29.8, 38.4, 40.9; HR—183, 180, 178; SV (ml)—163, 213, 230; arterial O_2 content (volume %)—19.6, 21.7, 22.2; and O_2 transport (liters/min)—5.8, 8.3, 9.1. Because these results were obtained 2-7 days postinfusion, they would not be due to a significant hypervolemia. Instead, the authors attributed the significant increase in SV and $\dot{Q}$ to an increased availability of O_2 to the myocardium. The increased O_2 transport, due to increases in both $\dot{Q}$ and arterial O_2 content, contributed to the increased $\dot{V}O_2$ max. It should be noted, however, that although the O_2 transport increased approximately 2.5-3.3 l/min, the $\dot{V}O_2$ max increased only 350 ml/min, assuming a 70-kg runner. Thus, the ability of the muscle cells to use the delivered O_2 may be another limiting factor to endurance capacity.

In an attempt to produce some practical results, Williams and others (1981) investigated the effect the infusion of 920 ml equivalent of autologous blood would have upon 5-mile time (5MT) and both local (RPE-L) and cardiovascular-respiratory (RPE-B) ratings of perceived exertion. Twelve long-distance runners undertook a series of four competitive 5MT trials on a treadmill. Four test conditions were utilized: presaline trial, postsaline trial after 920 ml saline solution, preblood trial, and postblood trial after 920 ml equivalent of whole blood. All subjects took all trials in this double-blind placebo crossover experimental design. Running time and RPE were recorded at each 0.5-mile split. Blood samples were taken before and after each trial. The data were analyzed via a repeated measures ANOVA. In general, the following results were noted following the blood infusion when compared with the other three trials: a significantly higher Hb concentration, a significantly lower RPE-L and RPE-B during the first 2 miles of the run, and a significantly faster 5MT. The authors concluded that the infusion of 920 ml equivalent autologous blood would increase performance capacity in an athletic event characterized by high levels of aerobic energy expenditure.

In another double-blind counterbalanced study, Goforth, Campbell, Hodgdon, and Sucec (1982), using six trained distance runners as subjects, reported that the infusion of 760 ml autologus RBC increased $\dot{V}O_2$ max by 0.46 l/min and the VO_2 at anaerobic threshold by 0.33 l/min. The time to run 3 miles also decreased by 23.7 seconds following the induced erythrocythemia. $\dot{V}O_2$ max returned to the preinfusion level 4 weeks after the blood infusion, even though the hematocrit was still slightly elevated. Hematocrit levels returned to normal in 8 weeks.

Nonsupportive Research Findings

Robinson, Epstein, Kahler, and Braunwald (1966) reported that the infusion of 1,000-1,200 ml of autologous blood into six subjects had no effect upon $\dot{V}O_2$ max during treadmill exercise. They indicated that all of the infused blood was accommodated in the venous compartments, the capacitance vessels.

Williams and his colleagues (1973) evaluated the effects of reinjected hematological components on endurance capacity and maximal HR. Twenty male athletes, mostly distance runners, were pretested on a maximal treadmill run and assigned to one of four groups: whole blood (500 ml), packed RBC (275 ml), plasma (225 ml), and control. Five hundred ml of blood was withdrawn from the subjects in the three experimental groups; the control group also went through the venipuncture protocol. All subjects were blindfolded during the withdrawal and reinfusion stages of the investigation; a double-blind design was utilized. Twenty-one days following withdrawal, the hematological components were infused into the appropriate groups. The maximal test was readministered approximately 2 hours postinfusion, 2 days postinfusion, and 6 days postinfusion. A two-way ANOVA revealed no significant effects due to treatments, and the authors concluded the infusion of whole blood, packed RBCs, or plasma, at least in the quantities utilized in their study, had no differential effect upon endurance capacity or maximal heart rate. However, the blood was not frozen and no hematological measures were recorded.

Frye and Ruhling (1977), using a single-blind design, randomly assigned 16 male and female volunteers to four groups following a modified Balke protocol pretest. The four groups were control, exercise, RBC infusion, and exercise and RBC infusion. All subjects experienced venipuncture with the latter two groups having 500 ml withdrawn. During the next 2 weeks, the exercise groups trained 5 days/week. Seventeen days after the initial withdrawal, all subjects experienced venipuncture again; the first two groups received normal saline and the infusion groups received their own packed RBC. Analysis of the data revealed no significant differences between groups relative to peak $\dot{V}O_2$.

Videman and Rytömaa (1977) withdrew 400-600 ml of blood from 10 trained men and stored it at $4°$ C for 2-3 weeks. After 2 weeks, the blood was infused into five men, and at 3 weeks the other five received their blood. During this time frame, the subjects undertook a 6-minute submaximal bicycle task three to four times weekly. Hb and $\dot{V}O_2$ max (predicted from heart rate response) were measured at each trial. The authors concluded there was no increase in physical performance following the transfusion.

Using a double-blind placebo design, Williams et al. (1978) studied the effect of blood infusion upon maximal endurance capacity and ratings of perceived exertion (RPE). Sixteen long-distance runners, 13 of whom were marathoners, undertook four trials of a maximal treadmill run to exhaustion over a 5-week period. Criterion measures were time to exhaustion (TE) and RPE during each trial. Data on Hb, Hct, and RBC were collected prior to each trial. Based on TE at Trial 1, subjects were matched and assigned to either the experimental or control group. One week after the first trial, all subjects had 500 ml blood withdrawn. The blood was then stored in a frozen state. Trial 2 was undertaken 2 weeks postwithdrawal. One week after trial 2, or 21 days postwithdrawal, the experimental group was infused with their own RBC while the control group received 500 ml normal saline. Trial 3 was taken 2 hours postinfusion and Trial 4 a week later. The results of the factorial repeated measures ANOVA revealed no significant differences between groups for either TE or RPE, even though the Hb level for the experimental group was significantly higher than the control group at Trials 3 and 4.

Pate, McFarland, Van Wyk, and Okocha (1979) studied the effects of blood reinfusion on physiological responses to endurance exercise in females. The subjects, all trained distance runners, were assigned to experimental and control groups after pair-matching for $\dot{V}O_2$ max. Each subject in the experimental group (n = 7) underwent removal of 450 ml of blood. Following storage for 21 days at 4° C, the packed red cells were reinfused. A double-blind design was employed with the control group (n = 8) undergoing sham procedures; no blood was removed from the control group. Hb concentration and physiological responses to submaximal and maximal treadmill running were observed prior to blood removal (Trial 1) and at 24 hours (Trial 2) and 7 days (Trial 3) after reinfusion. Results indicated that at Trial 2 and Trial 3, Hb varied only slightly from values observed at Trial 1 in both experimental and control groups. $\dot{V}O_2$, blood lactate, HR, $\dot{V}_E$, and respiratory quotient were essentially constant in both groups with the three exposures to submaximal and maximal exercise. There was no difference in time to exhaustion between the groups. Comparison of the groups' second and third trial performances using analysis of covariance (Trial 1 score as covariate) indicated that none of the observed differences between groups was statistically significant. These data show that the specific blood reinfusion procedure employed in this study does not significantly affect Hb or physiological response to endurance exercise in female distance runners.

Summary and Conclusions

The theory underlying the utilization of blood doping as an ergogenic aid has a strong physiological foundation. However, the research conducted thus far has been controversial in certain areas.

Several studies have revealed a beneficial effect of blood infusion upon submaximal exercise HR; however, others have evidenced no effect. Moreover, submaximal HR is not a valid indicator of maximal endurance capacity. In addition, maximal HR is not affected by blood infusion.

In general, the data support the conclusion that blood doping will increase $\dot{V}O_2$ max. Eight studies have reported increased $\dot{V}O_2$ max levels following an actual or modified blood doping methodology, although only one of these studies followed a double-blind placebo protocol. Of the three studies reporting no increased $\dot{V}O_2$ max levels, two infused only 500 ml of blood 21 days following withdrawal. Although the increased $\dot{V}O_2$ max was attributed primarily to the increased Hb level and resultant greater O_2-carrying capacity of the blood and not to increased cardiac output, the recent findings of Spriet and others (1980) suggest the latter also may make an important contribution to the increased $\dot{V}O_2$ max.

Performance time, either in time to exhaustion or a set distance for time, was benefited by blood infusion in seven studies, three of which used a double-blind protocol. A double-blind protocol also was used in the three studies that have noted no effect; however, only 500 ml of blood was infused 21 days post-withdrawal.

Two major distinctions between the supportive and nonsupportive findings should be noted. First, with one exception, in studies that infused whole blood volumes in the range of 800-1,200 ml, or the equivalent in packed RBC, increases were found in $\dot{V}O_2$ max and time to exhaustion. On the other hand, studies that have not evidenced such results uniformly used only 460-500 ml or the equivalent in packed RBC. Hence, the amount of blood infused may be a critical determinant of enhanced performance. The second factor was the time interval from withdrawal to infusion. Normally, it takes 5-6 weeks to restore hemoglobin levels following withdrawal of 500 ml. If the blood is frozen, there is no problem. However, if the blood is stored unfrozen in the conventional manner, law dictates that it must be used within 21 days. This time period may not be sufficient to allow for complete regeneration of lost RBC and Hb. Hence, the infusion, particularly if only 500 ml is used, may not create a highly significant erythrocythemia. In the three well designed double-blind studies that evidenced no significant increase in $\dot{V}O_2$ max or performance time, both of these limitations existed.

In conclusion, it appears that the infusion of 800-1,200 ml of whole blood, or the equivalent in packed RBC, into an endurance athlete with normal blood volume and Hb level, will significantly increase total RBC and Hb concentration. These increases will contribute to significant improvements in both $\dot{V}O_2$ max and endurance performance.

However, there may be several problems—medical, legal, and ethical—relative to its practical application. There appear to be no medical problems with the infusion of two units of autologous blood to a healthy individual; however, the withdrawal, storage and infusion must be done under strict medical protocol and supervision as developed by the American Red Cross Blood Donation Centers.

Legality of its use may be another problem. If any world-class runners are using the blood-doping technique, they probably would not admit it because admission could lead to possible reprisals. Whether or not the technique is illegal or not may depend upon the rules of the particular athletic governing body involved. For example, the Medical Commission of the International Olympic Committee (IOC) would probably consider it to be a violation of their doping law. Although primarily concerned with the use of drugs in sports, the IOC law also states that doping is the administration of or the use by a competing athlete of any substance foreign to the body or of any physiological substance taken in abnormal quantity or taken by an abnormal route of entry into the body, with the sole intention of increasing in an artificial and unfair manner his performance in competition. However, although it may be construed to be illegal, blood doping would be virtually impossible to detect under practical circumstances.

Some may contend that an athlete's victory would be tarnished if he or she used blood doping in competition, for it may be a breach of proper sportsmanship. On the other hand, others suggest it may be a practical alternative to altitude training by bringing about similar increases in Hb concentration without the expense of traveling to a distant state. In this sense, blood doping may not be considered unethical.

Blood doping appears to be an effective method to increase distance running performance, and whatever the problems may be, this issue should be addressed by the medical and rules governing bodies of the various athletic associations throughout the world.

References

AMDUR, N. Effect of drugs to aid athletes studied by U.S. *The New York Times*, August 22, 1976.

BALKE, B., Grillo, G., Konecci, E., & Luft, U. Work capacity after blood donation. *Journal of Applied Physiology*, 1954, **7**, 231-238.

BERNE, R., & Levy, M. *Cardiovascular physiology*. St. Louis: C.V. Mosby, 1967.

BLOOD bankers probe for the answer to oxygen release problem. *Medical Laboratory*, 1972, **8**, 14-15.

BLOOD doping. *Track and Field News*, November, 1971, pp. 2-3.

BUICK, F., Gledhill, N., Froese, A., Spriet, L., & Meyers, E. Effect of induced erythrocythemia on aerobic work capacity. *Journal of Applied Physiology*, 1980, **48**, 636-642.

BUNN, H., Forget, B., & Ranney, H. *Human hemoglobin*. Philadelphia: W.B. Saunders, 1977.

COTTRELL, R. British Army tests blood doping. *The Physician and Sports-medicine,* 1979, **7**, 14-16.

DEVRIES, H.A. *Physiology of exercise for physical education and athletics.* Dubuque: W.C. Brown, 1974.

EDINGTON, D., & Edgerton, V. *The biology of physical activity.* Boston: Houghton Mifflin, 1976.

EKBLOM, B., Goldbarg, A., & Gullbring, B. Response to exercise after blood loss and reinfusion. *Journal of Applied Physiology,* 1972, **33**, 175-180.

EKBLOM, B., Wilson, G., & Astrand, P.O. Central circulation during exercise after venesection and reinfusion of red blood cells. *Journal of Applied Physiology,* 1976, **40**, 379-383.

FAHEY, T., & Rolph, R. Venous and capillary blood hematocrit at rest and following submaximal exercise. *European Journal of Applied Physiology,* 1975, **34**, 109-112.

FRYE, A., & Ruhling, R. RBC infusion, exercise, hemoconcentration and $\dot{V}O_2$. *Medicine and Science in Sports,* 1977, **9**, 69.

GLEDHILL, N., Spriet, L., Froese, A., Wilkes, D., & Meyers, E. Acid-base status with induced erythrocythemia and its influence on arterial oxygenation during heavy exercise. *Medicine and Science in Sports and Exercise,* 1980, **12**, 122.

GOFORTH, H., Campbell, N., Hodgdon, J., & Sucec, A. Hematologic parameters of trained distance runners following induced erythrocythemia. *Medicine and Science in Sports and Exercise,* 1982, **14**, 174.

GREGERSEN, M., & Chien, S. Blood volume. In V.B. Mountcastle (Ed.), *Medical physiology.* St. Louis: C.V. Mosby, 1968.

GULLBRING, B., Holmgren, A., Sjostrand, T., & Strandell, T. The effect of blood volume variations on the pulse ratio in supine and upright positions and during exercise. *Acta Physiologica Scandinavica,* 1960, **50**, 62-71.

GUYTON, A. *Textbook of medical physiology.* Philadelphia: W.B. Saunders, 1981.

GUYTON, A., & Richardson, T. Effect of hematocrit on venous return. *Circulation Research,* 1961, **9**, 157-164.

HORSTMAN, D., Weiskopf, R., Jackson, R., & Severinghaus, J. The influence of polycythemia, induced by 4 weeks sojourn at 4300 M(HA), on sea level (SL) work capacity. In C. Bard, M. Fleury, & E. Waghorn (Eds.), *Abstracts of the International Congress of Physical Activity Sciences,* 1976.

HOWALD, H. Blut-Doping. *Schweiz Zeitschrift Sportsmedizin,* 1975, **23**, 201-203.

HOWELL, M., & Coupe, K. Effect of blood loss on performance in the Balke-Ware Treadmill Test. *Research Quarterly,* 1964, **35**, 156-165.

HUESTIS, D., Bove, J., & Busch, S. *Practical blood transfusion*. Boston: Little and Brown, 1976.

ITZCHAK, Y., Silverberger, A., Modan, M., Adar, R., & Deutsch, V. Hematocrit, viscosity and blood flow velocity in men and women. *Israel Journal of Medical Science*, 1977, **13**, 80-82.

KARPOVICH, P., & Millman, N. Athletes as blood donors. *Research Quarterly*, 1942, **13**, 166-168.

KLEIN, H. *Polycythemia*. Springfield, IL: C.C. Thomas, 1973.

LEAVELL, B., & Thorup, O. *Fundamentals of clinical hematology*. Philadelphia: W.B. Saunders, 1976.

MOLLISON, P. *Blood transfusion in clinical medicine*. Oxford: Alden and Mowbray, 1972.

OSCAI, L., Williams, B., & Hertig, B. Effect of exercise on blood volume. *Journal of Applied Physiology*, 1968, **24**, 622-624.

PACE, N., Lozner, E., Consolazio, W., Pitts, G., & Pecora, L. The increase in hypoxia tolerance of normal men accompanying the polycythemia induced by transfusion of erythrocytes. *American Journal of Physiology*, 1947, **148**, 152-163.

PATE, R., McFarland, J., Van Wyk, J., & Okocha, A. Effects of blood reinfusion on endurance performance in female distance runners. *Medicine and Science in Sports*, 1979, **11**, 97.

REPLOGLE, R., & Merrill, E. Experimental polycythemia and hemodilution: Physiological and rheologic effects. *Journal of Thoracic and Cardiovascular Surgery*, 1970, **60**, 582-588.

ROBERTSON, R., Gilcher, R., Metz, K., Bahnson, H., Allison, T., Skriner, G., Abbott, A., & Becker, R. Effect of red blood cell reinfusion on physical working capacity and perceived exertion at normal and reduced oxygen pressure. *Medicine and Science in Sports*, 1978, **10**, 49.

ROBERTSON, R., Gilcher, R., Metz, K., Casperson, C., Abbott, A., Allison, T., Skriner, G., Werner, K., Zelicoff, S., & Krause, J. Central circulation and work capacity after red blood cell reinfusion under normoxia and hypoxia in women. *Medicine and Science in Sports*, 1979, **11**, 98.

ROBINSON, B., Epstein, S., Kahler, R., & Braunwald, E. Circulatory effects of acute expansion of blood volume. *Circulation Research*, 1966, **29**, 26-32.

SHEPHARD, R. *Frontiers of fitness*. Springfield, IL: C.C. Thomas, 1971.

SPRIET, L., Gledhill, N., Froese, A., Wilkes, D., & Meyers, E. The effect of induced erythrocythemia on central circulation and oxygen transport during maximal exercise. *Medicine and Science in Sports and Exercise*, 1980, **12**, 122-123.

VIDEMAN, T., & Rytömaa, T. Effect of blood removal and autotransfusion on heart rate response to a submaximal workload. *Journal of Sports Medicine and Physical Fitness*, 1977, **17**, 387-390.

VON ROST, R., Hollman, W., Liesen, H., & Schulten, D. Uber den Einfluss einer Erthrozyten-Retransfusion auf die Kardio-pulmonale Leistungsfahigkeit. *Sportarzt und Sportmedizin*, 1975, **26**, 137-144.

WEISSE, A., Calton, F., Kuida, H., & Hecht, H. Hemodynamic effects of normovolemic polycythemia in dogs at rest and during exercise. *American Journal of Physiology*, 1964, **207**, 1361-1366.

WILLIAMS, M., Bocrie, J., Goodwin, A.R., & Perkins, R. Effect of blood reinjection upon endurance capacity and heart rate. *Medicine and Science in Sports*, 1973, **5**, 181-186.

WILLIAMS, M., Lindhjem, M., & Schuster, R. The effect of blood infusion upon endurance capacity and ratings of perceived exertion. *Medicine and Science in Sports*, 1978, **10**, 113-118.

WILLIAMS, M., & Ward, A.J. Hematological changes elicited by prolonged intermittant aerobic exercise. *Research Quarterly*, 1977, **48**, 606-616.

WILLIAMS, M., Wesseldine, S., Somma, T., & Schuster, R. The effect of induced erythrocythemia upon 5-mile treadmill run time. *Medicine and Science in Sports*, 1981, **13**, 169-175.

WILLIAMS, W., Beutler, E., Ersley, A., & Rundles, R. *Hematology*. New York: McGraw-Hill, 1972.

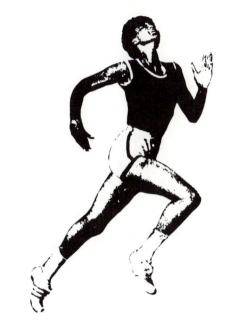

Part 4
Psychological Ergogenic Aids

9
Hypnosis

William P. Morgan
and David R. Brown

The inclusion of a chapter on hypnosis in a volume dealing with
ergogenics and sports seems appropriate for a number of reasons
that will be described in this chapter. Hypnosis, however, clearly
differs from other ergogens in two very important respects. First,
while recognized ergogenic aids such as water are known to facilitate muscular performance, the influence of hypnosis on sports
performance is somewhat unclear at this time. Therefore, this
chapter will be restricted largely to a review of the empirical research carried out in laboratory settings and selected theoretical
formulations. Second, although many ergogenic aids can be, and
are, administered by a variety of individuals who are not required
to possess specialized skills, the use of hypnosis within an ergogenic context does require specialized training on the part of the
practitioner. A cursory overview of this issue will be presented,
and additional details may be obtained by reviewing the ethical
codes of organizations such as the American Psychological Association (APA), Society for Clinical and Experimental Hypnosis

William P. Morgan, Ed.D., F.A.C.S.M., and **David R. Brown, Ph.D.,** are with
the Sport Psychology Laboratory at the University of Wisconsin in Madison.

(SCEH), and the American Society of Clinical Hypnosis (ASCH).

The first portion of this chapter explores the issue of qualifications, followed by a review of selected theoretical explanations as to why hypnosis might possess ergogenic properties, and the next section contains a review of clinical and experimental investigations dealing with the influence of hypnosis on muscular performance. The final section consists of a summary statement that includes recommendations for future research and clinical applications in the exercise and sport sciences.

Qualifications of Practitioners

The question of who is a qualified practitioner of hypnosis has been raised many times over the past several decades, and one of the most recent attempts to place this question in perspective was presented by Hilgard (1979). The question represents an extremely complex issue. Hilgard (1979) has noted, for example, that "Lack of advanced degrees does not necessarily mean incompetence and society memberships do not guarantee competence either" (p. 5). Hilgard (1979) goes on to point out, however, that broader professional training that extends beyond hypnosis *per se* has advantages, the main one being "that the true professional will know much more that is relevant about personality and individual differences than is implied by hypnosis" (p. 5). An advanced degree in psychology and membership in professional societies such as the SCEH, ASCH, and Division 30 of the APA should be viewed as *necessary* rather than *sufficient* evidence of competence. In other words, an advanced degree in psychology and membership in SCEH, ASCH, and APA does not qualify one as a hypnotist. Division 30 of APA, for example, was once a quasi-licensing group that required letters of recommendation, training in hypnosis, and experience in the use of hypnosis, but membership in the Division now requires only application and dues. In other words, Division 30 is now an interest unit of APA, and membership can no longer be viewed as a sign of special competence. It has recently been proposed by Levitt (1981) that the only realistic testimony to ability as a hypnotist is certification by the American Board of Psychological Hypnosis (ABPH).

The discussion thus far fails to answer the question of who is qualified to practice hypnosis. This question cannot be answered in our view, at least not to everyone's satisfaction, in a single chapter or even a volume devoted exclusively to the issue. It is possible, however, to offer some guidelines that should prove to be useful in most research and clinical settings within sports. First of all, a clear distinction is made between the use of hypnosis in research and clinical practice by all professional organizations concerned with the use of hypnosis. The use of hypnosis, for example, to manipulate an independent variable in an experiment usually involves a very different proposition than the hypnotherapeutic treatment of clinical problems such as depression, anxiety, obesity, insomnia, impotence, and drug addiction.

The recommendation to be advanced by the authors is that individuals who employ hypnosis as a research tool be members of Division 30 of the APA and SCEH. It is also recommended that those who employ hypnosis in their clinical practice hold membership in the appropriate APA Division(s) and adhere to state laws involving certification and licensing. Since all 50 states and the District of Columbia have enacted laws regulating the practice of psychology, this latter recommendation should be viewed within a legal context. Certification laws limit the use of the title "psychologist," and licensing laws both regulate the use of the title and limit the scope of the practice of psychology to areas of competence and training.

The question of who is a qualified practitioner of hypnosis needs to be amplified to include the question of purpose. Use of hypnosis in research and clinical practice represent related but, at the same time, quite different propositions. Although membership in organizations does not in itself ensure that hypnotists will stay within the bounds of their competence, it does increase the likelihood that hypnotists will be in compliance with existing ethical codes. One accepted principle is that hypnosis does not qualify a hypnotist to perform activities that he or she is not competent to perform without hypnosis. For example, an athlete, coach, or team physician who solicits the aid of a hypnotist might reasonably ask the hypnotist:

1. Are you a psychologist, and, if so, what kind of a psychologist?
2. Are you certified and/or licensed as a psychologist in this state?
3. Are your areas of training and competence related to my problems and needs?
4. Are you a member of APA, SCEH, or ASCH?
5. Are you certified by the ABPH?

Individuals who employ hypnosis in their research and clinical practice should be qualified to do so. Consumers, whether they be test subjects in an experiment, or clients in a clinical setting, have every right to know the answers to questions such as those listed above.

Theoretical Considerations

Maximal physical performance is limited by many factors, and one of the most important involves the individual's actual capacity. The ability and willingness to endure the discomfort and possible pain associated with all-out efforts represent other factors. Physical performance is limited, in part, by inhibitory mechanisms, and this has a protective effect from the standpoint of injury prevention. It has been pointed out by Gorton (1959), for example, that "the full contractile power of human muscle is known to be greater than is normally apparent as demonstrated by the fractures due to muscular contraction observed as complications in electric shock therapy (ECT)." In other words, if electrodes are improperly placed or if excessive voltage is employed in ECT, it is possible that bones will fracture or dislocate. Gorton has also theorized that reserves of muscular power probably exist but are not available under normal conditions.

Disinhibition of the inhibitory mechanisms that limit the expression of muscular activity should theoretically result in the transcendence of normal capacity. As a matter of fact, this mechanism represents one way of explaining the superhuman feats often described in the popular press. Also, it is noteworthy that superhuman physical feats have sometimes, although not always, been accompanied by injury such as single or multiple fractures.

It is also commonly believed that at least a portion of the gains in performance that accompany physical training result from the individual's developing higher pain tolerance, that is, becoming less sensitive to the discomfort associated with physical effort, and this results in the ability to perform at higher intensities. This explains, in part, why two individuals with identical aerobic power, for example, 60 ml/kg/min, perform differently on an endurance event. One individual, for example, might be able to perform at 80% of maximum, whereas the other might not be able to exceed 60% of maximum for a prolonged period. This, of course, relates in part to the point at which the onset of anaerobisis occurs in the two cases. That is, extensive clinical and anecdotal evidence suggests that individuals usually do not perform muscular activities at maximum. Attempts to elicit "maximal" physical performance probably result in "submaximal" efforts, which should be regarded as an "operational maximum"; that is, the effort usually represents a "pseudo-maximum," which is labeled as "maximum" for operational purposes. This point of view maintains that a reserve usually exists, and this reserve can theoretically be tapped in times of need.

The concept of a reserve is also supported by experimental laboratory evidence that indicates "maximal" muscular performance can be enhanced by disinhibition of inhibitory mechanisms. The process of disinhibition can be provoked by means of alcohol, drugs (e.g., amphetamine sulfate), loud noise, and hypnosis, according to Ikai and Steinhaus (1961). Actually, the report by Ikai and Steinhaus (1961) should be viewed as indicating that these treatments are superior to no treatment (i.e., control). Although their paper clearly reveals that all measures of maximal strength are actually submaximal and that performance can be enhanced above these operational levels, the enhancement via disinhibition probably results from *suggestion*, rather than the respective treatments. Because a placebo paradigm was not employed by Ikai and Steinhaus (1961), there is no way of knowing whether the effects were due to the treatments or to one or more behavioral artifacts such as the Hawthorne effect (Morgan, 1972). The important consideration, of course, is that *suggestion*, not the hypnotic or pharmacologic treatments, probably produced the ergogenic effect. Because suggestion plays a central role in the study of most hypnotic phenomena, the interactive confounding of hypnosis and suggestion represents a very significant problem when considering hypnosis research. Suggestion is especially crucial when attempting to transcend normal levels of physical performance. It should be noted, however, that this problem is not unique to hypnosis, and unless the impact of various behavioral artifacts can be specified, the efficacy of any ergogen remains questionable.

This methodological problem is illustrated in a report by Barber and Calverley (1964), who assessed the strength of grip and weight holding endurance of 60 female subjects who were randomly assigned to one of four groups: (a) task-motivating instructions, (b) hypnotic induction procedure, (c) hypnotic induction procedure plus task motivating instructions, and (d) control. None of the experimental conditions significantly affected strength of grip. The hypnotic induction condition depressed weight holding endurance, while task motivating instructions in both the hypnotic and waking states resulted in significant increases in endurance. This indicates that suggestion rather than hypnosis produced the ergogenic effect.

It has been demonstrated that expression of maximal muscular strength, as measured by the 1-repetition maximum (1-RM) bench press test, can be increased significantly in college males by means of stereotyped suggestion in the motivated waking state (Morgan, 1981). The test subjects who participated in this experiment had been trained for a period of 2 months, and therefore the strength gains were not simply due to the fact that untrained individuals who lacked experience, or "desensitization," were employed. In the same report, however, perceptual manipulation also resulted in significant gains in 1-RM performance even though verbal suggestion was not employed. The test subjects attempted to perform a 1-RM with a weight they assumed to be their 1-RM, but it was actually 5 pounds heavier in each case. This, of course, might be viewed as nonverbal suggestion.

One of the earliest studies dealing with the influence of suggestion *per se* on muscular strength was carried out by Manzer (1934). Groups of 50 male and 50 female subjects were tested on strength of grip, and 25 in each group were told that the dynamometer would be adjusted to tension loads of easy, medium, and hard. The purpose of the experiment was ostensibly to study the difference in performance on these trials in comparison to a "standard" condition. Control groups consisting of 25 males and 25 females also performed the same number of trials against the standard resistance. Suggestions of hard resistance resulted in strength gains of 5% in the males and 7% in the females when compared with the "standard" conditions. Because the dynamometer tension was maintained constant throughout all trials, the enhanced performance presumably resulted from differences in perceived task difficulty brought about by suggestion. The important point once again, however, is that baseline measures of maximum strength were enhanced in the waking state by means of suggestion.

Additional support for the view that suggestion *per se* may be the factor responsible for enhanced performance is provided in the report by Pomeranz and Krasner (1969), who evaluated the maximal isometric strength of the dominant hand in 18 male and 18 female subjects. Six trials were performed on a dynamometer, and the total force generated across the six measures served as the criterion score. An equal number of males and females were randomly assigned to placebo and control groups, and they were then administered six additional trials. The control subjects were merely retested after a standard rest period that was identical in duration with that followed by the placebo group. A salve consisting of neobase and red food coloring (i.e., inert substance) was administered to the hands of subjects in the placebo group with the suggestion that "they had been assigned to the 'drug' group and were given information concerning the 'drug' to the effect that the 'drug' had already undergone extensive testing and had proved very effective'' (p. 16).

Analysis revealed that the males and females did not differ, nor was there an interaction between sex and trials. There was a significant main effect, however, and the control group had a mean decrement of 11.0 kg, whereas the placebo group experienced an insignificant decrease of 1.9 kg. These results indicate that most of the fatigue effect associated with repeated dynamometer trials can be abolished by means of suggestion (i.e., placebo plus a rationale). This investigation reinforces the necessity of attempting to quantify the magnitude of the Hawthorne effect (Morgan, 1972) in research involving experimentation with various ergogenic aids. If this is not done, the possibility of "any" treatment versus "no" treatment (i.e., control group) becomes a tenable explanation. Use of a placebo plot in this type of experimentation is usually quite appropriate. It should be emphasized, however, that a placebo is far more likely to be effective when a theoretical rationale is presented to the test subject (O'Leary & Borkovec, 1978). This implies, of course, that suggestion is the crucial ingredient.

The research cited to this point has involved acute paradigms. A chronic design consisting of maximal two-legged isokinetic knee extensions was recently performed by Coyle, Feiring, Rotkis, Cote, Roby, Lee, and Wilmore (1982). Twenty-two college-aged males trained 3 days/week for 6 weeks on a slow, fast, or mixed (i.e., slow and fast) schedule, and improvements in peak torque were compared to results for control and placebo groups. The control subjects did not train, and the placebo subjects received muscle stimulation consisting of approximately 20 milliamps of current to the quadricep muscle group on training days. This stimulation resulted in a mild skin anesthesia, and the muscular contraction was less than 3% of that developed during a maximal contraction or maximal stimulation. Although the stimulation produced a distinct sensation, there is no reason to believe that a physiological training effect could result from such a sham.

In the study by Coyle et al. (1982), however, the subjects in the placebo group were told that the electrical stimulation was known to be effective, and the purpose of the experiment was to quantify the actual effect produced by the stimulation. Peak torque produced isometrically at a joint angle of 65° increased significantly for the slow (20.3%), fast (23.6%), and mixed (18.9%) training groups, whereas the control group decreased slightly (-1.5%). The placebo group, however, had a significant increase of 8.1% in peak torque, and this gain was significantly superior to that of the control group. More importantly, perhaps, was the finding that physical training was not significant to the placebo treatment for this specific task. The placebo subjects reported that they "felt stronger," and this may have provoked, or been the consequence of, disinhibition of inhibitory mechanisms. At any rate, this investigation offers further support that suggestion *per se* may enhance physical performance.

The investigations reviewed in this section are extremely important when considering the possible ergogenic effects of hypnosis, because presumed effects might be due to suggestion rather than hypnosis. The possible confounding of suggestion and hypnosis in research involving muscular performance was first emphasized by Barber (1966), who presented a critical review of research studies dealing with the effects of hypnosis and motivational suggestions on muscular strength and endurance. This review led to the conclusion that the hypnotic state, without suggestions for enhanced performance, did not facilitate muscular strength or endurance. Barber (1966) also noted that although motivational suggestions of enhanced performance in the hypnotic state are generally ergogenic, they are no more effective in this regard than similar suggestions in the motivated waking state. The methodological problem associated with comparing *suggestion* in the hypnotic state with *nothing* in the nonhypnotic state seems rather fundamental or obvious. Unfortunately, most of the existing research dealing with hypnosis and muscular performance has failed to employ experimental designs that control for the confounding of hypnosis and suggestion, and this represents an important design consideration.

Earlier Reviews

This chapter updates and extends earlier reviews involving the influence of hypnosis on muscular performance. The first published review of this topic was presented by Hull (1933) and this was followed by the reviews by Gorton (1959), Johnson (1961b), Weitzenhoffer (1963), Barber (1966), Morgan (1972), and Morgan (1980). Hull's review focused on hypnotic suggestibility and the transcendence of voluntary capacity, and the major conclusion was that the existing evidence was contradictory. Hull explained the conflicting evidence in terms of the design inelegancies which had characterized the available research. In many respects, one could easily arrive at the same conclusion today, a half century later. However, there has been some progress, and in those areas where direct empirical advances have not been made, theoretical principles can now be applied. These formulations will be considered in this chapter where possible.

The review by Gorton (1959) suggests that muscular performance can be enhanced by hypnosis, and Gorton has proposed that performance gains result from disinhibition of inhibitory mechanisms. Gorton indicates that reserves of muscular power exist, but these reserves are not available under normal circumstances. Hypnotic suggestion, however, is potentially capable of mobilizing these reserves, according to Gorton (1959).

The review presented by Johnson (1961b) concludes on a more conservative note, indicating that direct hypnotic suggestions designed to enhance muscular performance may work, but such suggestions cannot be relied upon to be effective. Johnson (1961b) also noted that negative suggestions designed to impair performance have consistently been observed to be effective.

Following a review of studies dealing with hypnosis and muscular strength, Weitzenhoffer (1963) concluded that few of the investigations were comparable in procedures. This led Weitzenhoffer (1963) to propose that the apparent contradictions in this research area reflect dissimilar designs. This particular review does not support the view that hypnosis improves muscular strength.

In a subsequent review, Barber (1966) concluded that hypnosis *per se* does not enhance muscular performance. Barber maintains that motivational instructions are usually effective in facilitating muscular performance whether administered in the hypnotic or waking state.

In a later review by Morgan (1972), it was concluded that attempts to decrease muscular performance by means of hypnotic suggestion are almost always effective, but one would intuitively expect similar success with cooperative individuals in the waking state. Although such an observation may not seem to be very provocative, the applied implications are quite important. An alleged case involving group hypnosis will be cited for the sake of illustration. Several years ago, a football coach from the Big Ten Conference enlisted the services of a hypnotist prior to the annual Rose Bowl game. The hypnotist presented hypnotic suggestions to the team prior to the game, and they were informed that they would not feel tense, but rather relaxed and calm, as they awaited the opening kickoff. Although the intention or motivation of the hypnotist was not disclosed, it might be argued that hypnotic suggestion of this type would be designed to impair the team's performance. Several theoretical positions would argue against a football team's being relaxed precompetitively, and there is empirical evidence bearing on the issue that challenges such an approach (Langer, 1966). The team in question lost the game, as one would predict, but whether or not the failure stemmed directly from the hypnotic suggestions cannot be stated. At any rate, the suggestion employed in this case represents the type one would employ in order to provoke a performance decrement. It is known, for example, that some athletes perform best when relaxed, others when slightly aroused, and still others appear to do their best when quite aroused (Hanin, 1978). The issue of arousal is also thought to be related to task complexity (Landers, 1978), and it is obvious that the division of labor on a football team consists of tasks that differ markedly in level of complexity.

In the earlier reviews mentioned above (Johnson, 1961b; Morgan, 1972) it was concluded that attempts to decrease muscular performance by means of hypnotic suggestion are almost always effective. In the review by Morgan (1972) it was also concluded that attempts to facilitate muscular performance by means of hypnotic suggestion have been successful where hypnotherapists have attempted to correct psychomotor problems, reduce pain, resolve aggression conflicts, and control (increase or decrease) anxiety states in the competitive athlete. However, the research literature bearing on this topic was found to be equivocal through the year 1970, and the situation has not changed over the past decade (Morgan, 1981). The equivocal nature of this literature can be explained in a number of ways. First, the physical characteristics of the participants in these experiments have seldom been presented. It is usually much more difficult to increase the physical performance of trained athletes who are performing at or near their physiological maximum than it is to facilitate the performance of untrained persons (Morgan, 1972). Hence, part of the equivocality of this literature can be explained on the basis of uncertainty concerning subject characteristics. Second, the actual physical task has often differed substantially in various experiments precluding direct comparisons of findings, and the nature of the task has not always been clearly described. In other words, negative versus positive findings in given studies may reflect the physical task rather than the effect, or lack of effect, of hypnotic suggestion. Third, the type of induction procedure has not always been specified, and this creates a significant problem. Inductions that are primarily ''relaxing'' in nature would theoretically have a different effect on physical performance than those that are primarily ''alerting'' in nature. Fourth, the type of suggestions used in the hypnotic state may be of an ''involving'' nature, or they may require little in the way of involvement (''uninvolving'') on the part of the person being tested (Morgan, 1972). Because research in the area of hypnosis and muscular performance has failed to consistently address these four issues, one is able either to conclude that the research evidence is equivocal, or to advance a qualified position. It is clear, for example, that hypnotic suggestions of enhanced physical ability are effective *if* subjects scoring high on hypnotizability and low on physical performance are administered "involving" instructions following an "alterting" induction. There is also evidence that phenomenal gains in physical performance can occur under controlled experimental conditions even when all of these conditions are not met. An example of this point will now be cited to illustrate the complex interaction of subject, task, induction, and suggestion.

One of the most convincing cases of a "psychological breakthrough" to be brought about by hypnotic suggestion was reported by Johnson and Kramer (1961). These investigators compared the effects of nonhypnotic, hypnotic, and posthypnotic stereotyped suggestion on strength, power, and endurance. Ten male subjects were tested under control, light trance, deep trance, and posthypnotic conditions. The tests included a grip dynamometer task (strength), the jump-and-reach task (power), and supine press of a 47-lb barbell to exhaustion (endurance). The testing extended over a 4-day period. The only statistically significant improvement observed was in endurance when the two hypnotic conditions were compared with the no-hypnosis treatments. Neither of the hypnotic conditions was consistently superior. One subject in this study, however, experienced what might be regarded as disinhibition of inhibitory mechanisms.

The subject was a professional football player who bench pressed the 47-lb barbell 130 times in the first testing session where suggestions were given but hypnosis was not utilized. Hypnosis was then introduced and on the next three testings his scores were 180 (when he was stopped by the investigator), 230, and 233, respectively. In contrast, the next strongest athlete began the study at 57 repetitions and eventually reached a maximum of 75. Since our own research has revealed that a performance of 100 repetitions is exceptionally high, it is reasonable to regard this subject's hypnotic performance as a superhuman feat. To determine whether the professional football player's performance was dependent on hypnosis, he was later retested without hypnosis and was stopped by the investigator after completing 350 repetitions with the same 47-lb weight.

There are several points of interest regarding this case. First, it is inconceivable that this weight-trained, mesomorphic, professional football player could almost double his initial performance in the hypnotic state, because such subjects are generally thought to perform at or near their maximums when tested in the waking state. Also, Johnson and Kramer (1961) have pointed out that this subject recovered quickly from each bout, and he did not report soreness at any time. Age regression was employed with this subject several months following the experiment, and he was led to relive the first test while in the trance state. He gave the impression that he had accepted the suggestions as vivid reality, and his performance became a matter of life and death. Under age regression he also reported that he would give up in complete fatigue and then watch in amazement as his arms seemingly lifted the weight by themselves. This case is an example of the type of performance cited to support the view that most individuals are capable of performing far above "maximal" levels under certain conditions.

The most recent review in this area dealt with the use of hypnosis in sports medicine (Morgan, 1980). This review revealed that hypnosis has not been employed on a systematic basis by researchers or clinicians in the field of sports medicine even though the potential for its application is seemingly limitless. There are numerous ways in which investigators in the exercise and sport sciences might employ hypnosis in their research as a means of manipulating independent variables and/or providing controls over various behavioral artifacts within an experimental setting. This particular point will be explored in a subsequent section, but the point is that a potentially useful research tool has not been systematically employed. One of the purposes of this chapter will be to illustrate how the hypnotic tool might be employed in exercise and sport sciences research. It is even more surprising, however, that hypnosis has not been employed more extensively in the clinical areas of sports medicine since its efficacy in the management of pain (Hilgard & Hilgard, 1975), and in psychosomatic medicine in general (Burrows & Dennerstein, 1980), has been well documented.

It is not entirely clear why hypnosis has not been employed more extensively as a research or therapeutic tool in the exercise and sport sciences. One possible explanation is that workers in these fields have traditionally not been trained in psychiatry or psychology, and there are simply very few clinicians or researchers who possess training in the use of hypnotic procedures (Morgan, 1980). This undoubtedly represents one plausible explanation. However, there has also been a tendency to equate the "use of hypnosis" with the "abuse of drugs" in sports, and this represents an unfortunate misconception. A paper presented at the 1975 Annual Meeting of the American Medical Association, for example, was titled "Hypnosis and Drug Abuse in Sports" (Rosen, 1976). In this particular paper Rosen (1976) stated that "Athletes frequently apply for hypnosis to increase physical performance. . . .

This is inadvisable and can be dangerous'' (p. 31). Although Rosen fails to explain why the application of hypnosis is ''inadvisable'' and evidence is not presented to support the contention that it ''can be dangerous'' when used in this manner, it is likely that such views have discouraged physicians and psychologists from using hypnosis in sports medicine settings.

It will be recalled that Barber (1966) has maintained that suggestion in the motivated waking state is just as effective as hypnotic suggestion in facilitating muscular strength and endurance. It is also known that a placebo, when accompanied by a theoretical rationale (i.e., suggestion), can be just as effective as many drugs (Morgan, 1972, 1981), so governing bodies that might elect to regulate the use of hypnosis in sports would be obligated also to consider the use of suggestion *per se* in sport.

The question should not be one of whether or not hypnosis should be used in sport (Morgan, 1980). The appropriate questions relate to who, how, and under what circumstances hypnosis should be employed in sport. The issue of who is a qualified hypnotist has already been addressed. The related concerns of how and under what circumstances hypnosis should be employed will be reviewed in the following section dealing with research and clinical applications.

Research Applications

Research dealing with hypnosis and muscular performance has generally relied on one of two paradigms. One approach has been to study a particular problem in exercise physiology or psychology and utilize hypnotic suggestion as a means of manipulating an independent variable or controlling the experimental setting. A second approach, by far the most frequently employed, has involved the use of various forms of hypnotic suggestion as a means of facilitating or improving physical performance.

Experimental Manipulations

An example of the first type of application is described by Massey, Johnson, and Kramer (1961), who were interested in controlling the influence of a specific attitudinal set on endurance performance. There has been a debate for many years about the optimal level of physical warm-up necessary prior to performance of a physical task, and this problem is later addressed in detail by Franks in chapter 13 of this volume. A recognized problem inherent in such a study is that subjects' past experiences with warm-up and their attitudes toward the value of warm-up is known to have an influence on physical performance. Smith and Bozymowski (1965), for example, studied the influence of attitude toward physical warm-up on physical performance. These investigators developed an attitude inventory and classified college female subjects as possessing favorable or unfavorable attitudes toward warm-up. The subjects were tested on an obstacle course without a warm-up and following a 3-minute warm-up period. Subjects who possessed a favorable attitude toward warm-up performed significantly better during the race when it was preceded by a warm-up than did those with less favorable attitudes. In other words, the efficacy of warm-up in this particular investigation was found to be governed by attitude towards warm-up, not the warm-up *per se.*

In order to control for this particular extraneous variable, Massey et al. (1961) conducted an experiment in which the subjects presumably were unaware of whether or not they had warmed up prior to performing a physical task that consisted of pedaling a bicycle ergometer 100 revolutions at a resistance of 26 lb. The subjects were 15 male college students, who performed a standardized warm-up under hypnosis on one day and rested while under hypnosis on another day. The warm-up and control days were counterbalanced, posthypnotic amnesia was employed, and the subjects performed the endurance task in the posthypnotic state. The standard warm-up procedure was found to have no influence on physical performance. It was also reported by these investigators that lack of warm-up was not associated with muscle soreness or injury.

Another example of how hypnosis can be employed in exercise research involves the study of perceived exertion. In an attempt to elucidate the physiological mechanisms involved in effort sense, some investigators have computed the bivariate correlation between perceived exertion ratings and physiological variables such as heart rate, ventilatory minute volume, skin temperature, rectal temperature, and lactate production. This approach has not proven to be fruitful for many reasons, the primary one being that simplistic correlational models lack explanatory power. Another approach has involved the alteration of physiological responses such as heart rate, ventilation, or lactate production by administration of beta blocking agents, elevated CO_2 levels of inspired air, or enriched O_2 concentrations, respectively. The problem with such approaches is that unintended physiological changes frequently result as well. Another research strategy, and one which relies on hypnosis, consists of altering the *product* (i.e., perceived exertion) and evaluating the effect of such perturbation on the *process* (i.e., heart rate, ventilation, etc.).

Examples of this research strategy are reported by Morgan, Raven, Drinkwater, and Horvath (1973) and Morgan, Hirota, Weitz, and Balke (1976). In the first investigation, subjects cycled a bicycle ergometer at a resistance of 100 watts under hypnotic and waking conditions following suggestions that exercise intensity would be moderate and under hypnotic conditions with suggestions of light and heavy work. Perception of effort was quantified with Borg's psychophysical scale (Borg, 1973), and the perceived exertion levels were congruent with the suggestion. In other words, standard work performed at a constant load of 100 watts was perceived as being easier or more difficult even though the actual workload remained unchanged. Heart rate was elevated with the suggestion of heavy work, but the major physiological changes observed to accompany the altered percept were associated with ventilatory parameters. Indeed, ventilatory minute volume increased about 20 ℓ/min following suggestions of heavy work. A similar investigation was carried out by Morgan et al. (1976), in which subjects exercised on a bicycle ergometer at a resistance of 100 watts for 20 minutes under control and hypnotic conditions with suggestions of "uphill" and "level" work presented for 5-minute blocks within the "steady state" condition. The findings were similar to those of the former experiment in that perception of effort was congruent with the hypnotic suggestion, and ventilatory minute volume was the primary physiological change noted. This research suggests that ventilatory parameters represent a primary input signal upon which an exercising subject's perceived exertion rating is based.

These examples of research involving warm-up and perceived exertion illustrate two types of experimental settings in which the hypnotic tool has proven to be quite effective. As mentioned earlier, the more common application of hypnosis has involved paradigms in which attempts have been made to directly manipulate physical performance, and these will be reviewed next.

Hypnosis and Muscular Performance

The research to be reviewed in this section has involved a variety of physical tasks. The most frequently employed task has been strength of grip as measured by the hand dynamometer. The usual approach in this research has consisted of having the subject perform between one and three maximal contractions, although some investigators have employed repeated trials to a point of exhaustion (Eysenck, 1941). This latter approach represents an attempt to measure muscular endurance as opposed to the more commonly studied muscular strength.

The second most frequently employed task has been arm endurance. In this task the subject maintains the arms at right angles to the body and parallel with the floor for as long as possible without weights or while holding and supporting weights. Investigators have utilized objects ranging in weight from several grams up to 20 kg.

Some of the earliest research involved the study of small muscle groups with the Mosso ergograph or finger ergometer. Strength of the entire arm, usually involving maximal isometric contractions of the elbow flexor muscles, has been studied by some investigators. Exercise has also been performed on bicycle ergometers, involving all-out sprints of a maximal nature or steady-state work performed at a moderate intensity (e.g., 100 watts) for periods ranging from 5 to 20 minutes. Explosive power has been assessed by means of the vertical jump test, and dynamic endurance of large muscle groups has been studied using the bench press. The influence of posthypnotic suggestions on treadmill running performance has been studied in two recent investigations.

A physical task frequently employed by stage hypnotists for the purpose of demonstrating the efficacy of hypnosis is the "human plank" test, or "feat," as it is often called. The authors, however, have been able to locate only one study in which this task has been studied experimentally (Collins, Note 1).

All of the published research located by the authors has been based upon controlled experiments carried out in laboratory settings with the single exception of a report by Simonson (1937) that involved running on an outdoor track. There is evidence that hypnosis has been employed with athletes who subsequently performed physical tasks in various athletic settings, and these clinical applications will be discussed in a separate section.

A summary of the physical tasks employed by investigators in the study of hypnosis and muscular performance appears in Tables 1, 2, and 3. These tasks have been classified as being primarily of an isometric, dynamic, or motor learning/performance nature. It is not possible to list the studies summarized in Tables 1-3 as being either positive or negative in outcome, because some of the investigations are both, whereas others have been equivocal. Furthermore, the specific outcomes of most of these studies have been described in earlier chapters (Morgan, 1972, 1980).

Strength and Endurance

Certain of the investigations listed in Tables 1, 2, and 3 dealt with the influence of hypnosis *per se* on muscular performance, whereas other studies have concentrated on the effect of various hypnotic, posthypnotic, and waking suggestions. Some studies have shown that hypnosis *per se* has no influence on muscular performance, whereas other studies have found performance increments or decrements. The literature is clearly equivocal regarding this area.

Although a number of investigators have reported that hypnotic suggestions designed to facilitate muscular strength and endurance are effective, an equal number of studies have found this not to be the case (Table 1). Also, there is some evidence that task-motivating instructions in the waking state are just as effective as the same suggestions in the hypnotic state.

There is limited evidence that suggestions of an "involving" nature are superior in the hypnotic state. It has also been found that subjects tend to depress waking performance in order to insure facilitated efforts under hypnosis conditions. The only point in the literature on which widespread agreement exists is that negative suggestions designed to impair muscular strength and endur-

Table 1
Summary of Isometric Tasks Employed by Investigators in the Study of Hypnosis and Muscular Performance

Task	Investigator(s)
Arm dynamometer	Ikai & Steinhaus (1961); Mead & Roush (1949); Roush (1951)
Hand dynamometer	Barber & Calverley (1964); Crane (1940); Evans & Orne (1965); Eysenck (1941); Hadfield (1924); Ito (1979); Johnson & Kramer (1961); London & Fuhrer (1961); Mead & Roush (1949); Nevski & Sryashchich (1929); Rosenhan & London (1963); Slater (1967); Slotnick & London (1965); Young (1925)
"Human plank"	Collins (Note 1)
Weight holding	Barber & Calverley (1964); Charcot (1889); Evans & Orne (1965); Hyvärinen, Komi, & Puhakka (1977); Levitt & Brady (1964); London & Fuhrer (1961); Moikin & Poberezhskaya (1976); Moll (1913); Orne (1959); Reiger (cited in Hull, 1933); Rosenhan & London (1963); Slotnick & London (1965); Slotnick, Liebert, & Hilgard (1965); Wells (1928); Williams (1930)

Table 2
Summary of Dynamic Tasks Employed by Investigators in the Study of Hypnosis and Muscular Performance

Task	Investigator(s)
Bicycle ergometry	Albert & Williams (1975); Johnson, Massey, & Kramer (1960); Levin & Egolinsky (1936); Massey, Johnson, & Kramer (1961); Morgan, Raven, Drinkwater, & Horvath (1973); Morgan, Hirota, Weitz, & Balke (1976)
Hallucinated exercise	Agosti & Camerota (1965); Berman, Simonson, & Heron (1954); Bevegård, Arvidsson, Åström, & Jonsson (1968); Bier (1930); Cobb, Ripley, & Jones (1967); Fulde (1937); Hilgard & Boucher (1967); Kosunen, Kuoppasalmi, Naveri, Rehunen, Närvänen, & Adlercreutz (1977); Levin & Egolinsky (1936); Marshall (1970); Nemtzova & Shatenstein (1936); Whitehorn, Lundholm, & Gardner (1930)
Mosso ergograph	Mierke (1954); Nicholson (1920); Williams (1929)
Running (track)	Simonson (1937)
Running (treadmill)	Jackson, Gass, & Camp (1979)
Vertical jumping	Johnson & Kramer (1961)
Weight lifting	Johnson & Kramer (1960); Johnson & Kramer (1961); Morgan (1970); Nemtzova & Shatenstein (1936)

Table 3
Summary of Motor Learning and Performance Tasks Employed by Investigators in the Study of Hypnosis and Muscular Performance

Task	Investigator(s)
Ball bouncing	Arnold (1971)
Mirror tracing	Arnold (1971)
Reaction time	Blum & Wohl (1971); Graham, Olsen, Parrish, & Leibowitz (1968); Ham & Edmonston (1971); Ito (1978)
Stylus maze	Edmonston & Marks (1967)
Hypnotic anesthesia and fine motor performance	Wallace & Hoyenga (1981)

ance are usually effective. Although hypnotic suggestions of enhanced muscular strength and endurance are sometimes effective, they cannot be counted upon to consistently facilitate performance. Decrements in functional capacity can be routinely evoked under hypnotic conditions; however, even the most credulous hypnotists would admit that the same effect would be possible in the waking state as well.

Hallucinated Exercise

A series of investigations (Table 2) conducted over the past 50 years has revealed that hypnotic hallucinations of exercise tend to produce an increase in heart rate, and these increases have usually been observed to be consonant with the suggested intensity of exercise. Several investigators have also reported increased respiratory rate, ventilatory minute volume, and oxygen consumption. It has also been reported that cardiac output increases during hallucinated exercise, and these increments are thought to reflect a centrally induced general vasodilation in muscle.

The question of whether or not metabolic changes can be induced during exercise by means of hypnosis represents a different issue. First, hypnosis *per se* seems to increase the energy cost of standard work under normal conditions, and this probably reflects a general increase in arousal during hypnosis. Second, although hypnotically hallucinated exercise in the "resting" subject is consistently associated with increased heart rate, cardiac output, respiration, and oxygen uptake, hypnotic suggestions of increased and decreased work in the exercising subject have not produced consistent results, with the possible exception of exercise ventilation.

Motor Learning and Performance

Hypnotic suggestions of *increased* reaction time have consistently been observed to slow performance. Suggestions designed to *decrease* reaction time have sometimes resulted in such an effect, but faster times have not been consistently observed (Table 3). In many respects these findings parallel the observations in research involving muscular strength and endurance; that is, one can consistently decrease, but not increase, performance. The same findings have been made where more complex skills such as maze or mirror tracings have been utilized. It appears, however, that the type of hypnotic suggestion represents a crucial variable. Alerting suggestions, for example, are more likely to facilitate motor performance than are traditional hypnotic induction procedures, and hypnotic anesthesia induced in the arm has resulted in decreased fine motor performance.

Clinical Applications

Many reports in the popular literature suggest that hypnotic suggestion has been effective in facilitating muscular performance, but the validity of these reports is difficult to confirm or refute. On the other hand, several systematic studies have dealt with the application of hypnosis in the resolution of specific sport related problems, and these reports will be summarized in this section. The specific problem areas and the names of investigators are presented in Table 4.

It is rather common for athletes in certain sports to suddenly become unable to perform at past levels of consistent successful performance. For example, a baseball player with a batting average of .325 may go hitless for a series of games, and such a performance decrement is usually labeled a "slump." Johnson (1961a) has described the successful treatment of such a problem in a baseball player who had requested hypnotic treatment of a batting slump. The player was unaware of the basis for his performance decrement, but in the hypnotic state presented a detailed analysis of his swing, citing specific problems throughout the analysis. Johnson (1961a) asked the player whether he wished to have immediate, conscious recall of his analysis in the waking state, or simply to have the information "just come to him gradually." The player responded that he would prefer to have the information return in time rather than at once. The player's performance improved, and he went on to complete the season with an outstanding average of .400.

There are a number of interesting dimensions associated with this case. First, since players often come out of slumps spontaneously, it would be difficult to argue that the hypnoanalysis caused the improvement. Second, the information was not consciously available to the player. Third, the player demonstrated unusual in-

Table 4
Summary of Reports Involving the Use of Hypnosis in the
Treatment of Selected Clinical Problems

Problem area	Investigators
Anxiety	Garver (1977), Naruse (1965), Uneståhl (1981)
Performance slump	Johnson (1961a), Johnson (1965)
Physical injury	Ryde (1964)
Staleness	Morgan (1980)

sight in preferring that the hypnoanalytically retrieved material return gradually. Otherwise, he might have experienced the proverbial "paralysis through analysis," which allegedly occurred when the frog asked the centipede "Pray tell, which foot do you move first?" It will be recalled that the centipede was supposedly unable to resume normal movement patterns once the question was contemplated! Fourth, the player later thanked the hypnotist for the excellent analysis that led to his subsequent success. He would not believe that he had actually performed the analysis himself until the hypnotist reminded him that he had never seen him play and therefore would not have been able to diagnose the psychomotor problem and present a corrective prescription under hypnosis.

Ryde (1964) has presented a discussion of 35 cases consisting mainly of minor trauma resulting from athletic competition, as well as similar injuries sustained in nonathletic settings. The report describes the successful hypnotic treatment of various conditions such as tennis elbow, shin splints, chronic achilles tendon sprain, bruised heels, arch sprains, and other common ailments of uncertain minor pathology. Ryde has reported that hypnosis has been so effective in the treatment of such injuries that he now offers "to treat these disabilities initially by hypnosis and only proceed with conventional methods, should hypnosis fail or be refused" (p. 244). Workers in the field of sports medicine, especially those in orthopedic medicine and rehabilitation, will find Ryde's report of special interest. It should be emphasized that the hypnotic treatment of medical problems should only be carried out by an appropriately trained physician. An exception to this view might be that of a competent hypnotist working under the supervision of a physician. At any rate, it appears that hypnotherapy is effective in mobilizing the disabled athlete, and to this extent, it possesses ergogenic properties.

Johnson (1965) summarized a series of case studies involving athletic performance decrements attributable to aggression blockage. The athletes were treated by means of hypnotic age regression, and retrieval of repressed material and psychoanalytic interpretation and treatment were then used. The aggression conflicts were resolved by using posthypnotic suggestion. In one case, Johnson (1965) described a classic aggression-guilt-aggression cycle: the athlete was initially aggressive and performed well; he later felt guilty because of repressed childhood incidents involving aggression, and his performances declined; in time he again became aggressive and achieved former successful levels of performance.

It is known that precompetition anxiety can reach levels so intense that athletes at times become incapacitated. As mentioned earlier, attempts to manage anxiety states by means of hypnosis should be carried out cautiously and at a personalized level. One of the most comprehensive discussions of this topic has been presented by Naruse (1965). Anxiety in the precompetitive setting may be rather mild or so intense that the athlete is incapacitated. Naruse has labeled this state "stage fright," and he likens it to the "war neurosis" described by military psychiatrists. Naruse (1965) has described the use of (a) direct hypnotic suggestions, (b) posthypnotically produced autohypnosis, and (c) self-hypnosis in conjunction with autogenic training and progressive relaxation in the treatment of anxiety states in elite athletes. The actual procedure employed with a specific athlete was determined on an individual basis, and adoption of a given approach was governed in part by the athlete's personality structure, as well as the unique nature of the "stage fright." Hypnotherapists who contemplate work with elite athletes should find the paper by Naruse (1965) to be helpful in developing a therapeutic model.

Enhancement of performance in selected sport activities by means of hypnotic control of arousal levels has also been described by Garver (1977), who has described a therapeutic method requiring athletes under hypnosis to establish a 1-to-10 arousal-level scale. The zero anchor represents the lowest possible arousal level of an athlete, and 10 represents the highest. The athlete is then taken up and down the hierarchy, experiencing different arousal intensities at different numerical points, and is supposed to feel optimal arousal level sensations at point 5. Athletes tend to develop conditioned responses, or a "feeling" for each level, which they can then employ posthypnotically during competition.

Garver presents two cases in which numerical arousal level, posthypnotic cues, and cognitive rehearsal were successfully employed to control debilitating arousal states. One case involved a gymnast whose performance during competition was adversely affected by nervousness and anxiety; the other involved a golfer whose performance was affected by his level of anger.

The use of hypnotic age regression as a means of understanding the performance decrement of a college distance runner following a record performance has been described by Morgan (1980). The analysis was carried out within a multidisciplinary framework, and it was possible to first rule out that the decrement was due to a loss of physiologic function or medical problems. The runner possessed an aerobic power of 70 ml/kg/min, which is equivalent to that reported for elite runners (Milvy, 1977), and a series of standard medical tests were all found to be negative. Also, the runner's personality structure and mood state were not found to be remarkable in comparison with values published for elite distance runners (Morgan & Pollock, 1977). The runner appeared to be highly motivated, and he reported that he was "willing to do anything to be able to once again perform at a high level" (p. 370).

The runner was capable of entering a deep trance state, and it was decided to further explore the problem with age regression because (a) there were no medical contraindications, (b) there was no evidence of psychopathology, and (c) he possessed the physiologic capacity to perform at the desired level. Age regression to the day of his record performance revealed that he had experienced what can best be described as excruciating pain. The discomfort associated with the race was so profound that it had been repressed. When asked whether he wished to have posthypnotic recall of this repressed material he replied in the affirmative and there was therefore no attempt to create amnesia for the experience. When asked if he wished to continue with the program of "insight training" he replied that he would prefer to give the matter additional thought. In point of fact, however, he did not continue beyond this point, which suggests that retrieval of the repressed material altered his conscious desire to achieve his former record-setting pace. Additional details concerning the case are outlined in the report by Morgan (1980).

A systematic approach to the use of hypnosis and various relaxation procedures with athletes and sport teams has been described by Unestähl (1981). There are three common components in the training program devised by Unestähl. One is the altered or alternative states of consciousness (ASC). A second is imagination with special emphasis on visualization, and the third is suggestion with emphasis on autosuggestive principles. This program places a great deal of emphasis on analysis of "the winning feeling," which Unestähl also labels "the ideal performing state," or IPS. Basic similarities between IPS and ASC have been observed in various sports. Unestähl emphasizes that athletes often "have selective or even total amnesia after perfect performance, which makes it difficult for them to describe or analyze the IPS afterwards." In other words, the movement experiences are not available at a level of conscious recall. Hypnosis (ASC) is employed as a means of defining the IPS in this model. The training program is based on the three components mentioned above (i.e., ASC, imagination, and suggestion). The first 3 months of the program focuses on Inner Mental Training (IMT). During this period the athlete is taught advancing levels of somatic and psychic relaxation (weeks 1-4), followed by training in dissociation and detachment procedures (weeks 5-6); goal programming, ideomotor training, and systematic desensitization (weeks 7-9); problem-solving techniques (week 10); and self-confidence and concentration training (weeks 11-12).

The training program described by Unestähl (1981) has a strong theoretical basis, and it is also supported by convincing empirical evidence. Research dealing with the influence of hypnotic and posthypnotic suggestion on maximal strength (elbow flexion and knee extension), heart rate, lactic acid production, electromyographic activity, and subjective ratings or perception appear to be congruent with predictions generated by the model. In one experiment, for example, Unestähl has demonstrated that the production of lactic acid following "mental" and normal cycling is almost identical. In another experiment it was demonstrated that three months of IMT resulted in a significant lowering of lactic acid concentration following maximal strain in comparison with controls who did not receive IMT. These findings offer experimental evidence in support of the clinical model which has been proposed by Unestähl (1981).

Summary

Hypnosis has been employed in the exercise and sport sciences for many years. Although the efficacy of this particular ergogenic aid will undoubtedly be debated for many years to come, it seems reasonable to conclude that hypnosis can facilitate the physical performance of selected individuals in specific circumstances. Also, the management of pain by means of hypnosis has been demonstrated in the practice of both general and sports medicine, and this has significant implications concerning rehabilitation from injury and return to competition. It is also apparent that hypnosis offers a unique research tool where the need exists to manipulate or control an independent variable in an experimental setting.

An important and complex concern associated with the use of hypnosis in sport settings, which is probably not a serious concern with respect to many ergogenics, relates to the matter of qualifications. This concern has been addressed in this chapter, and it is once again emphasized that individuals who elect to employ hypnosis in research and/or clinical settings should be properly trained and qualified to do so.

Reference Note

1. Collins, J.K. *Muscular endurance in normal and hypnotic states: A study of suggested catalepsy.* Unpublished honors thesis, University of Sydney (Australia), 1961.

References

AGOSTI, E., & Camerota, G. Some effects of hypnotic suggestion on respiratory function. *The International Journal of Clinical and Experimental Hypnosis,* 1965, **13**, 149-156.

ALBERT, I., & Williams, M.H. Effects of post-hypnotic suggestions on muscular endurance. *Perceptual and Motor Skills,* 1975, **40**, 131-139.

ARNOLD, J. Effects of hypnosis on the learning of two selected motor skills. *Research Quarterly,* 1971, **42**, 1.

BARBER, T.X. The effects of hypnosis and suggestions on strength and endurance: A critical review of research studies. *British Journal of Social and Clinical Psychology,* 1966, **5**, 42-50.

BARBER, T.X., & Calverley, D.S. Toward a theory of "hypnotic" behavior: Enhancement of strength and endurance. *Canadian Journal of Psychology,* 1964, **18**, 156-167.

BERMAN, R., Simonson, E., & Heron, W. Electrocardiographic effects associated with hypnotic suggestion in normal and coronary sclerotic individuals. *Journal of Applied Physiology,* 1954, **7**, 89.

BEVEGÅRD, S., Arvidsson, T., Åstrom, H., & Jonsson, B. Circulation effects of suggested muscular work under hypnotic state. *Proceedings of the International Union of Physiology,* 1968, **7**, 42.

BIER, W. [Contributions to the influence of psychic processes on the circulation.] *Zeitschrift fuer klinische Medizin,* 1930, **113**, 762. (*Psychological Abstracts,* 1932, **6**, No. 4737.)

BLUM, G.S., & Wohl, B.M. Monetary, affective, and intrinsic incentives in choice reaction time. *Psychonomic Science,* 1971, **22**, 69.

BORG, G.A.V. Perceived exertion: A note on "history" and methods. *Medicine and Sciences in Sports,* 1973, **5**, 90-93.

BURROWS, G., & Dennerstein (Eds.). *Handbook of hypnosis and psychosomatic medicine.* Amsterdam: Elsevier/North Holland Biomedical Press, 1980.

CHARCOT, J.M. [*Lectures on diseases of nervous system.*] (T. Savill, trans.) London: New Syclenham Society, 1889.

COBB, L.A., Ripley, H.S., & Jones, J.W. Role of the nervous system in free fatty acid mobilization as demonstrated by hypnosis. In M.J. Karvonen &

A.J. Barry (Eds.), *Physical activity and the heart*. Springfield, IL: Charles C. Thomas, 1967.

COYLE, E.F., Feiring, D.C., Rotkis, T.C., Cote, R.W., Roby, F.B., Lee, W., & Wilmore, J.H. The specificity of power improvements through slow and fast isokinetic training. *Journal of Applied Physiology*, in press.

CRANE, C.W. *Psychology applied*. Evanston, IL: Northwestern University Press, 1940.

DUDLEY, D.L., Holmes, T.H., Martin, C.J., & Ripley, H.S. Changes in respiration associated with hypnotically induced emotion, pain, and exercise. *Psychosomatic Medicine*, 1964, **26**, 46-57.

EDMONSTON, W.E., & Marks, H.E. The effects of hypnosis and motivational instructions on kinesthetic learning. *The American Journal of Clinical Hypnosis*, 1967, **9**, 252-255.

EVANS, F.J., & Orne, M.T. Motivation, performance, and hypnosis. *The International Journal of Clinical and Experimental Hypnosis*, 1965, **13**, 103-116.

EYSENCK, H.J. An experimental study of the improvement of mental and physical functions in the hypnotic state. *British Journal of Medical Psychology*, 1941, **18**, 304-316.

FULDE, E. [The influence of hypnotic states of excitation on gas exchange.] *Zeitschrift für die gesamte Neurologie und Psychiatrie*, 1937, **159**, 761-766. (*Psychological Abstracts*, 1939, **13**, No. 3646.)

GARVER, R.B. The enhancement of human performance with hypnosis through neuromotor facilitation and control of arousal level. *American Journal of Clinical Hypnosis*, 1977, **19**, 177-181.

GORTON, B.E. Physiologic aspects of hypnosis. In J.M. Schneck (Ed.), *Hypnosis in modern medicine*. Springfield, IL: Charles C. Thomas, 1959.

GRAHAM, C., Olsen, R.A., Parrish, M., & Leibowitz, H.W. The effect of hypnotically induced fatigue on reaction time. *Psychosomatic Science*, 1968, **10**, 223-224.

HADFIELD, J.A. *The psychology of power*. New York: MacMillan, 1924.

HAM, M.W., & Edmonston, W.E. Hypnosis, relaxation and motor retardation. *Journal of Abnormal Psychology*, 1971, **77**, 329-331.

HANIN, Y.L. A study of anxiety in sports. In W.F. Straub (Ed.), *Sport psychology: An analysis of athlete behavior*. Ithaca, NY: Movement Publications, 1978.

HILGARD, E.R. More about forensic hypnosis. *American Psychological Association Division 30 Newsletter*, April 1979.

HILGARD, E.R., & Boucher, R.G. *Hypnosis research memorandum 59*. Palo Alto, CA: Stanford University, Department of Psychology, 1967.

HILGARD, E.R., & Hilgard, J.R. *Hypnosis in the relief of pain*. Los Altos, CA: William Kaufmann, 1975.

HULL, C.L. *Hypnosis and suggestibility: An experimental approach.* New York: Appleton-Century-Crofts, 1933.

HYVÄRINEN, J., Komi, P.V., & Puhakka, P. Endurance of muscle contraction under hypnosis. *Acta Physiologica Scandinavica,* 1977, **100**, 485-487.

IKAI, M., & Steinhaus, A.H. Some factors modifying the expression of human strength. *Journal of Applied Psychology,* 1961, **16**, 157-163.

ITO, M. A mechanism of acquired anxiety and its effects on choice reaction time. *Japanese Journal of Physical Education,* 1978, **22**, 331-342.

ITO, M. The differential effects of hypnosis and motivational suggestions on muscular strength. *Japanese Journal of Physical Education,* 1979, **24**, 93-100.

JACKSON, J.A., Gass, G.C., & Camp, E.M. The relationship between posthypnotic suggestion and endurance in physically trained subjects. *The International Journal of Clinical and Experimental Hypnosis,* 1979, **27**, 278-293.

JOHNSON, W.R. Body movement awareness in the non-hypnotic and hypnotic states. *Research Quarterly,* 1961, **32**, 263-264. (a)

JOHNSON, W.R. Hypnosis and muscular performance. *Journal of Sports Medicine and Physical Fitness,* 1961, **1**, 71-79. (b)

JOHNSON, W.R. The problem of aggression and guilt in sports, In F.A. Antonelli (Ed.), *Proceedings, First International Congress of Sport Psychology,* 1965.

JOHNSON, W.R., & Kramer, G.F. Effects of different types of hypnotic suggestions upon physical performance. *Research Quarterly,* 1960, **31**, 469-473.

JOHNSON, W.R., & Kramer, G.F. Effects of stereotyped nonhypnotic, hypnotic and posthypnotic suggestions upon strength, power, and endurance. *Research Quarterly,* 1961, **32**, 522-529.

JOHNSON, W.R., Massey, B.H., & Kramer, G.F. Effect of posthypnotic suggestions on all-out effort of short duration. *Research Quarterly,* 1960, **31**, 142-146.

KOSUNEN, K.J., Kuoppasalmi, K., Näveri, H., Rehunen, S., Närvänen, S., & Adlercreutz, H. Plasma renin activity, angiotensin II, and aldosterone during the hypnotic suggestion of running. *Scandinavian Journal of Clinical Laboratory Investigations,* 1977, **37**, 99-103.

LANDERS, D.M. Motivation and performance: The role of arousal and attentional factors. In W.F. Straub (Ed.), *Sport psychology: An analysis of athlete behavior.* Ithaca, NY: Movement Publications, 1978.

LANGER, P. Varsity football performance. *Perceptual and Motor Skills,* 1966, **23**, 1191-1199.

LEVIN, S.L., & Egolinsky, I.A. [The effect of cortical functions upon energy changes in basal metabolism.] *Fiziologicheskii Zhurnal S.S.S.R.,* 1936, **20**, 979-992. (*Psychological Abstracts,* 1939, **13**, No. 4128.)

LEVITT, E.E. President's message. *American Psychological Association Division 30 Newsletter,* August 1981.

LEVITT, E.E., & Brady, J.P. Muscular endurance under hypnosis and in the motivated waking state. *The International Journal of Clinical and Experimental Hypnosis,* 1964, **12**, 21-27.

LONDON, P., & Fuhrer, M. Hypnosis, motivation and performance. *Journal of Personality,* 1961, **29**, 321-333.

MANZER, C.W. The effect of verbal suggestions on output and variability of muscular work. *Psychological Clinic,* 1934, **22**, 248-256.

MARSHALL, G.D. Heart rate responses in real and hallucinated exercise. *Hypnosis research memorandum 113.* Palo Alto, CA: Stanford University, Department of Psychology, 1970.

MASSEY, B.H., Johnson, W.R., & Kramer, G.R. Effect of warm-up exercise upon muscular performance using hypnosis to control the psychological variable. *Research Quarterly,* 1961, **32**, 63-71.

MEAD, S., & Roush, E.S. A study of the effect of hypnotic suggestion on physiologic performance. *Archives of Physical Medicine,* 1949, **30**, 700-704.

MIERKE, K. [Directional and motivational forces in the execution of tasks.] *Zeitschrift für experimentelle und angewandte Psychologie,* 1954, **2**, 92-135. (*Psychological Abstracts,* 1956, **30**, No. 4044.)

MILVY, P. (Ed.). The marathon: Physiological, medical, epidemiological and psychological studies. *Annals of the New York Academy of Science,* 1977, **301**, 1-1090.

MOIKIN, Y.V., & Poberezhskaya, A.S. Mechanism of work refusal through fatigue reflected in electromyographic changes under hypnosis. *Bulletin of Experimental and Biological Medicine,* 1976, **80**, 862-864.

MOLL, A. [*Hypnotism*] (A.F. Hopkirk, trans.). New York: Scribners, 1913.

MORGAN, W.P. Oxygen uptake following hypnotic suggestion. In G.S. Kenyon (Ed.), *Contemporary psychology of sport.* Chicago: Athletic Institute, 1970.

MORGAN, W.P. Hypnosis and muscular performance. In W.P. Morgan (Ed.), *Ergogenic aids and muscular performance.* New York: Academic Press, 1972.

MORGAN, W.P. Hypnosis and sports medicine. In G. Burrows & L.D. Dennerstein (Eds.), *Handbook of hypnosis and psychosomatic medicine.* Amsterdam: Elsevier/North Holland Biomedical Press, 1980.

MORGAN, W.P. The 1980 C.H. McCloy research lecture: Psychophysiology of self-awareness during vigorous physical activity. *Research Quarterly for Exercise and Sport,* 1981, **52**, 358-427.

MORGAN, W.P., Hirota, K., Weitz, G.A., & Balke, B. Hypnotic perturbation of perceived exertion: Ventilatory consequences. *American Journal of Clinical Hypnosis,* 1976, **18**, 182-190.

MORGAN, W.P., & Pollock, M.L. Psychologic characterization of the elite distance runner. In P. Milvy (Ed.), *Annals of the New York Academy of Science,* 1977, **301**, 382-403.

MORGAN, W.P., Raven, P.B., Drinkwater, B.L., & Horvath, S.M. Perceptual and metabolic responsivity to standard bicycle ergometry following various hypnotic suggestions. *International Journal of Clinical and Experimental Hypnosis,* 1973, **31**, 86-101.

NARUSE, G. The hypnotic treatment of stage fright in champion athletes. *International Journal of Clinical and Experimental Hypnosis,* 1965, **13**, 63-70.

NEMTZOVA, O.L., & Shatenstein, D.I. [The effect of the central nervous system upon some physiological processes during work.] *Fiziologicheskii Zhurnal S.S.S.R.,* 1936, **20**, 581-593. (*Psychological Abstracts,* 1939, **13**, No. 4129.)

NEVSKI, I., & Sryashchich, K. [Influence of hypnosis on muscular strength.] *Novoe V. Refleksologii fiziologii neronolsistemy,* 1929, **3**, 458-480. (*Psychological Abstracts,* 1930, **4**, No. 4290.)

NICHOLSON, N.C. Notes on muscular work during hypnosis. *Johns Hopkins Hospital Bulletin,* 1920, **31**, 89-91.

O'LEARY, K.D., & Borkovec, T.D. Conceptual, methodological, and ethical problems of placebo groups in psychotherapy research. *American Psychologist,* September 1978, 821-830.

ORNE, M.T. The nature of hypnosis: Artifact and essence. *Journal of Abnormal Psychology,* 1959, **58**, 277-299.

POMERANZ, D.M., & Krasner, L. Effect of a placebo on simple motor response. *Perceptual and Motor Skills,* 1969, **28**, 15-18.

REITTER, P.J. The influence of hypnosis on somatic fields of function. In L.M. LeCron (Ed.), *Experimental hypnosis.* New York: MacMillan, 1958.

ROSEN, H. Hypnosis and drug abuse in sports. In T.T. Craig (Ed.), *The humanistic and mental health aspects of sports, exercise and research.* Chicago: American Medical Association, 1976.

ROSENHAN, D., & London, P. Hypnosis: Expectation, susceptibility, and performance. *Journal of Abnormal Social Psychology,* 1963, **66**, 77-81.

ROUSH, E.S. Strength and endurance in the waking and hypnotic states. *Journal of Applied Physiology,* 1951, **3**, 404-410.

RYDE, D. A personal study of some uses of hypnosis in sports and sports injuries. *Journal of Sports Medicine and Physical Fitness,* 1964, **4**, 241-246.

SIMONSON, E. [Experiments on the physiology of foot racing.] *Travail humain,* 1937, **5**, 286-305. (*Psychological Abstracts,* 1938, **12**, No. 243.)

SLATER, C. Expectancy and hypnotic performance. (Doctoral dissertation, Washington State University, 1967). *Dissertation Abstracts International,* 1967, **28**, 2632B. (University Microfilms No. 67-15, 763)

SLOTNICK, R., & London, P. Influence of instructions on hypnotic and nonhypnotic performance. *Journal of Abnormal Psychology*, 1965, **70**, 38-46.

SLOTNICK, R.S., Liebert, R.M., & Hilgard, E.R. The enhancement of muscular performance in hypnosis through exhortation and involving instructions. *Journal of Personality*, 1965, **33**, 36-45.

SMITH, J.L., & Bozymowski, M.F. Effect of attitude toward warm-ups on motor performance. *Research Quarterly*, 1965, **36**, 78-85.

UNESTÅHL, L. New paths of sport learning and excellence. *Proceedings of the Fifth World Sport Psychology Congress*, 1981.

WALLACE, B., & Hoyenga, K.B. Performance of fine motor coordination activities with an hypnotically anesthetized limb. *The International Journal of Clinical and Experimental Hypnosis*, 1981, **29**, 54-65.

WEITZENHOFFER, A.M. *Hypnotism: An objective study in suggestibility.* New York: John Wiley and Sons, 1963.

WELLS, F.L. Reaction time and allied measures under hypnosis: Report of a case. *Journal of Abnormal and Social Psychology*, 1928, **24**, 264-275.

WHITEHORN, J.C., Lundholm, H., & Gardner, G.E. The metabolic rate in emotional moods induced by suggestion in hypnosis. *American Journal of Psychiatry*, 1930, **9**, 661.

WILLIAMS, G.W. The effect of hypnosis on muscular fatigue. *Journal of Abnormal and Social Psychology*, 1929, **24**, 318-329.

WILLIAMS, G.W. A comparative study of voluntary and hypnotic catalepsy. *American Journal of Psychology*, 1930, **42**, 83-95.

YOUNG, P.C. An experimental study of mental and physical functions in the normal and hypnotic states. *American Journal of Psychology*, 1925, **36**, 214-232.

10

Covert Rehearsal Strategies

John M. Silva III

Sports performance and skill enhancement are affected by a myriad of variables. One variable of central importance to skilled performance is practice. Most teachers, participants, and researchers are aware of the significant role physical practice plays when it is presented in an appropriate learning environment (Singer, 1971). Thus, several hours of practice time are usually devoted to the physical drilling or repetition of skills in order to engrain desired movement patterns and remove or refine inappropriate motor programs. Although such a traditional methodology certainly has its merit, it is somewhat curious that a profession that has long emphasized the unity of the body and mind devotes little, if any, formal practice time to the mental or covert rehearsal of skilled performance. Covert rehearsal, in the context of this paper, is defined as imagined, symbolic rehearsal of an activity. This covert rehearsal may be manifested as covert subvocalizations, visual display, or kinesthetic-visual stimulation. All forms of covert rehearsal, however, are characterized by a lack of major voluntary movement in the gross musculature of the rehearser.

John M. Silva, Ph.D., is with the Department of Physical Education at the University of North Carolina in Chapel Hill.

The neglect of covert rehearsal as a viable practice methodology for the preparation and execution of skilled performance is a somewhat Western phenomenon. For centuries Tibetan monks trained in "Lung-Gum" have used covert rehearsal and dissociative strategies along with physical training in preparation for long distance running (Watson, 1973). By integrating physical and mental practice these monks have repeatedly run extraordinary distances over hazardous courses with remarkably swift times. Such Eastern practices have generally been dismissed as too mystical for the technologically minded West. However, the basic premise operating in the training of these monks is that one must train the mind as well as the body. When placed in these terms, this is a position with which few contemporary coaches would argue. Indeed, when poor or inconsistent performance by an athlete is not attributable to a lack of ability but rather to an inability to perform up to expectation, psychological explanations are often given as the basis for the marginal performance.

The role of cognition in skilled performance has become more widely recognized not only by coaches, but also by researchers. Marteniuk (1976) has stated:

> Perceptual-motor skills, though their overt manifestations are motor in nature, have a large mental or cognitive component that influences much of the information processing activities concerned with the performance and learning of these skills. In fact, before these skills can be really understood, this writer believes that much more emphasis must be placed on attempting to understand the cognitive nature of these skills. (p. 224)

With Marteniuk's suggestions in mind, the purpose of this chapter is to provide the reader with foundational information on the theoretical basis concerning the link between covert mental activities and overt manifestations of skill performance. After the theoretical base of this relationship is established, a review of current research in mental practice, imagery, and covert rehearsal will be presented. An attempt will be made to provide the reader with literature that has been supportive, as well as nonsupportive, of the effects of covert rehearsal strategies and skilled performance enhancement. Following this review, a brief summary and suggestions for subsequent research will be provided in order to augment the continued inquiry into this relatively untapped area of sport psychology.

Covert Processes and Overt Behavior: Theoretical Foundations

The use of covert rehearsal strategies in sport settings is a relatively new application of a technique that dates back to the turn of the century. One of the earliest attempts to link the relationship between covert processes and overt behavior was advanced by James (1890a, 1890b). James maintained that perceptual images or the idea of an action or behavior initiates performance. James (1890a) stated, "my experience is what I agree to attend to" (p. 402). The key words in this often quoted passage are "I agree." These words connote a cognitive or conscious effort to select certain environmental stimuli that elicit images of response probabilities. The idea that cognition and images often premediate a response was the basis of James's (1890b) ideo-motor mechanisms theory. According to this theory, repeated experiences of stimulus-response chains result in conditioned anticipatory images of response feedback. These images then become anticipatory to actual performance, resulting in discriminative control over overt responses. If anticipatory cognitions are inappropriately conditioned, the probability of correct or appropriate overt responses is consequently diminished. In essence, what James was attempting to convey was the premise that our thoughts mediate our behavior; overt acts are not simply a stimulus-response chain unaffected by our experiences and expectations of future behavioral outcomes. During the period of rigid behaviorism in psychology (1910-1940s) James's theory fell into disrepute because it was dealing with processes that were subjective and not easily quantifiable. Thus, the potential influence of covert processes upon overt behavior lay dormant for several decades. The work of Wolpe (1958), a behavioristically trained therapist, reintroduced the idea that covert processes can influence overt behavior. His research resulted in the subjective experience regaining respectability in mainstream psychology. Wolpe carefully investigated how imagery and covert rehearsal assisted patients with various phobic reactions in overcoming well engrained fears. Wolpe (1958) carefully developed a technique known as systematic desensitization that is based upon covert practice and behavioral principles. Clients were led to imagine particular events in the therapist's office that were combined with overt instructions. Subsequently, Wolpe noticed that patients' covert and overt behavioral responses were changing in a constant and adaptive manner that was consistent with their new set of covert images, external expectancies, and self-instructions.

The theoretical principles underlying the work of James and Wolpe, outlined above, emanate directly from learning theory. Mahoney (1974) has used the term *continuity assumption* to clarify the learning theory foundation of many covert rehearsal strategies. Traditionally, behaviorism has been concerned with only the overt responses of the organism. The continuity assumption maintains that similar learning principles function at both the overt (behavioral) and covert (imaginal) levels. This assumption has been supported by staunch behaviorists such as Homme (1965) and Skinner (1953), who acknowledged the import of private events, but chose to study the "more accessible" overt behavior of subjects. Others as early as Jacobson (1930) and Miller (1935) have found continuity in physiological responses to overt as well as covert stimuli. Later work by Barber and Hahn (1964) and Craig (1968) also reported autonomic effects concomitant with covert or imagined experiences. Further evidence dismissing a duality notion regarding covert processes, physiological responses, behavior expectancies, and behavior outcomes has been reported in the research of Atkinson and Wickens (1971), Bauer and Craighead (1979), Bower (1972), Lang (1979), Mahoney, Thorensen, and Danaher (1972), Meichenbaum and Cameron (1974), and Meichenbaum and Goodman (1969). These studies serve as representative examples that attest to the argument that one's thoughts are directly related to and can actually initiate physiological reactions, expectancies of behavior outcomes, and actual overt behavioral responses. Meichenbaum (1978) has argued convincingly that it is not of central importance to maintain that specific covert visualizations or verbalizations are causative in maladaptive behavior or inappropriate behavior. What is of paramount interest, however, is the degree to which subjects have conditioned themselves to believe that these covert experiences realistically represent reality. An analogy for sport environments would argue that it is not necessarily the image of being negatively evaluated by 10,000 spectators that results in a player missing a crucial field goal kick in a football game or a pivotal foul shot in basketball, but rather it is the belief that the athlete maintains regarding the reality or likelihood of this image that may influence one's performance capability. Surely, all athletes periodically engage in covert imagery that has negative connotations for performance expectancy. Although these covert images may be a source of distraction from the task in and of themselves, it is perhaps, as noted by Meichenbaum (1978), the belief system and coping ability of the athlete that determines the effective power of the image.

Psychological Processes and Covert Rehearsal

On the basis of the brief theoretical review presented above, a summary of the psychological processes that function in the use of covert rehearsal strategies can be outlined. Cautela (1977) has detailed these processes by paralleling operant and social learning procedures with covert conditioning procedures. Cautela (1977) described in depth how overt behavior can be influenced by covert positive reinforcement, covert negative reinforcement, covert sensitization (punishment), covert extinction, covert response (response cost), and covert modeling processes. Because covert learning is assumed to parallel overt learning principles, many advantages can be accrued from covert strategies directed toward behavior change, performance expectancies, or actual athlete performance. According to Meichenbaum (1977, 1978), these include an increased sense of control due to the development of careful monitoring of functional and dysfunctional covert images and dialogue, the rehearsal of relevant images, the modification of inappropriate images or covert dialogue that may contribute to undesired overt responses, and the development of rational coping skills facilitated by repeated covert rehearsal of behavioral strategies. Obviously, each of these mental preparations can be of potential benefit to a wide range of sport activities and to some extent high-caliber athletes in various sports have been found to engage in such preparatory mental activity to a greater extent than their non-elite counterparts (Highlen & Bennett, 1979; Mahoney & Avener, 1977). As research continues to probe the effects of systematic covert rehearsal upon skilled performance, both the scientist and the practitioner will be provided with greater insight concerning often-asked questions such as (a) How important is the subject's level of skill (novice performer vs. elite performer), (b) What is the relationship between imagery control and clarity with performance enhancement, (c) How much time should be spent on imagery and covert rehearsal strategies, and (d) What type of integrated program of mental and physical practice optimizes performance improvement? In the following section classic and current research will be reviewed in order to provide an indication of the present state of research in the field of covert rehearsal and skill performance.

Research on Covert Rehearsal and Skill Performance

Research in the general area of covert rehearsal spans at least a 50-year period (e.g., Washburn, 1916). Comprehensive reviews of past literature are offered in the articles by Corbin (1972) and Richardson (1967a, 1967b). Rather than present the reader with a lengthy and perhaps redundant review, the focus of this section will be primarily on research conducted during the 1960s to the present.

Studies Supportive of Covert Rehearsal
Strategies and Skill Performance

Studies supportive of various covert rehearsal strategies are characterized by tremendous variations in research methodology and the experimental techniques employed. Early research by Vandell, Davis, and Clungston (1943) and Twining (1949) provided significant impetus to the specific study of mental practice and motor skill performance. Both of the studies cited above found that mentally rehearsing a motor skill resulted in considerable performance improvement that was virtually equivalent to the performance of groups utilizing physical practice. The motor tasks utilized in each of these studies were skills that were relatively familiar to the subjects (e.g., basketball throw, ring toss). Although both of these studies possessed notable methodological flaws, the heuristic value of this early work is not to be underestimated. During the 1950s and 1960s, several studies were conducted on the effects of "prepractice activities" on skill performance (e.g., Ammons, 1951), mental practice and muscular endurance (e.g., Kelsey, 1961), mental practice effecting skill development (e.g., Clark, 1960), and mental training effecting the acquisition of motor skills (e.g., Ulich, 1967). Clark's (1960) study of 144 high-school-aged male basketball players equated subjects on factors such as arm strength, intelligence, and level of competitive experience. The athletes were evaluated on free-throw-shooting proficiency according to whether they had been assigned to a 14-day physical practice group or a 14-day mental practice group. Clark found that for the more experienced groups (varsity and junior varsity teams), mental practice was as effective as physical practice. This result was not found, however, for the novice group that experienced an average gain of 44% improvement in shooting proficiency using physical practice compared to an improvement of 26% for the mental practice group.

Ulich (1967) reported on a series of six studies designed to assess the effects of observation and mental training on various tasks of finger and manual dexterity. Ulich took physiological measures while subjects engaged in active training periods or passive training periods (observation or mental practice). Active practice resulted in the greatest increments in pulse rate, respiratory rate, and myographic activity, as expected. However, notable increases were also recorded in these measures for subjects in the mental practice condition and to a lesser extent for subjects engaging in the observational condition. Comparisons of subject performance across the studies conducted led Ulich to conclude that (a) motor skills can be learned actively or passively, (b) mental practice is as effective as physical practice and more effective than observational practice for tasks of manual dexterity, (c) mental practice can facilitate the retention of motor skills, and (d) passive training techniques tend to elicit similar but less intense physiological responses in subjects.

Research on the effect of mental practice and skill performance continued to be popular during the late 1960s and 1970s. Jones (1965), Surburg (1968), Shick (1970), and White, Ashton, and Lewis (1979) all conducted studies designed to evaluate the role of mental practice in facilitating sport skills performance. Jones (1965) found that both directed and undirected mental practice resulted in improved tennis skills. Surburg (1968) varied audio, visual, and audiovisual instruction with either no mental practice or with concurrent engagement in mental practice sessions. He found that the three experimental groups who engaged in mental practice in conjunction with stimulation via a second modality improved significantly more than the experimental groups not using mental practice. The greatest improvement was achieved by the experimental group exposed to audio information about the forehand tennis drive combined with 10 minutes of mental practice time. Shick (1970) found mental practice was effective in improving the sport skill of volleyball serving, but not effective in improving wall volleying. Significant differences in performance were also recorded as a function of the length of time a subject engaged in mental practice. Three minutes of mental practice was found to be significantly more effective in improving the serve than was 1 minute of mental practice. White et al. (1979) studied the effects of mental practice and physical practice on the action-reaction swimming start. Subjects were assigned to either a physical practice condition, a mental practice condition, or a combined physical-mental practice condition. Subjects using mental practice visualized their skill from detailed instruction charts that illustrated the skill; they were requested to practice mentally 5 minutes each evening. The authors found that subjects in the physical-mental practice combination group demonstrated the greatest improvement. Mental or physical practice alone also resulted in significant improvement over a control group that showed no change. Improvement was also significantly related to a subject's ability to use kinesthetic imagery.

A recent well controlled study by Ryan and Simons (1981) attempted to investigate questions raised in previous research on covert practice strategies. Ryan and Simons were interested in determining the effects of mental practice on tasks that differed in their cognitive-motoric content. The authors also assessed two other commonly raised issues: (a) Do individual differences in the vividness and controllability of images influence performance, and (b) What is the influence of the relative frequency of mental practice on skill acquisition? Subjects were randomly assigned to conditions of physical practice (PP), mental practice (MP), or a no-practice control (NP). Subjects in the experimental groups learned two novel tasks that differed in task demand along a cognitive-motoric continuum. Subjects in the PP condition were provided with 12 actual trials; each trial was separated by a 30-second rest interval. Subjects in the MP condition received one physical trial followed by nine mental rehearsal trials 30 seconds in duration, separated by 30-second rest intervals. The NP condition consisted of one physical trial followed by 9 minutes of rest and two final physical trials of 30 seconds. The results demonstrated that for the motoric stabilometer task, PP was significantly superior to either MP or NP, while no differences between MP and NP were found for this task. On the cognitive dial-a-maze task, however, MP and PP subjects performed equally well and both significantly exceeded the performance of subjects in the NP condition. The authors found no significant relationship between vividness or controllability and performance on the stabilometer task, but for the dial-a-maze cognitive task found a significant correlation between vividness and performance. The frequency of MP and subject performance was evaluated only for MP subjects and only on the dial-a-maze task. No significant relationships were found for this analysis.

In the studies reviewed above the authors utilized what could be classified as a global mental imagery program with subjects. That is, subjects mentally practiced a general image of what or how the skill should be performed. The imagery was in no way individually suited to particular performance needs or performance problems experienced by a subject. Given the general nature of the imagery programs employed in these studies, it is indeed impressive that significant improvement in performances were found across various types of motor and sport skills.

During the early 1970s, mental practice and the use of imagery began to be employed in a more specific manner. Researchers, drawing upon relaxation techniques (Wolpe, 1958) and cognitive behavior modification principles (Meichenbaum, 1977), tailored intervention strategies with imagery components to specific performance problems. In this approach an objective component or several components of a skill are identified and baseline measures of performance are recorded preintervention. Program implementation often consists of cognitive restructuring, relaxation instruction and practice, and the implementation of self-instructional imagery or mental practice programs. Objective evaluations of the skill are then recorded during the postintervention period, allowing for an evaluation of intervention effectiveness. In some studies (e.g., Silva, 1982) skill improvement is assessed during actual competition in which the subject is engaged. This change in methodology represents a significant test of the efficacy of mental practice programs because improvement or performance gain is evaluated during the pressure of organized competition. Some of the earliest published reports describing the use of cognitive intervention in a sport setting are found in the work of Suinn (1972, 1976) with Olympic skiers. Using "on site" psychological interventions, Suinn has reported enhancing the performance of elite skiers using a program called visuo-motor behavior rehearsal (VMBR). The VMBR program involves developing progressive relaxation and covert visualization of specific images selected on the basis of their importance in enhancing a subject's skill performance. Several studies have appeared in the literature recently that have utilized VMBR techniques as an intervention strategy designed to improve performance. Titley (1976) reports case study information on a place kicker trained in VMBR. No preintervention data was reported for comparison purposes, but impressive postintervention data was reported with the subject, in competition, kicking nine out of nine extra-point attempts and one out of one field-goal attempts in the game following the first three treatment sessions. The subject went on to kick consistently throughout the season, including a 1974 NCAA record-setting field-goal kick of 63 yards.

Lane (1980) employed VMBR techniques with a small group of high school basketball players ($n = 3$). The athletes trained in VMBR increased their foul shooting proficiency by 10% at home games and by 15% at away games based upon comparisons with their previous year's statistics. Similar improvement for the nonparticipating team members was not achieved over the same competitive interval. Lane (1980) reports several case study results of the successful implementation of VMBR with athletes competing in various sports at competitive levels ranging from elementary school through professional.

Noel (1980) conducted a more controlled study of the effectiveness of VMBR with male tennis players involved in a tennis tournament. A group of 14 subjects was equated for skill level and divided into two groups of 7; one group received VMBR while the control group did not receive any VMBR training or rehearsal. The VMBR program utilized in this study focused on the tennis serve under tournament conditions. A coping strategy of imagery was employed that made VMBR subjects aware that errors may occur and that they should deal with any errors calmly and make the necessary adjustments. Subjects practiced VMBR 7 days prior to the first tournament match. The first 3 days involved practicing a relaxation technique, and during the final 4 days both relaxation and visualization was practiced following typed instructions that were provided to the subjects. The results indicated that the serving performance of high-ability players improved with VMBR while the performance of low-ability players actually decreased with VMBR practice.

The performance of karate participants engaged in a program of VMBR was evaluated in a study by Weinberg, Seabourne, and Jackson (1981). Subjects were matched for skill and assigned to either VMBR, relaxation, imagery, or an attention-placebo control condition. Performance measures and a measure of trait anxiety were given to all subjects prior to the start of the experimental program. Subjects were requested to employ the appropriate covert strategy for 20 minutes/day for a 6-week period. At the conclusion of the 6-week period, subjects were readministered the performance and anxiety measures. The results of this study demonstrated a significant reduction in trait anxiety for all the experimental groups engaged in a covert rehearsal strategy. Significant performance differences were found in the area of sparring proficiency; the experimental group employing VMBR scored higher than the other comparison groups. The authors noted that a combination of reduced anxiety and covert rehearsal may maximize appropriate concentration strategies.

The covert strategies utilized in VMBR represent one method of cognitive intervention that appears to have the potential to facilitate skill performance in competitive settings. Another technique that has been reported in the psychology and sport psychology literature applies more emphatically cognitive behavior modification (CBM) techniques. These techniques differ from VMBR in that a significant emphasis is placed upon cognitive restructuring and self-instructional imagery. That is, specific thought patterns of subjects that are potentially dysfunctional to optimal performance are identified and subjects are instructed not only in imagery directed toward appropriate self-talk and performance but also in techniques designed to stop and replace dysfunctional ruminations. In effect, programs are geared to individual thought patterns, and subjects are trained through restructuring to modify inappropriate patterns and to engrain appropriate and adaptive cognitive chains.

Desiderato and Miller (1979) utilized a CBM-based program to improve the tennis performance of a competitive female player. By utilizing relaxation techniques, self-instructional covert verbalization, and imagery for a 3-week period, the subject improved her ability to win deuce point games in match play. Prior to intervention, baseline data indicated that the subject had won 29% of the deuce games in which she was involved during competitive play and 49% of the deuce games in which she was involved during noncompetitive play. Following the CBM program, postintervention data indicated that the subject had won 60% of her competitive deuce games (an increase of 31%) and 55% of her noncompetitive deuce games (an increase of 6%), resulting in an overall increase of 37% in deuce games won.

A similar CBM approch was used by Meyers and Schleser (1980) with a collegiate basketball player who was having difficulty concentrating on field-goal shooting. The athlete was provided with seven sessions over a 3-week period during which relaxation procedures and imagery sequences were developed. A coping strategy of imagery used with the subject involved the imagined presentation of a scene five times for 30 seconds. The subject's scenes were arranged in a hierarchical order; successful performances were imagined first, and problematic situations introduced later in the four-scene set. Coping self-instructions were introduced to the subject for the problematic situations imagined. These covert vocalizations were task-oriented and attempted to minimize self-critical statements for performance errors. The subject's performance during seven postintervention games was compared to performance during seven preintervention games that were matched according to subject playing time. The results indicated a significant improvement in field-goal percentage (42.4% vs. 65.6%) and a significant improvement in the subject's points/game average (11.3 vs. 15.3). These improvements occurred for the subject while the performance of other regular playing teammates showed no significant change over the same seven-game period.

DeWitt (1980) conducted two studies that involved cognitive training techniques. Study 1 was conducted with a group of university football players who had been classified by their coach as having high levels of stress that debilitated performance. Electromyographic (EMG) readings were taken for subjects under nonthreatening imaginal situations and under stressful imaginal situations. When exposed to stressful imaginal situations, subjects were given biofeedback concerning their EMG readings and were required to use relaxation techniques when readings exceeded the baseline measurements by 10% or greater. When subjects were able to initiate and maintain a decrease back to baseline readings,

the experimenter moved on to the next imaginal scene in the hierarchy and followed the procedure identified above. Subjects participated in this program for 12 sessions, and comparisons based on
the coaches' standard 10-point performance scale were made for
preintervention and postintervention periods. The results indicated a significant decrease in EMG recordings across treatment
sessions, indicating the athletes were adapting to the imaginal situations and perceiving them as less threatening. Player performance
also improved significantly; coaches' mean ratings of experimental
players' performance increased from 3.67 preintervention to 7.17
postintervention on the 10-point scale. Study 2 was conducted
with members of a male university basketball team. Subjects were
randomly assigned to a treatment or contact-control group. The
treatment group engaged in 11 1-hour sessions that involved the
development of relaxation techniques, imagery, coping techniques, thought-stopping techniques, and other psychological
skills commonly used in CBM research. Preintervention performance was compared with postintervention performance for both
the treatment and control groups. The results indicated a significant reduction in EMG and heart rate levels of treatment subjects
across the 11-session period. Subjects receiving the CBM program
also demonstrated a significant gain in performance ratings while
control subjects showed no gain in performance over the same
time interval.

Silva (1982) has reported the successful use of CBM techniques
with university-level hockey and basketball players. Subjects are
exposed to a three-phase intervention program that is tailored to
the unique needs of each participant. Phase 1 involves an identifi-
cation phase where athletes identify the specific performance problem in need of modification and establish the situational and behavioral boundaries of this problem. Once a boundary has been
satisfactorily established, subjects are asked to overtly verbalize
any covert verbalizations that may be experienced immediately
before, during, and/or after the undesired behavior is performed.
The second phase involves the restructuring of inappropriate
cognitive chains being manifested by the subject. The final phase
pairs adaptive and coping self-instructional imagery with concen-
trative cues of a covert verbal nature. In Study 1, data are reported
on a collegiate hockey player who accumulated 52 minutes of
penalty time over an 11-game interval for an average of 4.72 minutes of penalty time/game. Intervention was employed with the
subject over the remainder of the season (6 weeks) and penalty
time statistics were compared with the preintervention statistics.
During the 10-game intervention period, the subject's penalty time

was reduced to 22 minutes for an average of 2.20 minutes/game. A similar program is reported as having positive results in reducing the fouling behavior of a collegiate basketball player and increasing the foul-shooting performance of a college basketball performer. In Study 2, the athlete had committed an average of 4.30 fouls/game over a 13-game period while teammates had committed only 2.96 fouls over the same period. Following intervention, the subject reduced fouling during the remainder of the season (10 games) to an average of 3.40 fouls/game while teammates committed an average of 2.70 fouls per game during the same interval. The third study reported was conducted with a college basketball player who chronically suffered from poor free-throw shooting throughout his college career. Prior to intervention, the subject was shooting 53.86% (first 7 games) while teammates were shooting 63.50% from the foul line. Following 14 days of intervention, performance data were recorded for the last 16 games of the season. During this period the subject shot 74.91% from the foul line for an improvement of 21.05%. Teammate performance during the same interval was 66.20% for an increase of 2.7%.

Studies Nonsupportive of Covert Rehearsal Strategies and Skill Performance

Although an impressive number of studies utilizing covert rehearsal techniques have reported performance improvement in motor and sport skills, it would be remiss not to report various published studies that have not found any beneficial effects due to covert practice methods. Certainly fewer studies reporting no effect from covert rehearsal can be located in the literature. One plausible explanation for this quantitative imbalance may be that authors and journal editors are often more reluctant to submit and publish research that finds no significant differences between treatment groups. Thus, an accurate reflection of the ratio of studies finding covert rehearsal strategies beneficial to performance compared to those not finding any effect or finding a negative effect is clearly unattainable. The determination of the efficacy of covert rehearsal strategies should not be relegated to a simple comparison based on the quantity of supportive to nonsupportive literature. Such an assessment would be of dubious and superficial value and thus the reader is advised not to draw such a conclusion from this review of nonsupportive literature.

One of the earlier studies finding a negative effect is Gilmore and Stolurow's (1951) research on motor versus mental practice and performance on a ball-and-socket task. Thirty-six subjects were assigned to one of six different groups. Half the subjects were pre-tested and then engaged in a relatively massed practice session of mental rehearsal or physical rehearsal while the third pretested group engaged in an activity unrelated to the criterion task. The other half of the subjects were not pretested but also experienced one of the three experimental sessions described above. All sub-jects were posttested and the results of pretest to posttest improve-ment were analyzed. Subjects in the physical practice and no-practice groups demonstrated an improvement; the physical prac-tice group was superior to either mental practice or no practice. The mental practice group actually showed a decline in perfor-mance and overall performance was significantly inferior to both the physical practice and no-practice groups. Unfortunately, no ex-planation of these interesting results is advanced by the authors.

Corbin (1967) conducted a comprehensive study designed to determine what effects covert rehearsal, overt rehearsal, or a covert-overt rehearsal combination may have upon the learning of a novel complex motor skill called wand juggling. In addition to this research question he also investigated two additional hypoth-eses: (a) Does the initial skill level of a subject differentially affect the mode of learning (covert versus overt), and (b) Is retention or the longevity of skill performance a function of the mode of learn-ing a subject is exposed to? On the basis of pretreatment testing, subjects were assigned to high, medium, or low skill groups. Sub-jects within each skill group were randomly assigned to control, covert rehearsal, overt-covert rehearsal, or overt rehearsal groups. Subjects practiced over a 21-day period and were posttested on the 23rd day of the experiment and then again on the 54th day of the experiment. The results indicated no differences in performance between the control and covert rehearsal group. The overt-covert and the overt groups were significantly better than the control but did not significantly differ from each other. Corbin concluded that although physical practice was the single most effective modality, mental practice seemed to be better utilized when based on experi-ence and when actual practice preceded performance of the skill (p. 148). According to Corbin, it is possible that the extreme novel-ty of the task made it difficult for subjects to visualize the task, and thus the effect of covert practice may have been minimized.

Smyth (1975) conducted a study that also utilized tasks relatively unfamiliar to the subjects. In Experiment 1, subjects were assigned to either an active practice group, mental practice group provided with time, a mental practice group provided with mental practice "trials," or a no-practice control group. Subject performance on a mirror-tracing task was then evaluated according to error time and average completion time. The results showed that subjects who had active practice improved significantly over the other groups, and the mental practice group provided with time differed from the no-practice group by a small but significant amount. The author concluded that for the mirror-drawing task mental practice is only of minimal usefulness during initial learning stages, and experience with the task and more explicit instructions may have resulted in mental practice being more effective. It should be noted that subjects in the mental practice conditions did not have any actual physical trials or experience with mirror tracing prior to engaging in the mental practice of the task. Experiment 2 investigated the use of mental practice in conjunction with varying amounts of physical practice. A pursuit rotor task was selected with a square track and a 2-cm-square target light that moved clockwise at 30 rpm. Subjects were assigned to a no-practice group, a 4-minute continuous practice group, a 4-minute mental practice group, an alternate active-practice no-practice group, an alternate active-practice mental-practice group, a group having 1 minute of active practice followed by 3 minutes of rest, or a group having 1 minute of mental practice followed by 3 minutes of rest. Following this 4-minute period subjects performed a 50-second test trial, during which time "on target" was recorded. The results indicated that all groups experiencing physical practice performed significantly better than the no-practice and mental-practice-only groups. There were no significant differences between the no-practice group and the mental practice group nor were there any significant differences between any of the physical practice groups. Smyth concluded that the distribution of mental practice with or without actual physical practice did not affect subject performance, and mental practice did not appear to facilitate performance during any stage of learning.

Meyers, Schleser, Cooke, and Cuvillier (1979) conducted two experiments designed to assess the effects of covert practice upon the performance of selected gymnastic skills. Female gymnastic participants in a local YMCA program served as subjects. All subjects were given introductory instructions that described cognitive practice and were then assigned to a treatment group. Four groups were established: (a) positive self-instruction, (b) coping instruction, (c) negative instruction, and (d) neutral self-talk. Subjects practiced their appropriate instructional set and the physical skill over a period of 2 to 4 weeks. Pretest scores for performance of a front flip and a front walkover indicated no significant differences between the experimental groups. Analysis of the posttest data indicated that all four groups experienced significant pretraining to posttraining improvement. However, no significant differences in performance were found among the four groups. Neutral self-talk was, in effect, as productive as coping self-talk or any of the other cognitive strategies in enhancing pretraining to posttraining performance. In Study 2, the authors followed procedures similar to those utilized in Study 1, but assigned subjects to experimental groups as follows: (a) physical practice, (b) cognitive practice, (c) cognitive and physical practice, and (d) no-practice control. Three gymnastic tasks were performed pretraining and posttraining by all subjects. Analysis of posttraining scores demonstrated that both the physical practice group and the cognitive-physical group improved on all three tasks. The cognitive-alone group improved on the high and low difficulty task while the no-practice group showed improvement on the low difficulty task and the moderate difficulty task. Additional analysis indicated that physical practice was the superior method of training. The authors cited the younger age of their subjects as potentially responsible for the lack of a more positive cognitive training effect. They also referred to the possible detrimental effect cognitive training may have had on a fine motor skill. Because the cognitive training was not suited to any specific skill deficiency but was general in nature, this argument may be plausible. The cognitive training imposed upon the athletes may have even disturbed their own cognitive set prior to and during performance.

The effect of internal versus external mental practice strategies were assessed in a study of female collegiate basketball players conducted by Shelton and Mahoney (Note 1). Members of a college varsity basketball team were blocked according to pre-experimental free throw accuracy and then randomly assigned to either an internal imagery group or an external imagery group. Subjects in the internal group mentally practiced free throws with the emphasis being on kinesthetic involvement. This is sometimes referred to as the first person perspective. Subjects in the external group mentally practiced free throws using the third person perspective, which emphasizes watching oneself perform as if in a movie. Baseline shooting accuracy was calculated for all subjects and posttraining performance was compared to baseline performance. Training occurred over 15 mental practice sessions. As in the Meyers et al. (1979) study, covert intervention was a general nontailored content analysis of the skill. Results of this study indicated that subjects utilizing external imagery performed more accurately than those using internal imagery. This difference was found to be related to a nonsignificant deterioration in performance by subjects practicing internal imagery rather than a significant improvement by subjects practicing external imagery. An analysis of change scores as a function of baseline skill demonstrated that highly skilled athletes actually decreased slightly in accuracy while lower skilled athletes improved significantly in performance. The authors conclude that the results imply that an internal mental practice strategy may not be optimal for all athletes or skills. A second conclusion offered is that less skilled performers may benefit from mental practice to a greater extent than more skilled performers. Several studies (e.g., Corbin, 1967; Noel, 1980; Smyth, 1975) have previously shown, however, that the relationship between skill level and mental practice strategies is in no way a simple linear relation.

Epstein (1980) also conducted a study designed to evaluate internal and external imagery strategies on skilled motor performance. Subjects were randomly assigned to an internal imagery condition, an external imagery condition, or a control condition. All subjects were given various preexperimental tests to determine their "natural imagery style." Following this assessment subjects were provided with 30 trials of dart throwing used to determine baseline ability. Subjects were then given either internal imagery instructions, external imagery instructions, or were asked to engage in a backward-counting task. Performance on dart throwing was then recorded for two trials, each trial consisting of 30 dart throws. Results showed no significant differences in performance as a function of mental rehearsal. Males' performance on the dart-throwing task was superior to females' performance while females using imagery demonstrated greater variability in performance scores. The authors speculated that lower skill levels possessed by the female subjects may have been responsible for a distracting effect of the imagery. This is, of course, in direct opposition to the suggestion of Shelton and Mahoney (Note 1), who proposed that lower skilled female basketball players may benefit more from mental practice strategies. These opposing explanations of nonsignificant results demonstrates the potential problems that exist when a researcher attempts to explain a nonsignificant result, especially when the explanation is devoid of any theoretical base.

Epilogue

The contemporary sport scientist is still most likely wondering if the efficacy of mental practice and covert strategies has been reliably established. Even the most recent literature in this area tends to indicate that several issues remain to be resolved before the true significance of covert rehearsal techniques can be determined. It should be clear to the reader, however, that researchers in the area of covert practice have tested the "usefulness" of this potential aid with basically four dissimilar methodological approaches. One approach conceptualizes mental practice as a skill that needs little introduction to a naive subject. Thus, subjects participating in these studies generally receive no formal training, may engage in imagery for relatively short periods of time (3 to 30 minutes), and may be provided with only one session of "practice" prior to an evaluation of performance. A second and common methodology involves reading general skill content information to subjects and then allowing them to formulate images based on the information they were provided. The third methodology, which may inadvertently be the ultimate test of efficacy, involves having untrained subjects engage in general content imagery for a skill or task they have never physically performed. The final methodology, which has been used with increasing frequency during the last decade, involves teaching subjects imagery and relaxation techniques over a period of days or weeks and providing subjects with specific self-instructional imagery that has relevance to some performance dimension in need of improvement or modification. The fact that some studies using imagery methods as those described in the first three illustrations have found performance enhancement via imagery perhaps attests to the robustness of covert practice. Research that has used a simple paradigm of acute exposure to mental practice strategies as a methodology does not provide an adequate test of effect. An adequate test of covert practice must insure that (a) the subject is trained in the technique, (b) the subject practices covertly, (c) the performance task has some relevance to the subject, (d) comparison and control groups are established, and (e) performance is evaluated over a relatively long period of time in order to assess the stability of any performance change.

As cognitive intervention programs become more popular it will be of scientific and practical significance to address two major research questions that remain unanswered: (a) What are the mechanisms responsible for performance improvement when imagery and covert practice strategies are used in an intervention program, and (b) How significant are individual differences in influencing the relationship between covert rehearsal strategies and performance enhancement?

Basic research that isolates imagery and covert rehearsal strategies from other component parts of an intervention program will assist in answering the first question posed. Girodo and Wood

(1978) have demonstrated the importance of subject expectancy in mediating pain tolerance. Ness (1979) also found subject expectancy to be a potent influence upon performance on a strength task. Is expectancy or improved self-efficacy the mechanism of change and imagery the reinforcer? Others may investigate physiologic-motoric mechanisms potentially responsible for performance improvement via imagery based programs. At any rate, a better understanding of the underlying mechanisms of change whether psychological, physiological, motoric, or some combination will facilitate the development of future intervention programs.

Systematic programs of research are also needed in the area of individual differences. Studies remain to be designed where factors such as subject skill level, imaginal style, and nature of the task are carefully varied and comprehensively evaluated in relation to performance.

In closing, there appears to be ample literature to support the position that imagery and covert rehearsal strategies can be viewed as realistic aids to performance when utilized in conjunction with systematic intervention programs. To maintain that covert strategies are not potentially useful performance aids would be a myopic view. However, additional supportive research emphasizing controlled comparisons and the evaluation of performance change stability are needed. Until such information is available, a cautious conditional endorsement seems justified.

Reference Note

1. Shelton, T.O., & Mahoney, M.J. *Mental practice with varsity basketball players: Parameters of influence*. Paper presented at The 14th Annual Convention of the Association for the Advancement of Behavior Therapy, New York, November 1980.

References

AMMONS, R.B. Effects of prepractice activities on rotary pursuit performance. *Journal of Experimental Psychology*, 1951, **41**, 187-191.

ATKINSON, R.C., & Wickens, T.D. Human memory and the concept of reinforcement. In R. Glaser (Ed.), *The nature of reinforcement*. New York: Academy Press, 1971.

BARBER, T., & Hahn, K. Experimental studies in "hypnotic behavior": Physiological and subjective effects of imagined pain. *Journal of Nervous & Mental Disease*, 1964, **139**, 416-425.

BAUER, R.M., & Craighead, W.E. Psychophysiological responses to the imagination of fearful and neutral situations: The effects of imagery instructions. *Behavior Therapy*, 1979, **10**, 389-403.

BOWER, G.H. Mental imagery and associative learning. In L. Gregg (Ed.), *Cognition & learning in memory*. New York: Wiley, 1972.

CAUTELA, J.R. Covert conditioning: Assumptions and procedures. *Journal of Mental Imagery*, 1977, **1**, 53-64.

CLARK, L.V. Effect of mental practice on the development of a certain motor skill. *Research Quarterly*, 1960, **31**, 560-569.

CORBIN, C.B. The effects of covert rehearsal on the development of a complex motor skill. *Journal of General Psychology*, 1967, **76**, 143-150.

CORBIN, C.B. Mental practice. In W.P. Morgan (Ed.), *Ergogenic aids & muscular performance*. New York: Academic Press, 1972.

CRAIG, K. Physiological arousal as a function of imagined, vicarious, and direct stress experiences. *Journal of Abnormal Psychology*, 1968, **73**, 513-520.

DESIDERATO, O., & Miller, I.B. Improving tennis performance by cognitive behavior modification techniques. *Behavior Therapist*, 1979, **2**, 19.

DEWITT, D.J. Cognitive and biofeedback training for stress reduction with university athletes. *Journal of Sport Psychology*, 1980, **2**, 288-294.

EPSTEIN, M.L. The relationship of mental imagery and mental rehearsal to performance of a motor task. *Journal of Sport Psychology*, 1980, **2**, 211-220.

GILMORE, R.W., & Stolurow, L.M. Motor and "mental" practice of ball and socket task. *American Psychologist*, 1951, **6**, 295.

GIRODO, M., & Wood, D. Talking yourself out of pain: The importance of believing that you can. *Cognitive Therapy & Research*, 1978, **3**, 23-34.

HIGHLEN, P.S., & Bennett, B.B. Psychological characteristics of successful and nonsuccessful elite wrestlers: An exploratory study. *Journal of Sport Psychology*, 1979, **1**, 123-137.

HOMME, L.E. Perspectives in psychology: XXIV. Control of coverants, the operants of the mind. *Psychological Record*, 1965, **15**, 501-511.

JACOBSON, E. Electrical measurements of neuromuscular states during mental activities. *American Journal of Physiology*, 1930, **95**, 694-712.

JAMES, W. *Principles of psychology*, (Vol. 1). New York: Holt, 1890. (a)

JAMES, W. *Principles of psychology*, (Vol. 2). New York: Holt, 1890. (b)

JONES, J.G. Motor learning without demonstration of physical practice, under two conditions of mental practice. *Research Quarterly*, 1965, **36**, 270-276.

KELSEY, I.B. Effects of mental practice and physical practice upon muscular endurance. *Research Quarterly*, 1961, **32**, 47-54.

LANE, J.F. Improving athletic performance through visuo-motor behavior rehearsal. In R.M. Suinn (Ed.), *Psychology in sports: Methods & applications*. Minneapolis: Burgess, 1980.

LANG, P.J. A bio-informational theory of emotional imagery. *Psychophysiology*, 1979, **16**, 495-511.

MAHONEY, M.J. *Cognitive & behavior modification*. Cambridge, MA: Ballinger, 1974.

MAHONEY, M.J., & Avner, M. Psychology of the elite athlete: An exploratory study. *Cognitive Therapy & Research*, 1977, **1**, 135-141.

MAHONEY, M.J., Thorensen, C.E., & Danaher, B.G. Covert behavior modification: An experimental analogue. *Journal of Behavior Therapy & Experimental Psychiatry*, 1972, **3**, 7-14.

MARTINIUK, R.G. *Information processing in motor skills*. New York: Holt, Rinehart & Winston, 1976.

MEICHENBAUM, D. *Cognitive behavior modification: An integrative approach*. New York: Plenum, 1977.

MEICHENBAUM, D. Why does using imagery in psychotherapy lead to change? In J.L. Singer & K.S. Pope (Eds.), *The power of human imagination: New methods in psychotherapy*. New York: Plenum, 1978.

MEICHENBAUM, D., & Cameron, R. The clinical potential of modifying what clients say to themselves. *Psychotherapy: Theory, Research & Practice*, 1974, **11**, 103-117.

MEICHENBAUM, D., & Goodman, J. The developmental control of operant motor responding by verbal operants. *Journal of Experimental Child Psychology*, 1969, **7**, 553-565.

MEYERS, A., & Schleser, R. A cognitive behavioral intervention for improving basketball performance. *Journal of Sport Psychology*, 1980, **2**, 69-73.

MEYERS, A., Schleser, R., Cooke, C.J., & Cuvillier, C. Cognitive contributions to the development of gymnastics skills. *Cognitive Therapy & Research*, 1979, **3**, 75-85.

MILLER, N.E. *The influence of past experience upon transfer of subsequent training*. Unpublished doctoral dissertation, Yale University, 1935.

NESS, R.G., & Patton, R.W. The effects of beliefs on maximum weightlifting performance. *Cognitive Therapy & Research*, 1979, **3**, 205-212.

NOEL, R.C. The effect of visuo-motor behavior rehearsal on tennis performance. *Journal of Sport Psychology*, 1980, **2**, 221-226.

RICHARDSON, A. Mental practice: A review and discussion: Part I. *Research Quarterly*, 1967, **38**, 95-107. (a)

RICHARDSON, A. Mental practice: A review and discussion: Part II. *Research Quarterly*, 1967, **38**, 263-273. (b)

RYAN, E.D., & Simons, J. Cognitive demand, imagery, and frequency of mental rehearsal as factors influencing acquisition of motor skills. *Journal of Sport Psychology*, 1981, **3**, 35-45.

SHICK. J. Effects of mental practice on selected volleyball skills for college women. *Research Quarterly*, 1970, **41**, 88-94.

SILVA, J.M. Performance enhancement in competitive sport environments through cognitive intervention. *Behavior Modification*, 1982, **6**, 443-463.

SINGER, R.N. *Motor learning & human performance*. New York: Macmillan, 1971.

SKINNER, B.F. *Science & human behavior*. New York: Macmillan, 1953.

SMYTH, M.M. The role of mental practice in skill acquisition. *Journal of Motor Behavior*, 1975, **7**, 199-206.

SUINN, R.M. Behavior rehearsal training for ski racers. *Behavior Therapy*, 1972, **3**, 519-520.

SUINN, R.M. Body thinking: Psychology of Olympic champs. *Psychology Today*, 1976, **10**, 38-43.

SURBURG, P.R. Audio, visual, and audio-visual instruction with mental practice in developing the forehand tennis drive. *Research Quarterly*, 1968, **39**, 728-734.

TITLEY, R.W. The loneliness of a long-distance kicker. *The Athletic Journal*, 1976, **57**, 74-80.

TWINING, W.E. Mental practice and physical practice in the learning of a motor skill. *Research Quarterly*, 1949, **20**, 432-435.

ULICH, E. Some experiments on the function of mental training in the acquisition of motor skills. *Ergonomics*, 1967, **10**, 411-419.

VANDELL, R.A., Davis, R.A., & Clungston, A. The function of mental practice in the acquisition of motor skill. *Journal of General Psychology*, 1943, **29**, 243-250.

WASHBURN, M.F. *Movement & mental imagery*. Boston: Houghton, 1916.

WATSON, L. *Supernature*. New York: Doubleday, 1973.

WEINBERG, R.S., Seabourne, T.G., & Jackson, H. Effect of visuomotor behavior rehearsal, relaxation and imagery on karate performance. *Journal of Sport Psychology*, 1981, **3**, 228-238.

WHITE, K.D., Ashton, R., & Lewis, S. Learning a complex skill: Effects of mental practice, physical practice, and imagery ability. *International Journal of Sport Psychology*, 1979, **10**, 71-78.

WOLPE, J. *Psychotherapy by reciprocal inhibition*. Palo Alto, CA: Stanford University Press, 1958.

11

Stress Management Procedures

Rod K. Dishman

Even a cursory review of the contemporary scientific and professional literature in sport psychology reveals an accelerated interest in stress management procedures as potential ergogenic interventions (e.g., Hanin, 1981; Klavora & Daniel, 1979). This interest has also been evidenced by the inclusion of stress management symposia in recent meetings of national exercise and sport science groups such as the American College of Sports Medicine and the Sport Psychology Academy of the American Alliance for Health, Physical Education, Recreation and Dance. Moreover, the edited proceedings (Sime & Zaichkowsky, 1982) of the 1981 meeting of the Sport Psychology Academy has been published as a guide for the exercise and sport practitioner. The published annual proceedings of the North American Society for the Psychology of Sport and Physical Activity has also typically contained papers related to stress management. In addition, a substantial portion of the program for the recently held Fifth World Congress of the Internation-

Rod K. Dishman, Ph.D., is with the Department of Health and Physical Education at Southwest Missouri State University in Springfield.

al Society for Sport Psychology was devoted to the control of stress in top-level athletes, and the final day of the meeting consisted of professional workshops that dealt exclusively with application of stress management techniques.

The increased attention to stress management topics in North American sport science has apparently paralleled or followed developments in other related fields. These have included popularization in the allied health sciences of the concept of stress; the growth of professional organizations such as the Association for Advancement of Behavior Therapy, the Society of Behavioral Medicine, the Behavior Therapy and Research Society, the American Association for the Advancement of Tension Control, and the Biofeedback Society of America, each of which is wholly or partially concerned with the control of stress; the cognitive-behavioral therapy resurgence in clinical psychology (Kendall & Hollon, 1979; Meichenbaum, 1977); and the recent trend in professional sport psychology toward the use of applied interventions designed to facilitate athletic excellence (Mahoney, 1979; Nideffer, 1981; Rushall, 1975; Suinn, 1972). These developments support the timeliness of an overview of research on the effectiveness of stress management as an ergogenic practice in sport.

The timeliness of this review appears, however, as much a function of contemporary clinical or applied trends in sport psychology as it is indicative of a growing base of knowledge. The two fundamental assumptions that underlie the practice of stress management in sport settings illustrate this point. First, stress is directly related to sport and exercise performance. Second, stress can be manipulated in a reliable manner. Although these assumptions have intuitive appeal and form the basis of much of the current practice in sport psychology, the actual empirical literature at both basic and applied levels is not convincing. In fact, despite additional study, little research (Landers, 1980) conducted since the early 1970s is available to notably challenge Martens' (1972, 1974) earlier conclusion that empirical evidence in this area appears equivocal. The recent adoption of an applied focus by North American sport psychologists is therefore noteworthy. Applied interventions in stress-related ergogenics have been employed by European and Asian sport psychologists for some time (Vanek & Cratty, 1970), but this practical approach was selectively rejected by North American scholars roughly 15 years ago. It now appears to be gaining acceptance despite the fact that the level of empirical explanation regarding the stress/performance relationship that existed then remains essentially unchanged today (Dishman, 1982; Landers, 1980).

This seems largely the result of methodological problems encountered in the conceptualization, measurement, and manipulation of stress in applied settings that will be addressed in this paper. Competing explanations for results of applied intervention will also be introduced; suggestions for future study are implied throughout. The overall purpose of the following review is the introduction of a potential stress management technology for sport ergogenics and the characterization of applied procedures as they relate to existing theoretical and empirical knowledge.

The Theory of Stress

Because of the encompassing nature of stress and the diversity in techniques for its assessment and management, it is necessary to provide a definitional overview before the ergogenic potential of stress interventions can be meaningfully interpreted. Stress is an abstract concept that, in its broadest and most conventional use, describes the rate of biological wear and tear associated with life (Selye, 1976). It is defined by the patterning of a specific syndrome of symptoms (the stress response) with nonspecific precipitating events (stressors). The stress response is a biological adaptation process that incorporates two major subsidiary stages: resistance (mobilization) and exhaustion (depletion) of biological resources. These stages are also syndromic, and the relevance of each for stress management in sport will provide the basis for much of the following review.

Stress is a *biological* concept, and whether it is viewed as psychological or as physiological is simply a function of the measurement paradigm a sport scientist elects to adopt. Acute or chronic adjustments in the ability to tolerate (resist) a standard stressor with a less pronounced stress reaction (e.g., low arousal) are conceptually identical in both the physiological and psychological case. An individual who is physically fit is able to tolerate a relatively intense metabolic (concrete) stressor while an individual who is emotionally fit can tolerate a relatively intense psychologic (abstract) stressor. In both acute and chronic instances, effective resistance precludes exhaustion. The biological nature of chronic stress is further reinforced when a system breakdown does occur. The clinical patient suffering a reactive depression presents a symptom profile essentially identical to that of the stale or overtrained athlete (Morgan, Note 1). The overstress syndrome is the same whether the precipitating stressor has been principally psychogenic or metabolic in nature.

Selye's conceptualization of stress as a syndrome is noteworthy because it implies reliability. Moreover, it has been adopted as the conventional view in the biomedical sciences, and it satisfies criteria of accuracy and parsimony for theory development. It is also based upon nearly 2,000 technical papers produced during a 40-year research career and has long been recognized by exercise physiologists as an effective framework within which to view systemic adaptations to the demands of acute and chronic exercise. Surprisingly, however, this encompassing view has infrequently been adopted in the sport psychology literature. As a result, several apparent incongruities have emerged between what is sometimes practiced in contemporary sport psychology as stress management and the theoretical/empirical base from which stress interventions might logically emanate.

The theoretical advantage of a concept such as stress can thus become a clinical liability. Because stress is an abstract construct, it must be operationalized into specific assessable symptoms before it can be of practical use. This is a necessity for measurement and application. However, selected symptoms may subsequently be regarded as synonyms for stress. This can create rather profound problems of theoretical and clinical interpretation. Although stress appears to represent a pattern of response that is relatively reliable across individuals and is thus generalizable, this may not be the case for specific symptoms. The practical significance of this rests with the precision with which generalized intervention techniques may be expected to affect specific stress correlates and with inferences that may be drawn about the impact of controlling specific stress-related variables upon the generalized stress syndrome.

Measurement

In basic sport psychology research, the variable most identified with stress has been arousal (Martens, 1974; Landers, 1980). This has presented the potential for measurement problems of construct validity and reliability. Arousal is best viewed as only a component of the stress response (primary stress) and is thus a symptom of stress (Selye, 1976). In an acute sense it is characteristic of Selye's stage of resistance and can contribute a source of wear and tear (transient autonomic responsivity in the presence of a stressor, as can be found in an anxiety state). From a chronic perspective it can serve as a symptom of exhaustion (prolonged sympathetic dominance in the presence of a stressor, as can be found in reactive depression). In other words, the meaning of arousal cannot be evaluated independently of its origin. It can signal a response that is adaptive in one instance or maladaptive in another, but it is not the equivalent of stress.

From the perspective of an acute response, the origin of arousal can assume an added significance. Metabolically induced arousal during acute exercise is characterized by an autonomic responsivity of endocrine and vascular systems that appears quite homogeneous across individuals when energy demand is at an equivalent percentage of each person's metabolic capacity (Astrand & Rodahl, 1977). Psychogenic, or centrally induced, arousal has also historically been viewed as a generalized homogeneous state (Duffy, 1972). Subsequent views (Lacey & Lacey, 1958) have, however, challenged the generalized nature of the arousal concept and have proposed that it can more meaningfully be differentiated into three distinct components, (a) activation of the cerebral cortex (electrocortical), (b) peripheral physiologic responsivity (autonomic), and (c) observable behavior. Moreover, arousal originating in the thought process (e.g., anxiety) has been distinguished into cognitive, physiological, and behavioral components (Borkovec, 1976). These views are consistent with low correlations that can be observed between measures of each domain under a standard stressor. In some individuals, for example, heart rate and blood pressure might decrease while electrocortical and electrodermal conductance increases. Although these low correlations have frequently been dismissed as measurement imprecision (Duffy, 1972), they are now viewed as indications that specific aspects or patterns of arousal may respond similarly or dissimilarly depending upon the stimulus encountered. This is not only consistent with the distinction just outlined between metabolically and psychologically induced arousal, but also with the known existence of anatomic pathways within both the reticular formation (the neurological control center for arousal) and the hypothalamus (the principal glandular control center for arousal), which have competing functions. The posterior hypothalamus influences sympathetic dominance of autonomic responsivity and results in peripheral arousal, while the anterior hemisphere exerts an antagonistic or parasympathetic influence. The reticular formation is also dimorphic. Brainstem reticular fibers interface the brain cortex, the posterior hypothalamus, and the thalamus, so sympathetic influence on arousal can originate from both internal and external sense organs and from the cortex itself (e.g., a thought). The thalamic reticular system, on the other hand, does not directly project to the cortex. It can effect both a sympathetic and a parasympathetic function but it is apparently subordinate to the brainstem reticular system.

These paradoxical structures and functions within the CNS provide anatomic support for differentiation and dissociation of the arousal response and highlight the importance of distinguishing its origin. In a broad sense, centrally induced arousal can apparently result from an internal learned source (a thought) or an external unlearned source (the orientation reaction to novel surroundings). Moreover, an acquired arousal response can be cognitively learned or it can be conditioned in a classical manner (Orne & Paskewitz, 1974). Depending upon both the person and the setting in which responsivity is elicited, there may be a significant differentiation of symptoms (Davidson, 1978). This has recently been supported in exercise settings by neurophysiological, biochemical, and psychometric studies. Sime (1977) observed a reduction in frontalis activity (EMG) following 10 minutes of light exercise (heart rate averaged 110 bpm) in trait anxious subjects exposed to a psychological stressor. No change was seen in subjective state anxiety, however. Because metabolic arousal was relatively low in this study, it is possible that a somatic relaxation occurred while the anxiety cognition remained. This would be consistent with findings by Schwartz, Davidson, and Goleman (1978), which implied that somatic relaxation associated with exercise was related to less somatic but more cognitive anxiety when compared with meditation, a more cognitively oriented relaxation procedure. However, when the metabolic demands of exercise are more intense (>70% maximum aerobic capacity), state anxiety has been found to be reduced in a manner quantitatively comparable to reductions following meditation (Morgan, 1981a). This suggests that metabolic arousal of an adequate intensity may compete with anxiety arousal to diminish its subjective evaluation or that metabolic arousal may distract attention from anxiety-provoking thought. This is certainly feasible, because the converse is known to occur in high-level performance. That is, cognitive relaxation patterns can be associated with diminished arousal (as measured by O_2 uptake) at a standard exercise stressor (Morgan & Pollock, 1977; Suinn, Morton, & Brammel, Note 2). The relative explanatory appeal of each alternative is, however, subordinate to the issue of an apparent differentiation in the arousal response. Likewise, it has been found that neither a maximum nor a submaximum 6-minute exercise tolerance test conducted on a bicycle ergometer influenced frontalis tension levels (EMG), although alpha patterns (EEG) indicated a central deactivation (Farmer, Olewine, Comer, Edwards, Coleman, Thomas, & Hames, 1978). This supports clinical and psychometric evidence for the subjective sense of calm and relaxation that is frequently reported during the elevated peripheral arousal of prolonged steady-state exercise (Morgan, 1981a).

Even within differentiated components of arousal there apparently can be a dissociation of specific symptoms. A reduction of CNS electrical activity has been observed centrally in both cortical (Farmer et al., 1978) and spinal (deVries, Wiswell, Bulbulian, & Moritani, 1981) regions and peripherally in the skeletal musculature (deVries, 1968). However, in cognitively nonanxious subjects, tension levels in other more proximal striated groups (e.g., frontalis) have been resistant to exercise arousal during both intense work of short duration (Farmer et al., 1978) and light work of long duration (Balog, in press). Differences in responsivity appear to exist even between skeletal muscle groups. Findings indicate greater responsivity to a psychological stressor (Pinel & Schultz, 1978) and a more sensitive management response to a metabolic stressor (deVries, 1968), for voluntary groups located cephalically more proximal (e.g., forearm flexors) than distal (e.g., quadriceps femoris). These findings are consistent with the view that tension in skeletal muscle is mediated by biofeedback loops within the CNS different from those of other voluntary groups (deVries et al., 1981) and that this can be a function of anatomic structure and learning. This dissociation of symptoms within a differentiated arousal response has also been supported in exercise at a biochemical (Ismail & El-Naggar, 1982) level and in sport at psychometric (Hamm, 1982) and behavioral (Martens, 1977) levels. In each case, the anticipated homogeneity of response within a given domain has not been observed. If measurement imprecision is dismissed as a less reasonable explanation, these findings collectively challenge the appropriateness for humans of classic animal models that propose that central alpha and peripheral gamma activity are reliably processed through a common CNS pathway. In other words, human subjects present a much less predictable arousal response than can be anticipated under a strictly physiological model, and in a comparative sense it appears this can largely be attributed to an exaggerated involvement of cortical influence in humans. This also helps account for the seemingly more homogeneous autonomic arousal response observed under metabolic stress, because abstract cortical influence may be overridden by more concrete subcortical control.

These findings have important implications for clinical or applied practice in sport because innate characteristics and the learning history of an individual can dictate the most appropriate technique chosen as an intervention, and because evidence supports that different stress management procedures can effect distinct arousal patterns (Schwartz et al., 1978). For example, the use of a physiologically based procedure such as progressive relaxation (Jacobson,

1938) might be expected to effectively influence a specific arousal correlate of an anxiety neurosis that is conditioned (e.g., muscular tension), whereas a cognitively or behaviorally based approach (Bandura, 1977; Meichenbaum, 1977) designed to restructure anxiety-provoking thought or reduce avoidance behavior might be innocuous because arousal is not cognitively or behaviorally based. Conversely, an anxiety arousal founded in irrational thought would not likely be responsive to a physiologically based procedure if the anxiety-provoking thought remains (Borkovec, 1976). In either case, the compatibility of the intervention pathway with the source of the target response is a critical clinical consideration (Wolpe, 1981).

Anticipated Performance Benefits

Although there appears to be sufficient homogeneity within the arousal response to justify a *theoretical* advantage for viewing it as a generalized biological mediator or construct, its utility for guiding specific *clinical practice* in sport is less clear. Moreover, it appears that the cognitive-neurophysiologic interface of arousal may provide a better model for evaluating the ergogenic potential of specific stress management procedures than a singularly psychological or physiological perspective. This possibility is noteworthy because two classic views of infrahuman motivation have been most prominent in providing models for stress research and application in sport ergogenics. Application of both Hullian drive theory (performance is a linear monotonic function of arousal) and the Yerkes-Dodson law (performance is a curvilinear, biphasic function of arousal) incorporates the concept of generalized arousal as the principal behavioral mediator. Both models were formulated on the basis of *behavioral* description in which arousal was an *inferred biological* state, but in the typical sport and exercise research paradigm designed to test these models, arousal has been operationally defined in *cognitive* or *subjective* terms and measured by self-reports of anxiety (Landers, 1980; Martens, 1972, 1974). Thus, a generalized physiological construct has been equated with a generalized psychological construct despite evidence that each is characterized by a substantial heterogeneity of response patterning.

Recent developments suggest that controversy over selectively adopting a drive or an inverted U or V model for sport and exercise has subordinated more basic or explanatory influences on performance. Current thinking (Landers, 1980) has suggested that a critical underlying issue in the arousal and performance relationship concerns the degree to which the sport setting imposes a heavy information processing load on the performer and the degree to which the skill performed is essentially dependent upon energy mobilization and/or the expression of maximum force, as opposed to skill requiring relatively complex motor integration or precision. Thus, attention and muscular tension levels are viewed as critical performance mediators. A moderate degree of arousal is believed to enhance performance when the setting is relatively demanding in terms of information processing and the skill requires relatively complex motor integration. The width of this moderate arousal band is viewed as a function of the complexity of the skill; complex performance is facilitated by a comparatively narrow or precise range of arousal. There is, on the other hand, support for a drive relationship in settings where success is largely dependent on energy mobilization (peripheral arousal) or force expression (central arousal) somewhat independent of heavy information loads or complex integrated movement (Genov, 1970; Ikai & Steinhaus, 1961).

Clinical Interventions

A model of sport stress must be accurate in accounting for the demands that sport settings impose on the athlete and characteristics of the athlete that determine whether these are met. This is a necessary prerequisite for predictable manipulations of critical stress/performance mediators and for the introduction of an intervention technology when a maladaptive response inhibits typical performance or when typical performance might be enhanced by a response made more adaptive. Based on these criteria, a generalized arousal model of stress, although parsimonious in its simplicity, has appeared neither accurate nor practically useful in sport. Basic research and clinical sport observation have subsequently implicated specific correlates of stress as more pertinent to sport demands. These include attentional focus, neuromuscular tension, confidence in ability and outcome expectancies, state anxiety, and metabolic arousal. Each of these variables has been shown to covary with psychological and physiological interventions in nonsport populations, and management procedures emanating from clinical psychology have become the adopted technology in applied sport settings. Most notable among these are specific procedures that focus principally on symptom reduction through neuromuscular relaxation (Jacobson, 1938); cognitive distraction (Benson, 1975) and restructuring (Beck, 1970; Ellis, 1962); behavioristic reinforcement (Lewis, 1974); or hybrid

approaches that combine neurophysiologic relaxation and/or behavioral control with cognitive/emotional modes (Bandura, 1977;
Meichenbaum, 1977; Schultz & Luthe, 1959; Smith, 1980; Wolpe,
1958). Variations apparently most appealing to sport practitioners
have involved strategies including biofeedback (EMG) assisted tension control (Zaichkowsky, 1982) and derivatives of Attention Control Training (Nideffer, 1981) and Visuo-Motor Behavior Rehearsal
(Suinn, 1972).

Biofeedback

The practice of biofeedback is based on the fundamental learning
principle that acquisition of a voluntary skill requires, or is enhanced by, knowledge about performance results. Biofeedback
essentially involves a technological interface between external
senses, the voluntary central nervous system, and the autonomic
nervous system to provide typically inaccessible information about
biological states to the individual. This theoretically enables the
learning of self-regulatory skills that would be ordinarily under exclusive autonomic control. Biofeedback-assisted learning in sport
has primarily involved neuromuscular control and tension reduction (EMG) (Zaichkowsky, 1982). Its overall effectiveness appears
specific to the symptom and its control pathway in the CNS (Blanchard & Epstein, 1977; Tarter-Benlolo, 1978). However, learning
guidelines for application are not empirically well founded at present (Miller, 1978).

Attention Control Training (ACT)

This approach combines the learning of selective attention to
critical performance/setting cues with anxiety control in order to
offset dysfunctional shifts in attention. It is an outgrowth of clinical
observation (Nideffer, 1981) and psychometric investigation
(Nideffer, 1976) and has been adapted to sport with an extension to
muscular tension control. This model conceptualizes attention
along orthogonal, but not exclusive, continua of narrow-broad
width and internal-external locus. The empirical base underlying
its use in sport is, however, principally cross-sectional, directed at
validating the Test of Attentional and Interpersonal Style (TAIS)
(Nideffer, 1976) as a screening device for applied use in tailoring attention training to specific athletes in a given sport (Kirschenbaum
& Bale, 1980; Landers, Furst, & Daniels, 1981; Richards & Landers,
1981; Zaichkowsky, Jackson, & Aronson, 1982; Jackson, Note
3). Adaptations of the general psychometric model to specific sport

settings have also occurred (Etzel, 1979; Van Schoyck & Grasha, 1981). Applied research verifying an intervention/performance relationship is as yet limited. However, attentional shifts are known to be self-induced in endurance sports, and these have been manipulated to facilitate performance in simulated settings (Morgan, 1981b; Suinn, 1981).

Visuo-Motor Behavior Rehearsal (VMBR)

Coined by Suinn (1972), this is an extension of imagery and relaxation skills, underlying systematic desensitization (Wolpe, 1958), to less phobic responses. Its cognitive dimension relates more directly to performance enhancement through imagery and behavioral cuing of performance execution (Suinn, 1982), and this is discussed by Silva in Chapter 10. An underlying component, however, is concerned with self-regulation of autonomic and behavioral responsivity to a stressor and essentially involves anxiety management (Suinn, 1981). The uniqueness of VMBR for stress management in sport lies in its theoretical comprehensiveness, its clinical adaptability to athlete and setting, and its heuristic impetus for applied sport research. Moreover, it is somewhat unique in emphasizing that stress management may effectively incorporate symptom inducement (e.g., increased arousal) rather than exclusive reduction. It is thus explicitly an interactional clinical model that can be specifically tailored to athlete characteristics and critical setting demands in a manner similar to Nideffer's (1981) Attention Control Training.

Adjunctive Procedures

The relationships between motor performance and additional stress adjuncts have been reviewed elsewhere for hypnosis (see Chapter 9 by Morgan & Brown); meditation (Layman, 1978); social facilitation (Landers, 1980); and life stress (Bramwell, Masuda, Wagner, & Holmes, 1975). Exercise-induced metabolic arousal (e.g., physiological warm-up, see Chapter 13 by Franks) has also previously been alluded to as an ancillary stress management procedure (Martens, 1972; Nideffer, 1981), and this is noteworthy for several reasons. Both acute and chronic exercise are known to covary with several stress-related variables such as subjective moods, including anxiety, central (cortical) and peripheral (muscle tension) neural excitability, attention, and elevations in neuroendocrine and brain monoamines (Morgan, 1981a). These relationships typically have been viewed from a preventive medicine perspective, however. Although the extension of habilitative psychological and behavioristic interventions to an ergogenic purpose has been eagerly received by sport psychologists under the stress management umbrella, exercise-induced stress has been tacitly viewed as merely adjunctive. This is notable because introduced evidence suggests that stress responsivity associated with both acute and chronic metabolic arousal is more homogeneous than "psychogenically" induced arousal, except when it is subordinated by abnormal cognitive or perceptual influence. Thus, performance facilitating changes in anxiety, tension, or attention may frequently occur as natural by-products of metabolic arousal. At any rate, it is likely that ergogenic alterations in performance mediating stress will be more effectively viewed within a biologic model as opposed to a singular psychologic or physiologic paradigm.

Applied Study

Applied research on stress management procedures in sport is rather limited, and this reflects the recency of an applied focus by North American sport psychologists. Overviews of much of this work can be found in edited volumes by Hanin (1981) and Sime and Zaichkowsky (1982) and in a paper by Suinn (1982). To facilitate economy of space and illustration of content in this paper, a resource outline of supportive and nonsupportive clinical research is provided in Table 1. This tabular presentation should also enhance ready comparison of procedures, method, and pattern of performance effects. Both refereed and nonrefereed (including theses) sources are included because there appears to be no systematic difference in the scientific quality of these studies. This approach should provide a more representative view of contemporary developments. Also, because of the area's youth, methodological issues which mitigate results are frequently common across several studies, and therefore a critical evaluation of research method and conceptualization will follow in categorical rather than annotated form.

Competing Explanations

Ergogenic effects have frequently been inconsistent across case studies and controlled group comparisons. When discrepancies are observed, several alternative interpretations can account for much of the apparent indeterminancy of results. These may contribute sources of both systematic and random error that inflate intragroup

Table 1
Applied Stress Management Research in Sport

Autonomic

Procedure	Reference	Subjects/Skill	Design	Mediator	Results
Oral ingestion of Oxprenolol (80 mg) (beta blocker)	Antal & Good, 1979	22 male British national pistol shooters/team selection	double-blind placebo within subjects counterbalanced	↓anxiety ↓BP ↓HR (ECG) CA no change self-report ↑attention ↑well-being ↓tension (implied)	Slow fire improved No change in rapid fire
(1) Biofeedback (EMG) assisted relaxation (frontalis) (1 10-min session) (2) Same as above plus cognitive restructuring (4 10-min sessions)	Bennett & Hall, Note 5	Novice archers/target accuracy	pre-post factorial treatment 1 treatment 2 control	↓tension (EMG)	No performance effects
Biofeedback (EMG) assisted relaxation (frontalis)	Blais, 1978	Trait anxious (SCAT) males (10-15 yrs)/balance time on stabilometer	pre-post placebo	↓tension (EMG)	No performance effects
Biofeedback (auditory) (HR & respiration)	Daniels & Landers, 1981	8 male national level rifle shooters	pre-post placebo	synchrony of autonomic patterning with performance	Increased reliability of patterning

Table 1 (Continued)
Applied Stress Management Research in Sport

Treatment	Author, Year	Subjects	Design	Dependent measures	Results
Progressive relaxation & cognitive rehearsal	Decaria, 1977	5 novice and 5 intermediate female high school gymnasts	multiple baseline across subjects no control no reversal	↓self-report of anxiety (no validity or reliability data)	Intermediates improved; no change for novice
Biofeedback (EMG) assisted relaxation (frontalis, masseter, trapezius) & cognitive restructuring (12 1-hr sessions)	DeWitt, 1980	6 college football (American) players/competitive performance	pre-post no control	↓anxiety (implied) ↓tension (EMG)	Coaches' rating improved (not blind)
Same as above plus HR feedback (11 1-hr sessions)	DeWitt, 1980	12 college basketball players/competitive performance	pre-post control	↓anxiety (implied) ↓tension (EMG) ↓HR (ECG)	Ratings improved (blind)
(1) Biofeedback (EMG) assisted systematic desensitization (2) Progressive relaxation and systematic desensitization (2 sessions/wk/6 wks)	Dorsey, 1977	25 college male gymnasts/competitive performance	pre-post factorial treatment 1 treatment 2 control	↓frontalis tension (EMG) for both treatments. State anxiety (STAI) did not decrease under competition.	No performance effects (NGJA scoring)
Biofeedback (EMG) assisted relaxation (frontalis) (3 hrs)	French, 1977	30 undergraduate males/ balance time on stabilometer and contact time on pursuit rotor	pre-post control	↓tension (EMG)	Performance improved and was correlated with tension

(1) Biofeedback (EMG) assisted relaxation (frontalis) (2) Meditation	Griffiths et al., 1981	50 novice underwater divers/underwater assembly task	pre-post factorial treatment 1 treatment 2 placebo	↓anxiety (STAI) no change in respiration ↑tension (EMG)	No effects for either treatment; pre-dive STAI negatively correlated with performance
Progressive relaxation (cued; 6 sessions)	Kukla, 1977	51 male high school baseball players/hitting a pitching machine	posttest control placebo	↓anxiety (STAI)	Treatment group performed better under social evaluation
Biofeedback (EMG) assisted systematic desensitization (4 1-hr sessions)	Teague, 1977	20 undergraduates/balance time on stabilometer	pre-post placebo	Setting-induced anxiety (STAI) was not reduced.	Performance increases for treatment group exceeded those for control
(1) Progressive relaxation (2) Biofeedback (EMG) assisted relaxation (frontalis) (6 hrs)	Tsukamoto, 1979	24 female age-level gymnasts (10-15 yrs)/ competitive performance	pre-post factorial treatment 1 treatment 2 placebo	no differences on anxiety (SCAT & STAI)	No performance effects (IGFC scoring)

Behavioral

Behavioral modeling	Feltz et al., 1979	60 female novice divers/1 meter platform back dive	posttest factorial client aided live model videotape	↑self-efficacy (assessed) ↓anxiety (implied)	Client aided modeling better than others; live and videotape equal

Table 1 (Continued)
Applied Stress Management Research in Sport

Behavioral modeling	Gould & Weiss, 1981	150 college females/ muscle endurance (lab)	posttest factorial (2 × 3) *model* × *talk* alike pos. unalike neg. control none	↑self-efficacy (assessed)	Alike model, using either positive or no statements, improved performance
Self-efficacy inducement	Weinberg et al., 1979	30 female and 30 male undergraduates/muscle endurance in competition (lab)	pre-post factorial high efficacy low efficacy	↑confidence self-talk (assessed)	High self-efficacy had greater performance; sex interaction
Self-efficacy inducement	Weinberg et al., 1980	56 female and 56 male undergraduates/muscle endurance in competition (lab)	posttest factorial (2 × 2) self-efficacy high, low expectancy public, private	↑self-efficacy (assessed)	High self-efficacy had greater performance; no public-private effects
Cognitive					
"Psych-up" time interval	Caudill et al., 1981	40 college females/ leg strength (lab)	pre-post factorial 15 sec 30 sec self-initiated yoked to self-initiated	↑central arousal (implied)	No time effects

Same as above plus mental preparation strategy	Caudill et al., 1981	60 male and female undergraduates/absolute muscle endurance (lab)	pre-post; within subjects counterbalanced factorial *time × strategy* 15 sec arousal 30 sec imagery 60 sec attention control group	↑implied by treatments	No time effects No difference among strategies All strategies better than control
Thought stopping (1 1½-hr session)	Chance, 1980	72 age-level swimmers/ competitive times	pre-post control	↓anxiety (implied)	No performance effects
Mental preparation strategies	Gould et al., 1980	15 female and 15 male undergraduates/ leg strength (lab)	posttest Latin Square factorial, within subjects attentional focus imagery preparatory arousal control-rest control-distraction	↑anxiety ↑confidence (both assessed)	Preparatory arousal and imagery were equally better than others No sex interaction

Table 1 (Continued)
Applied Stress Management Research in Sport

Cognitive coping	Meyers et al., 1979	30 female and 30 male undergraduates/leg strength (lab)	pre-post factorial preparatory arousal imagery control-rest	No influence on anxiety and psychometric activation. ↑confidence (all assessed)	Preparatory arousal better than control. Sex interaction
		40 female age-level novice gymnasts/front walkover front flip	pre-post factorial pos. self-talk neg. self-talk placebo	none implied	No performance effects
Cognitive distraction	Morgan et al., 1983	28 males/treadmill endurance at 80% max VO^2	pre-post control	no physiological differences ↑tolerance of discomfort (implied)	Increased endurance
		18 males/treadmill endurance decrement from 80% to 90% max VO^2	pretest—80% posttest—90% factorial distraction control placebo (experimenter blind)	same as above	No differences

Technique	Study	Subjects/task	Design	Psychological effects	Performance effects
"Psych-up" time interval	Weinberg et al., 1981	40 female and 40 male undergraduates/ leg strength (lab)	pre-post factorial 15 sec 30 sec self-initiated yoked to self-initiated	no change on a psychometric measure of CNS activation	No time effects, all intervals better than baseline, sex effects
Combined cognitive/emotive/autonomic					
VMBR plus cognitive restructuring	Bennett & Stothart, 1980	44 college gymnasts, archers, wrestlers, & badminton players/ competitive performance	pre-post control	↓anxiety (STAI)	No performance effects (coaches' ratings)
VMBR plus Stress Inoculation (Meichenbaum, 1977) (1 wk)	Desiderato & Miller, 1979	Case of a male amateur tennis player/ competitive performance	single baseline no control	↓anxiety ↑confidence (each implied)	Improved match play
VMBR plus cued thought stopping (150 min/3 sessions)	Gravel et al., 1980	9 male and 3 female college cross-country skiers/competitive performance	pre-post, follow-up placebo	cognitions (assessed) ↓anxiety ↑self-efficacy (each implied)	No performance data, self-reported improvement and less maladaptive thoughts
Progressive relaxation plus cognitive restructuring	Horton & Shelton, 1978	4 male college wrestlers/ competitive performance	pre-post single baseline no control	none implied	Improved won-lost record
VMBR	Kirschenbaum & Bale, 1980	Case of a male college golfer/competitive performance	posttest no control	↓tension ↑attention ↑self-efficacy (all implied)	Match play improved by one stroke
		3 male college golfers/ competitive performance	multiple baseline with a control subject	same as above	Improved match play

Table 1 (Continued)
Applied Stress Management Research in Sport

Method	Author	Sample	Design	Effects (implied)	Results
VMBR (15 10-min sessions)	Kolonay, 1977	72 male college basketball players (8 teams)/competitive free-throw percentage	pre-post factorial VMBR relaxation imagery control	↓anxiety ↑attention (each implied)	VMBR group improved No change for others
Cognitive coping muscle relaxation desensitization cued attention (7 sessions/3 wks)	Meyers & Schlesser, 1980	Case of a male college basketball player/competitive performance	pre-post matched baseline no control	↑confidence ↑attention (each implied)	Scoring average and shooting percentage improved
Coping imagery relaxation self-instruction (15 to 23 sessions across 5 to 6 wks)	Meyers et al., 1982	2 female college basketball players/competitive free-throw and field goal percentage	multiple baseline across subjects. reversal on one subject non-treatment skill variable as control	↑confidence ↑concentration ↓anxiety (all implied)	Improved performance
VMBR	Nelson, 1980	College golfers & runners/competitive performance	pre-post	none implied	No effects

Technique	Author	Subjects	Design	Results	Performance
VMBR (6 hrs/10 days)	Noel, 1980	14 male amateur tennis players/service in tournament play	pre-post control	↓tension (EMG) ↑attention (implied)	No performance effects
VMBR	Titley, 1976	Case of a male college placekicker (American football)/game performance	pre-post (observation) no control	↑anxiety ↑confidence ↑motivation (all implied)	Improved game performance, record setting
VMBR (20 min/day for 6 wks)	Weinberg et al., 1981	32 male college Karate club members/competitive performance	pre-post factorial (matched subjects, nonrandom) VMBR relaxation imagery placebo (experimenter blind)	↓trait anxiety ↓(STAI) HR no change ↓state anxiety ↓(STAI) (no performance relationship)	VMBR better than others for competitive sparring; no difference for "skill" and "combinations"; Rater reliability, .92, .90, .95, respectively
(1) Stress Inoculation (Meichenbaum, 1977) (2) Stress Management (Smith, 1980) (2 sessions/wk for 5½ wks)	Ziegler, 1982	8 male college cross-country runners/metabolic and autonomic response to 20-min treadmill run at 50% $\dot{V}O_2$ max	pre-post factorial treatment 1 treatment 2 control	↓oxygen uptake (submaximal) ↓HR at submax (both treatments)	No performance data

BP—blood pressure, CA—catecholamines, CNS—central nervous system, ECG—electrocardiogram, EMG—electromyogram, HR—heart rate, IGFC—International Gymnastics Federation Council, NGJA—National Gymnastic Judges Association, SCAT—Sport Competition Anxiety Test, STAI—State Trait Anxiety Inventory, VMBR—visuo-motor behavior rehearsal.

variability, diminish treatment effects, retard replication and comparison of results, and preclude generalizability. In various instances, experimental confounds have included heterogeneity in singular stress definitions and manipulative strategies, uncertain validity and reliability of behavioral assessments, selection of an intervention with apparent disregard for athlete characteristics or setting/performance demands, nonexplanatory methodology, and a possibly inappropriate psychometric model in some instances.

Individual Differences in Stress Response

There is well established interindividual variation in generalized biological response to a standard stressor (Astrand & Rodahl, 1977; Eysenck, 1967), and this has formed the basis for fundamental principles guiding research and clinical practice in applied human physiology (e.g., in exercise and sport). Although individual differences have also been noted by sport psychologists (Kroll, 1982; Landers, 1980; Martens, 1972; Morgan, 1980), with few exceptions (e.g., Mahoney, 1979; Nideffer, 1981; Suinn, 1981) they have been frequently ignored in applied research and practice, particularly in North America. This has occurred despite substantial supportive evidence that psychological traits can be of use when predicting and explaining stress-related behavior in sport settings (Morgan, 1979, 1980). Thus, a personality confound appears inherent in stress management studies that do not consider stress-related traits at the outset (Martens, 1972; Weinberg, 1978; Weinberg & Ragan, 1978). The lack of group differences in a controlled intervention can thus reflect real variability as well as error. For example, individuals who demonstrate a time-urgent, hard-driving, behavior pattern have been shown to experience a less pronounced central deactivation (smaller alpha amplitude) following exercise stress than their typically more "relaxed" counterparts (Farmer, et al., 1978). Alpha production differed across individuals even when the stressor employed was relative to biological tolerance for stress.

A series of field studies conducted in sport settings adds a more practical dimension to this basic research. Athletes have been observed to naturally employ a variety of self-inducement procedures to both raise and lower precompetitive arousal (Genov, 1970; Highlen & Bennett, 1979; Kauss, 1978; Shelton & Mahoney, 1978; Weinberg, Gould, & Jackson, 1980). These have been shown to be associated with actual strength performance in both laboratory and sport settings, and selected attempts to enhance their effectiveness by additional intervention procedures have not been successful (Gould, Weinberg, & Jackson, 1980). Other naturalistic sport research has indicated inherent habituative and/or adaptive responses by athletes in autonomic activity (Fenz & Epstein, 1967), cognitive appraisal (Mahoney & Avener, 1977; Meyers, Cooke, Cullen, & Liles, 1979; Morgan & Pollock, 1977), and attentional focus (Morgan & Pollock, 1977; Shelton & Mahoney, 1978; Van Schoyck & Grasha, 1981). Athletes have also typically scored in the extraverted range on standard psychometric measures of personality (Morgan, 1979, 1980), have been observed to reduce the perceptual magnitude of an objective stressor (Ryan & Foster, 1967), and have manifested a high pain tolerance (Ryan & Kovacic, 1966), when contrasted with the nonathlete. These psychophysical traits innately enhance arousal management by either facilitating habituation to the stress response or by directly diminishing sensory input. Additional psychometric findings have consistently supported that the successful world-class or elite athlete is reliably disposed to a stable emotional response to stress-provoking situations when compared with less successful athletes and nonathletic populations (Morgan, 1979). Moreover, both generalized and sport-specific measures of trait anxiety have predicted athletes' precompetitive anxiety states (Gerson & Deshaies, 1980; Klavora, 1979; Martens, 1977; Scanlan & Passer, 1979; Weinberg & Genuchi, 1980). More importantly, perhaps, experienced and successful athletes have been shown to be consistent in the pattern of their stress response under variable setting conditions (Fenz & Epstein, 1967; Langer, 1966; Morgan, 1970).

Results such as these suggest that through both learning (adaptive experience) and by natural selection (adaptive traits), a substantial portion of the athletic population may already possess certain stress management skills. Thus, the degree to which they may be expected to benefit from externally induced procedures or from further learning appears unclear. Moreover, evidence predicts that in certain athletes the targeted stress correlates may be relatively insensitive to an intervention technique. In addition, it appears that among individuals most likely to be affected by a management procedure, there can be a notable variation in both the quantity (magnitude) and the quality (specific symptoms) of the arousal or stress response that may best facilitate performance. Applied research indicates that different athletes have different levels of optimal responsivity (Klavora, 1979), and the patterning of the symptom complex manifested can vary significantly across athletes (Landers, 1981). For example, world-class rifle shooters, as a group, experience a 30% elevation in precompetitive heart rate above a resting baseline, but individually, some shooters perform better with a relatively low heart rate. Moreover, although elite women shooters manifest higher precompetitive heart rates than their male counterparts, no differences have been found in psychometrically measured state anxiety (Landers, 1981).

Intervention Specificity. Concerns regarding the reliability of both generalized and isolated measures of stress highlight the dilemma of selecting a management procedure that is both appropriate to the stress correlate assessed and to the patterning of that correlate for a given individual. Although pharmacologic agents can produce a rather homogeneous stress response and performance effect (Antal & Good, 1979), there can be a notable risk for errors of misapplication when employing psychological and behavioral interventions based on generalized principles. This is inherent in the notion of stress management because of the implied control of a generalized syndrome of symptoms. A syndromic view can misleadingly reinforce the use of intervention procedures that focus exclusively on a specific symptom with inferences then drawn about generalized effects or that focus on a comprehensive treatment package designed to manage several symptoms irrespective of individual variability in response patterning. Such practice is tantamount to viewing stress and arousal as situational variables that are independent of personal characteristics. This is noteworthy in view of the recent attention in sport psychology (Morgan, 1980) to the advantage of assessing both psychological traits and states in the prediction of behavior. It seems that endogenous and acquired traits of both a generalized and a sport-specific nature can interact with a standard stressor to determine the stress response observed. However, in applied sport psychology, arousal and stress-related concepts have frequently been viewed as state variables that respond in a reliable manner essentially independent of the individual, and this view has complemented situationist approaches to psychoergogenics in sport (e.g., Rushall, 1975).

Setting Demands

Individual differences apparently can be compounded by the particular demands a sport may place on specific stress correlates. It is well established, for example, that different sports require unique metabolic responses. Basic psychological research on perceptual motor skills (Landers, 1980) and clinical observation in applied sport psychology (Nideffer, 1981; Morgan, 1981b) have reinforced this uniqueness for movement precision and for information processing. However, much of the stress management work in sport appears largely atheoretical in the sense that it has either applied basic research or practice from general psychology or has involved applied sport research with selective disregard for relevant sport literature. Relatively few approaches (Mahoney, 1979; Nideffer, 1981; Suinn, 1981) have systematically incorporated procedures that are complemented by theoretical and empirical study in naturalistic sport settings. Moreover, few applied studies are available to provide empirical support. A field/laboratory study by Pinel and Schultz (1978) is noteworthy in this regard. Biofeedback (EMG) assisted increases in neuromuscular tension spanning a discrete ordinal range of low (0.5-1.0 nV), moderate (4.5-5.5 nV), and high (9.5-10.5 nV) amplitudes were associated in a negative monotonic fashion with both the force and precision of subsequent voluntary muscle contraction, but described a biphasic function (V relationship) with fatigue, in small muscle groups of the wrist flexors. Choice-reaction time did not covary with the same alterations in tension, however. Because the tasks selected can be viewed as representative of skills underlying complex athletic performance, basic support was provided for differential arousal demands across sport tasks.

Intervention Specificity. A more provocative interpretation of the Pinel and Schultz study supports that a neurophysiologically based intervention mode (EMG tension control) altered neurophysiologically dependent skills but did not influence a relatively more "cognitive" skill dependent upon decision making. This view is consistent with findings in other clinical settings (Weinberg, Gould, & Jackson, 1980) and supports the efficacy of interventions specific to the stress correlate to be manipulated. It also reinforces the apparent advantage of matching an intervention to the common mode underlying stress and performance.

From an applied perspective, however, the most innovative aspect of this study relates more to method than to results. The tension levels were not only self-regulated (with EMG feedback) in a reliable manner, but they were initially selected on the basis of naturally induced tension increases observed in collegiate wrestlers immediately prior to actual competition. This is an important methodological point because the issue of a clinically meaningful change, above baseline, in stress correlates has for the most part not been addressed at a measurement level in the applied sport literature (Klavora, 1979; Morgan, 1979; Suinn, 1981). Moreover, laboratory-induced changes in state anxiety (across similar levels of arousal), known to covary with performance altering tension (Weinberg, 1978), have paradoxically produced a nonmonotonic (V) relationship with performance requiring both precision and information processing, but not endurance. This again highlights the issue of sport specificity. However, the stress management technology used in sport settings is a direct outgrowth of clinical procedures initially designed for abnormal symptom populations under normal metabolic demands. Although these techniques appear applicable to many sport-related skills, controlled evidence of an applied nature is limited (Landers, 1981). This is ironic, considering repeated calls by North American sport psychologists for the abandonment of generalized personality tests and abnormal psychometric diagnostics in favor of more sport and situation specific measures. It seems sport psychology has selectively rejected generalized psychometrics (e.g., Kroll, 1982; Martens, 1977; Rushall, 1975) while selectively embracing generalized stress management procedures (Martens, 1981; Smith, 1980).

Although naturalistic stress testing may appear futuristic and pragmatically infeasible at the present, it is already occurring for selected sports when setting characteristics complement contemporary assessment techniques (Bard & Fleury, 1976; Landers, 1981), and an advancing technology in information processing may facilitate its practicality for hypothesis testing under competitive conditions. Moreover, it is likely that the description of actual responsivity under naturalistic circumstances represents a necessary step in applied methodology before practically significant setting demands and athlete response can be determined in many instances. This may better permit testing of explanatory models derived from basic research and more precise tailoring of selected management procedures to specific sports and to the individual athlete.

The Measurement/Methodology Interface

It is not readily apparent if the inconsistency that characterizes much of the stress management literature in sport can be attributed to unreliable measures of stress and performance, to the selection of inappropriate behavioral models (e.g., drive vs. inverted U arguments), or to an inappropriate psychometric model in some instances (linearity and interval scaling). The significance of this uncertainty is intimately tied to applied methodology, because issues of explanatory measurement might be dismissed as unnecessarily reductionistic (Peele, 1981) if the clinical efficacy of the procedures employed were empirically demonstrated to be clear and reliable (Anderson & Shanteau, 1977).

Stress management procedures that have appeared most effective in facilitating sport performance combine both cognitive and neurophysiologic components (e.g., Nideffer, 1981; Suinn, 1981).

This approach seems intuitively reasonable considering the multi-dimensionality of stress and the psychobiological nature of sport. However, support for clinical effectiveness has been largely anecdotal, involving descriptive group contrasts or case research in the absence of controls. Only a few studies have permitted speculation about the underlying mechanics implicitly responsible for performance effects (see Sime & Zaichkowsky, 1982, and Suinn, 1981), and a single refereed study (Weinberg, Seabourne, & Jackson, 1981) has actually assessed proposed mediators in a systematic and controlled manner. Even within controlled group designs that attempt to discount placebo effects, controls have typically been inadequate because they were innocuous and did not offer potential for competing explanations. That is, they have discounted the issue of *any* versus *no* treatment, but have not distinguished specific treatment effects from generalized setting effects. Moreover, available designs for single-case experimentation (Kazdin, 1980) can permit confidence in the descriptive dimension of internal validity. They can demonstrate that a stress management procedure is associated with a performance increment or decrement, but they cannot explain why the intervention works or predict for whom and in what setting it can be expected to work. This is conventionally viewed as a limitation in external validity or the generalizability of findings. However, an explanatory dimension to internal validity exists that also limits external validity, and this highlights the significance of the measurement model selected for method assessment. It is well recognized that when there is room for a change (no performance ceiling or floor is known) a variety of interventions can be effective regardless of content (Morgan, 1972). Social cues, therapist effects, and treatment expectations are known to be potent ingredients of a generalized placebo potential in behavioral interventions, regardless of whether the procedural mode is viewed as cognitive, neurophysiologic, or behavioristic (Blanchard & Epstein, 1977; Kazdin, 1980). Many procedures attempt to capitalize on these as complementary effects (Miller, 1978; Nideffer, 1981); they can be viewed as facilitative from a clinical or applied perspective. However, from the perspective of basic and applied research, they confound explanation and the measurement of competing explanatory mechanisms must subsequently be attempted. Thus, measurement can be considered a confounding factor in applied methodology.

Scaling. Issues over an appropriate psychometric model subsequently become salient because of the multidimensional and apparently differentiated nature of acute stress. The appropriateness of interval measurement in accurately describing stress represents a primary question. Because some stress correlates are directly indicated by a physical reality, it can be demonstrated that measurement intervals are equivalent. There is little argument over the assumption of linearity for physical indicators of stress such as oxygen consumption, heart rate, skin temperature and electroconductance, sweat rate, muscular tension, or catecholamine levels. Moreover, attention can be viewed as objective when assessed behaviorally (Bard & Fleury, 1976) rather than psychometrically (Silva, 1979). The appropriateness of a linear model for subjective stress is less clear, however, since arousal, anxiety, or expectations are abstract constructs.

From a *theoretical* standpoint, this can present a measurement dilemma when results of sport studies that differentially define stress in an abstract or in a concrete manner are contrasted. The discrepancy, for example, between a nonmonotonic relationship for performance observed when stress is assessed by self-reports of state anxiety (e.g., Weinberg, 1978) and a monotonic performance function for stress defined as muscular tension (e.g., Pinel & Schultz, 1978) might accurately be explained by differentiation of arousal, task specificity, or setting/sport demands. On the other hand, it is a measurement possibility that subjective estimates of state anxiety actually follow a function not described by an interval scale and that the discrepancy noted reflects measurement error. An elevation in state anxiety of a given scale unit might be practically insignificant in influencing arousal, attention, or tension for performance in a normal functional range of neurologic and metabolic demand, but might be critical at the limits of human performance that characterize top-level athletics. It might also have different consequences for different individuals. The apparent consensus that an inverted U function for stress is dependent on performance complexity (Landers, 1980; Martens, 1974) illustrates these points. It not only implies inadequate prediction and explanation for a bivariate model, but the existence of distinct band widths of optimal arousal for different levels of performance would suggest that corresponding intervals on an arousal or anxiety continuum actually represent nonequidistant measures of motor integration and attention. Because arousal and anxiety have no physical form and are constructed by their covariation with physiological and behavioral intervals, their function defines their form. A curvilinear relationship (Landers, 1980) in each case is thus as consistent with an ordinal or a ratio scale as for one that is interval.

The *clinical* significance of this largely depends upon the psychological or behavioral advantage stress-related assessments can offer (Grossberg & Grant, 1978). When scaling people, the essential goal is the measurement of attributes for the purpose of interindividual comparisons or rankings. No clinical advantage is available, however, when variability is reduced. For example, tolerance of metabolic stress (i.e., maximum VO_2) can explain and predict endurance performance across a diverse population, but it is of no practical use among a homogeneous group of elite distance runners (Pollock, Jackson, & Pate, 1980). In a like manner, intervally scaled attributes of subjective stress tolerance (i.e., trait and state anxiety) have not consistently predicted motor performance (Martens, 1972) unless combined in a mental health model in which scores reflect enough variation to be viewed within a pathological context (Morgan, 1979). Because it is estimated that only 10% of athletes will score within a pathologic range at a given time, empirical validity of intervally scaling athletes on subjective stress is not clear. It is conceivable that scaling the response itself may offer a clinically significant alternative (Weingarten, 1980). By scaling the stress response, scales could be developed for individual athletes (Klavora, 1979), and this might promote a more precise matching of stress management procedures to the individual case.

Moreover, the notion that feelings of stress (e.g., anxiety) may grow at a constant (power) or variable (exponential) proportion of total tolerance rather than at a constant proportion of the stress-provoking stimulus (logarithmic) is supported by basic and applied research in nonsport settings (see Grossberg & Grant [1978] for a review). Furthermore, it has been demonstrated (Sjoberg, Svensson, & Persson, 1979) that both activation and pleasure continua of mood are biphasic and do not fit a linear psychometric model, although polar extremes do. Thus, quantity aspects of stress-related mood might be rated according to physical indicators that are internal rather than external in locus. Although largely undocumented, this possibility is consistent with the implied role of catecholamines and indoleamines in mood (McGeer & McGeer, 1980) and behavior (Zuckerman, Buchsbaum, & Murphy, 1980) and the endorphins (Farrell, Cates, Maksud, Morgan, & Tseng, 1981) in subjective stress adaptation. Systemic levels of epinephrine and norepinephrine, for example, are known to accelerate positively during psychologically and metabolically induced stress and to covary with ratio estimates of subjective stress (Frankenhauser, 1971). A nonmonotonic alternative also offers phenomenological appeal and suggests a psychological parallel to physical stress tolerance; it is well supported that interindividual comparisons in stress response to metabolic demand are more meaningfully evaluated in terms relative to total capacity (i.e., % $\dot{V}O_2$ max).

The relative merits and liabilities of additive (i.e., interval) and multiplicative (i.e., ratio) models for psychological scaling have been discussed in detail elsewhere (Cliff, 1973; Ekman & Sjoberg, 1965; Nunnally, 1978; Stevens, 1975). Both have been used in psychophysical studies of exercise stress (Morgan, 1981b; Morgan & Horstman, 1978; Ryan & Foster, 1967; Ryan & Kovacic, 1966), and different functions can emerge in each case. Perceived exertion (Borg, 1978), for example, is a positive linear function of increasing metabolic demand when an interval category scale is used, but it describes a classic power function when assessed by magnitude estimation or production techniques (Morgan, 1981b). In the "psychophysical" case of perceived exercise stress, a measurement model of linearity (category scaling) has been selectively adopted on the basis of clinical and statistical efficacy rather than empirical accuracy (Morgan, 1981b). That is, the scaling of people rather than the exercise stimulus has become the principal interest. However, the actual practical impact of this approach has been limited (Gutmann, Squires, Pollock, Foster, & Anholm, 1981). This analogy is drawn to suggest that a similar situation may exist for sport "psychometrics" when subjective estimates of stress-related phenomena are assessed. Scales that complement the apparent limitations of singular logarithmic and power approaches might be refined (e.g., Borg, 1978).

Cognition vs. Perception. The preferred psychometric scaling model may also depend upon whether subjective stress is viewed in cognitive (thinking) or perceptual (feeling) terms. It can be argued that stress-related expectations (Scanlan & Passer, 1979) or anxiety thoughts, in the absence of direct physiological or behavioral events, lack quantity but can be ordinal. A linear measurement model can thus be imposed (Stevens, 1975) to provide an informational advantage in determining performance relationships (Fisher, 1980). This is noteworthy because of an increasing cognitive orientation in applied sport psychology (Mahoney, 1979; Martens, 1981; see Chapter 10 by Silva) and in stress management (Nideffer, 1981; Smith, 1980; Suinn, 1981). It remains unclear, however, whether a clinical or measurement advantage exists for viewing subjective stress in a cognitive, perceptual, or behavioral mode. That is, does thinking or does feeling motivate and impair performance, and are cognitive or perceptual estimates the most reliable measures? An analogous issue has fueled contemporary arguments in behavior therapy (Kendall & Hollon, 1979); general psychology (Zajonc, 1980); and sport psychology (Morgan, 1981b). A central issue in each case is the precedence of either thinking or feeling in the control of behavior. It appears, however, that either one can both precede and disrupt the other and the determination of this in high-level sport is basic to evaluating the implied effectiveness of stress management procedures that combine or singularly adopt a cognitive, somatic, or behavioristic orientation. This will require assessment of both thinking and feeling, and it is possible that different measurement models may be required in each instance (Anderson, 1974a, 1974b).

A Psychometric Adjunct: Monitoring Training Stress

Because measures of stress have not been shown to relate in the same way to sport performance, they cannot be considered as defining the same construct. That is, *acute* stress does not appear internally consistent as a sport predictor. Although it offers theoretical parsimony, its accuracy and clinical efficacy appear limited from an ergogenic standpoint. In an acute sense, therefore, it may be more accurate to characterize specific interventions as tension control or attention training rather than as stress management. When more global terms are used, such as relaxation, self-regulation, anxiety management, autogenic training, or stress inoculation, it appears beneficial to consider the need for specificity rather than generality of application (Suinn & Deffenbacher, 1980).

Evidence is available, however, which suggests that an alternate model of *chronic* stress may be more consistent with a syndromic view and may better satisfy criteria for theoretical and applied use. Two recent symposia sponsored by the American College of Sports Medicine (Morgan, Note 1; Dishman, Note 4) have illustrated a clinical utility for the psychometric monitoring of stress-induced mood shifts across time in a preventive rather than corrective model of sport stress.

Biological adaptations to training stress follow a negatively accelerating function, so the volume of training required to produce a fitness gain increases progressively as an athlete's total tolerance for stress is approached (Astrand & Rodahl, 1977). This creates a practical dilemma for the coach and athlete because attempts to maximize conditioning effects (stress adaptation) risk overtraining (exhaustion), and this is particularly a problem in endurance sports characterized by a large training volume. The overtrained or stale athlete typically presents symptoms nearly identical to those of the clinical patient suffering a reactive depression, and this is to be expected if each instance represents an exhaustion syndrome. When it occurs in athletics, it typically is associated with an objective performance decrement, and reduced training or complete rest is required. Thus, prevention is highly desirable. In a prognostic sense, standard biomedical indicators of stress have demonstrated considerable lability and have been less precise than psychometrically assessed mood. Mood has closely followed the clinical profile characteristically presented by the stale athlete and has reflected actual biologic adaptations to some degree. Moreover, when employed in naturalistic settings to diagnose a pathologic response, this model has predicted athletic performance in a practically significant manner (Morgan, 1979).

A chronic model is noteworthy for several reasons, and in each instance it appears to offer an advantage over a singularly acute paradigm. First, it views stress as a biological adaptation that can be manifested in psychometric symptoms of exhaustion, and this is consistent with either a psychologic or a physiologic perspective. Second, stress is regarded as a specific syndrome resulting from nonspecific sources. This permits generalization across athletes and sport settings in which training stress might be expected to be excessive. That is, a chronic model does not appear as confounded by individual differences or setting demands because of its interactional nature. Third, the chronic model introduced is an empirical outgrowth of clinically based research in sport settings (Morgan, Note 1) and is therefore not merely an attempt to fit applied data to an explanatory model. Fourth, although responses are intervally scaled and are based on interindividual variability assumed to be linear, issues of scaling appear subordinated by the consistency and practical effectiveness promised for both group- and single-case instances. In other words, this approach not only permits interindividual comparisons according to a known clinical range, but also permits a diagnostic function based on intraindividual variability. It is essentially a pathologic model in that transient responses are compared to a typical or baseline response obtained in the absence of training stress. Therefore, variability appears to represent a practically significant magnitude independent of scaling issues. The model assumes that chronic pathologic stress (a reliable state) can be reliably prevented by psychometric methods, rather than assuming that pathologically oriented interventions can reliably correct or enhance nonpathologic correlates of acute stress (an unreliable state).

Learning. A psychometric approach to monitoring chronic sport stress also avoids problems of learning that tend to characterize an acute paradigm. Because it is not clear that precompetitive interventions will endure during the dynamic context of ongoing competition, one acute approach centers on self-regulation of arousal correlates in which the intervention focus is shifted from the practitioner to the athlete (Martens, 1981). However, the process of learning stress-coping skills is not well understood (Jaremko, 1979). For example, the necessary time commitment is unclear. Although a maladaptive stress response can be conditioned with a single exposure, it is more typically a gradual adaptation to repeated incidents. Adaptive relearning might require, at the least, a commensurate time period, but this has not been addressed in most of the applied sport research. Moreover, some evidence (Fenz & Epstein, 1967; Mahoney & Avener, 1977; Meyers, Cooke, Cullen, & Liles, 1979) suggests that an exclusive focus on precompetitive states may result in misleading inferences about preferred stress alterations, because precompetitive states may be quite different from those naturally adopted by the athlete during successful performance. The learning of stress management skills has subsequently become a principal argument in applied sport psychology regarding the preferred locus of ergogenic procedures (Danish & Hale, 1981) and the professional qualifications required of a practitioner (Harrison & Feltz, 1979; Nideffer, DuFresne, Nesvig, & Selder, 1980). It appears straightforward that a performance or health-debilitating competitive crisis would benefit from intervention by a clinically trained sport psychologist, while acquisition of many self-regulatory skills could be equally well facilitated by a sport psychologist or an informed coach whose principal functions are educational (Martens, 1981; Nideffer, 1981). These issues are as yet unresolved, however, because evidence does not clearly support that clinical effects are dependent upon clinical training (Durlak, 1979) and because no empirical base is available to reliably guide the teaching of self-regulatory skills in either sport (Landers, 1981) or nonsport (Miller, 1978) settings. In any case, however, prevention precludes the need for intervention, and evidence suggests this may more reliably occur for chronic as opposed to acute stress management.

Conclusions

In a collective sense, the ergogenic effects of stress management procedures are difficult to interpret, and they exemplify the difficulty of effectively merging theory and practice. Several conventional techniques have been associated with performance increments. On the other hand, numerous studies have shown no influence, and when group data are involved, this implies individual decrements. This inconsistency can in part be attributed to several theoretical and methodological issues. Stress has typically been conceptualized as an acute concept, and interventions have focused on either specific symptom correlates, with inference drawn about the total stress concept, or on the source/symptom complex, with inference drawn about the influence of specific correlates or intervening factors. That is, considerable heterogeneity has existed across studies in the manner adopted for its operation and manipulation. Thus, the apparent indeterminancy of generalized stress or arousal as a performance influence may, in part, be attributable to what Messick (1981) has termed nomological noise. This results from the use of single indicants in different studies as reflections of the same construct (Martens, 1974). Because measures of stress each contain error variance as well as construct variance, comparisons across studies of performance relationships may reflect overlapping variance due to error rather than to the common construct, and this can seriously confound interpretation when research is principally descriptive or predictive. However, large within-group variability has been common in the absence of group effects, and this supports that innate and acquired differences in individual stress responsivity may combine with sport-specific setting demands to reduce the reliability of the stress construct and its performance effects. In many cases, this can preclude a predictable clinical benefit for both specific and generalized interventions applied in an across-the-board manner. A predictive advantage is likely to be gained by matching interventions and stress correlates that share the same biological or behavioral mode and that fit setting/performance demands. Moreover, procedures have generally focused on stress reduction. The converse may be more appropriate in certain instances because some athletes are known to naturally employ stress inducing strategies to an apparent performance advantage.

Applied approaches promising the greatest practical dividend have emanated from a cognitive-neurophysiologic model that appears adaptable to a given sport and athlete and that facilitates self-regulation rather than continued dependence on a clinical practitioner. Although this approach seems sound in theory, the actual empirical base is not conclusive. This is due largely to limited prospective research in applied sport settings, descriptive rather than explanatory research designs, use of behavioral assessments with questionable reliability and validity, infrequent integration and replication of field and laboratory research, and the possible adoption of inappropriate measurement models in some instances.

Furthermore, intervention strategies have been modeled after techniques designed for clinical nonsport populations, and it is theoretically unclear that a procedure that is effective in returning adaptive function to a normal behavioral and psychological range can be expected to facilitate performance in sport settings that impose extreme biological demands. It is also not known the degree to which changes can be effected for individuals already relatively skilled, confident, and nonanxious. Moreover, intervention effects have not typically been evaluated against a reliable stress or performance baseline. Applied sport research as yet cannot explain how an apparently successful intervention works or predict when or for whom it may work in the future. It is generally possible only to speculate about the stress and performance mediators actually responsible. When room for improved performance is present, various factors tied to an athlete's belief system can provide indirect alternative explanations that are equally as defensible as mechanisms purported to directly underlie the intervention. Although a generalized treatment effect can in itself offer a practical benefit, it is not one that is explainable or predictable in the individual case. In other words, stress management research supports what most informed coaches and athletes have learned by experience; stress correlates can impair and can enhance performance. Reliable effects of stress manipulations cannot, however, be assured at this point. Therefore, the appropriateness of available procedures rests largely on the intended purpose of the application and the willingness of the practitioner or consumer to accept the cost of risking misapplication in the individual case for benefits potentially available for the fictional average response. This can present a rather profound decision when a specific athlete's performance or well-being is of principal interest. On the other hand, procedures can also be innocuous.

Pragmatic issues inhibit applied stress management research, however. Randomization, manipulation, and effective placebo control comparisons are difficult to implement in naturalistic sport settings. Dynamic assessments are restricted by measurement technology, and in many instances applied sport science is limited by its inability to measure and describe sport performance and its context. Moreover, the sheer number of athletes in certain sports and levels of competition precludes screening and precision when implementing individualized interventions. These problems appear to have less potential when training stress is viewed in a chronic preventive framework. Diagnosis of a maladaptive response by monitoring psychometric mood shifts from a typical baseline appears to promise a more reliable and generalizable ergogenic adjunct.

On the basis of available evidence, stress management as an ergogenic aid must be regarded as an art that can be effective in qualified and skilled hands. However, its status as a generalizable science requires well conceived and controlled manipulation of stress and sport performance relationships such as those outlined. A decade ago, Martens (1972), in a related review of the ergogenic properties of anxiety, concluded, "We are a long way from knowing how to effectively use substances and phenomena for this purpose" (optimize "stress" for sport performance) (p. 63). This statement appears largely appropriate at the present as well. However, we seem to be substantially closer. Although not providing explanatory answers, the contemporary clinical or applied movement in stress management does appear to have helped define questions that may eventually provide a practical dividend. However, for application error to be reduced to the point that stress management can specify a nonrandom ergogenic advantage, rigorous research in both laboratory and field settings is necessary.

Reference Notes

1. Morgan, W.P. (Chair) *Sports psychology: Stress monitoring and management with athletes*. Symposium presented at the Pan American Congress and International Course on Sports Medicine and Exercise Science, Miami, Florida, May 23-26, 1981.
2. Suinn, R., Morton, M., & Brammell, H. *Psychological and mental training to increase efficiency in endurance athletes*. Technical report to Developmental Subcommittee, US Olympic Women's Athletics, 1980.
3. Jackson, C.W. *The relationship of swimming performance to measures of attentional and interpersonal style*. Paper presented at the annual meeting of the American Alliance for Health, Physical Education, Recreation and Dance, Boston, April, 1981.
4. Dishman, R.K. (Chair) *Overstress syndromes in sport and exercise*. Symposium presented at the annual meeting of the American College of Sports Medicine, Las Vegas, Nevada, May 28-30, 1980.
5. Bennett, B.K., & Hall, C. *Biofeedback training and archery performance*. Unpublished manuscript, University of Western Ontario, London, 1979.

References

ANDERSON, N. Algebraic models in perception. In E.C. Carterett & M.P. Friedman (Eds.), *Handbook of perception* (Vol. 2). New York: Academic Press, 1974. (a)

ANDERSON, N. Cognitive algebra. In L. Berkowitz (Ed.), *Advances in experimental social psychology* (Vol. 7). New York: Academic Press, 1974. (b)

ANDERSON, N., & Shanteau, J. Weak inference with linear models. *Psychological Bulletin*, 1977, **84**, 1155-1170.

ANTAL, L.C., & Good, C.S. The effects of oxprenolol on pistol shooting under stress. In R.W. Elsdon-Dew, C.A.S. Wink, & G.F.B. Birdwood (Eds.), *The cardiovascular, metabolic, and psychological interface*. London: Royal Society of Medicine and Academic Press, 1979.

ÅSTRAND, P-O., & Rodahl, K. *Textbook of work physiology: Physiological bases of exercise* (2nd ed.). New York: McGraw-Hill, 1977.

BALOG, L. The effects of exercise on muscle tension and subsequent muscle relaxation training. *Research Quarterly for Exercise and Sport*, in press.

BANDURA, A. Self-efficacy: Toward a unifying theory of behavioral change. *Psychological Review*, 1977, **84**, 191-215.

BARD, C., & Fleury, M. Analysis of visual search activity during sport problem situations. *Journal of Human Movement Studies*, 1976, **3**, 214-222.

BECK, A.T. Cognitive therapy: Nature and relation to behavior therapy. *Behavior Therapy*, 1970, **1**, 184-200.

BENNETT, B., & Stothart, C. The effects of a relaxation based cognitive technique on sport performances. In P. Klavora and K.A.W. Wipper (Eds.), *Psychological and sociological factors and sport*. Toronto: University of Toronto Press, 1980.

BENSON, H. *The relaxation response*. New York: William Morrow, 1975.

BLAIS, M. *EMG biofeedback for control over precompetitive anxiety within a laboratory controlled environment*. Unpublished master's thesis, University of Ottawa, 1978.

BLANCHARD, E., & Epstein, L. The clinical usefulness of biofeedback. In M. Hersen, R. Eisler, & P. Miller, *Progress in behavior modification* (Vol. 4). New York: Academic Press, 1977.

BORG, G. Subjective aspects of physical and mental load. *Ergonomics*, 1978, **21**, 215-220.

BORKOVEC, T.D. Physiological and cognitive processes in the regulation of anxiety. In G.E. Schwartz & D. Shapiro (Eds.), *Consciousness and self-regulation: Advances in research*. New York: Plenum, 1976.

BRAMWELL, S., Masuda, M., Wagner, N., & Holmes, T. Psychosocial factors in athletic injuries: Development and application of the social and athletic readjustment rating scale (SARRS). *Journal of Human Stress*, 1975, **1**, 6-20.

CAUDILL, D., Weinberg, R., Gould, D., & Jackson, A. The effects of the length of the psych-up interval on strength and endurance performance. *Psychology of Motor Behavior and Sport—1981* (Abstracts), NASPSA. Davis, CA: University of California, May 1981, p. 78.

CHANCE, J.P. The effects of thought stopping and covert assertion on performance of nine through eighteen year old swimmers (Doctoral dissertation, Mississippi State University, 1980). *Dissertation Abstracts International*, 1980, **41**(4-A), 3199.

CLIFF, N. Scaling. *Annual Review of Psychology*, 1973, **24**, 473-506.

DANIELS, F.S., & Landers, D.M. Biofeedback and shooting performance: A test of disregulation and systems theory. *Journal of Sports Psychology*, 1981, **4**, 271-282.

DANISH, S., & Hale, B. Toward an understanding of the practice of sport psychology. *Journal of Sport Psychology*, 1981, **3**, 90-99.

DAVIDSON, R.J. Specificity and patterning in biobehavioral systems: Implications for behavior change. *American Psychologist*, 1978, **33**, 431-436.

DECARIA, M.D. The effect of cognition rehearsal training on performance and on self-report of anxiety in novice and intermediate female gymnasts (Doctoral dissertation, University of Utah, 1977). *Dissertation Abstracts International*, 1977, **38**(1-B), 351.

DESIDERATO, O., & Miller, I. Improving tennis performance by cognitive behavior modification techniques. *The Behavior Therapist*, 1979, **2**, 19.

deVRIES, H.A. Immediate and long term effects of exercise upon resting muscle action potential. *Journal of Sports Medicine*, 1968, **8**, 1-11.

deVRIES, H.A., Wiswell, R., Bulbulian, R., & Moritani, T. Tranquilizer effect of exercise. *American Journal of Physical Medicine*, 1981, **60**, 57-66.

DE WITT, D. Cognitive and biofeedback training for stress reduction with university athletes. *Journal of Sport Psychology*, 1980, **2**, 288-294.

DISHMAN, R.K. Contemporary sport psychology. In R. Terjung (Ed.), *Exercise and sport sciences reviews* (Vol. 10). Philadelphia: Franklin Institute Press, 1982.

DORSEY, J.A. The effects of biofeedback-assisted desensitization training on state anxiety and performance of college age male gymnasts (Doctoral dissertation, Boston University, 1976). *Dissertation Abstracts International*, 1977, **37**(9-A), 5680.

DUFFY, E. Activation. In H. Greenfield & R. Sternbach (Eds.), *Handbook of psychophysiology*. New York: Holt, Rinehart and Winston, 1972.

DURLAK, J.A. Comparative effectiveness of paraprofessional and professional helpers. *Psychological Bulletin*, 1979, **86**, 80-92.

EKMAN, G., & Sjoberg, L. Scaling. *Annual Review of Psychology*, 1965, **16**, 451-474.

ELLIS, A. *Reason and emotion in psychotherapy*. New York: Stuart, 1962.

ETZEL, E.F., Jr. Validation of a conceptual model characterizing attention among international rifle shooters. *Journal of Sport Psychology*, 1979, **1**, 281-290.

EYSENCK, H.F. *The biological basis of personality*. Springfield, IL: Charles C. Thomas, 1967.

FARMER, P., Olewine, D., Comer, D., Edwards, M., Coleman, T., Thomas, G., & Hames, C. Frontalis muscle tension and occipital alpha production in young males with coronary prone (type A) and coronary resistant (type B) behavior patterns: Effects of exercise. *Medicine and Science in Sports*, 1978, **10**, 51.

FARRELL, P., Cates, W., Maksud, M., Morgan, W.P., & Tseng, L. Plasma beta-endorphin/beta lipotropin immunoreactivity increases after treadmill exercise in man. *Medicine and Science in Sports and Exercise*, 1981, **13**, 134.

FELTZ, D.L., Landers, D.M., & Raeder, U. Enhancing self-efficacy in high-avoidance motor tasks: A comparison of modeling techniques. *Journal of Sport Psychology*, 1979, **1**, 112-122.

FENZ, W.D., & Epstein, S. Changes in gradients of skin conductance, heart rate and respiration rate as a function of experience. *Psychosomatic Medicine*, 1967, **29**, 33-51.

FISHER, A.C. Thurstonian scaling: Application to sport psychology research. *Journal of Sport Psychology*, 1980, **2**, 155-160.

FRANKENHAUSER, M. Behavior and circulating catecholamines. *Brain Research*, 1971, **31**, 241-262.

FRENCH, S.N. Electromyographic biofeedback for tension control during fine and gross motor skill acquisition (Doctoral dissertation, Oregon State University, 1977). *Dissertation Abstracts International*, 1977, **37**(9-A), 5681.

GENOV, F. Peculiarity of the maximum motor speed of the sportsman when in mobilized readiness. In G.S. Kenyon (Ed.), *Contemporary psychology of sport*. Chicago: The Athletic Institute, 1970.

GERSON, R., & Deshaies, P. Competitive trait anxiety and performance as predictors of pre-competitive state anxiety. *International Journal of Sport Psychology*, 1978, **9**, 16-26.

GOULD, D., Weinberg, R., & Jackson, A. Mental preparation strategies, cognitions and strength performance. *Journal of Sport Psychology*, 1980, **2**, 329-339.

GOULD, D., & Weiss, M. The effects of model similarity and model talk on self-efficacy and muscular endurance. *Journal of Sport Psychology*, 1981, **3**, 17-29.

GRAVEL, R., Lemieux, G., & Ladouceur, R. Effectiveness of a cognitive behavioral treatment package for cross-country ski-racers. *Cognitive Therapy and Research*, 1980, **4**, 83-89.

GRIFFITHS, T.J., Steele, D.J., Vaccaro, P., & Karpman, M.B. The effects of relaxation techniques on anxiety and underwater performance. *International Journal of Sport Psychology*, 1981, **12**, 176-182.

GROSSBERG, J., & Grant, B. Clinical psychophysics: Applications of ratio scaling and signal detection methods to research on pain, fear, drugs and medical decision making. *Psychological Bulletin*, 1978, **85**, 1154-1176.

GUTMANN, M., Squires, R., Pollock, M., Foster, C., & Anholm, J. Perceived exertion-heart rate relationship during exercise testing and training in cardiac patients. *Journal of Cardiac Rehabilitation*, 1981, **1**, 52-59.

HAMM, H. Competitive anxiety: Assessment and prescriptions. In T. Orlick, J. Partington, & J. Salmela (Eds.), *Mental training for coaches and athletes*. Ottawa, Canada: The Coaching Association of Canada, 1982.

HANIN, Y. (Ed.). *Stress and anxiety in sport*. Moscow: Physical Culture and Sport Publishers, 1981.

HARRISON, R., & Feltz, D. The professionalization of sport psychology: Legal considerations. *Journal of Sport Psychology*, 1979, **1**, 182-190.

HIGHLEN, P.S., & Bennett, B.B. Psychological characteristics of successful and nonsuccessful elite wrestlers: An exploratory study. *Journal of Sport Psychology*, 1979, **1**, 123-137.

HORTON, A., & Shelton, J. The rational wrestler: A pilot study. *Perceptual and Motor Skills*, 1978, **46**, 882.

IKAI, M., & Steinhaus, A. Some factors modifying the expression of human strength. *Journal of Applied Physiology*, 1961, **16**, 157-161.

ISMAIL, A.H., & El-Naggar, A.M. Effect of exercise on multivariate relationships among selected psychophysiological variables in adult men. In J. Partington, T. Orlick, & J. Salmela (Eds.), *Sport in perspective*. Ottawa, Canada: The Coaching Association of Canada, 1982.

JACOBSON, E. *Progressive relaxation*. Chicago: University of Chicago Press, 1938.

JAREMKO, M. A component analysis of stress inoculation: Review and prospectus. *Cognitive Therapy and Research*, 1979, **3**, 35-48.

KAUSS, D. An investigation of psychological states related to the psycho-emotional readying procedures of competitive athletes. *International Journal of Sport Psychology*, 1978, **9**, 134-145.

KAZDIN, A. *Research design in clinical psychology*. New York: Harper and Row, 1980.

KENDALL, P.C., & Hollon, S.O. (Eds.). *Cognitive-behavioral interventions: Theory, research and procedures*. New York: Academic Press, 1979.

KIRSCHENBAUM, D., & Bale, R. Cognitive-behavioral skills in golf: Brain power golf. In R. Suinn (Ed.), *Psychology in sports: Methods and applications*. Minneapolis: Burgess, 1980.

KLAVORA, P. Customary arousal for peak athletic performance. In P. Klavora & J. Daniels, (Eds.), *Coach, athlete and the sport psychologist*. Champaign, IL: Human Kinetics, 1979.

KLAVORA, P., & Daniel, J. (Eds.). *Coach, athlete and the sport psychologist*, Champaign, IL: Human Kinetics, 1979.

KOLONAY, B. *The effects of visuo-motor behavior rehearsal on athletic performance.* Unpublished master's thesis, Hunter College, The City University of New York, 1977.

KROLL, W. Competitive athletic stress factors in athletes and coaches. In W. Sime & L. Zaichkowsky (Eds.), *Stress management in sport.* Reston, VA: AAHPERD Publications, 1982.

KUKLA, K.J. The effects of progressive relaxation training upon athletic performance during stress (Doctoral dissertation, Florida State University, 1976). *Dissertation Abstracts International*, 1977, **37**(12-B), 6392.

LACEY, J., & Lacey, B. Verification and extension of the principal of autonomic response-stereotypy. *American Journal of Psychology*, 1958, **71**, 50-73.

LANDERS, D.M. The arousal-performance relationship revisited. *Research Quarterly for Exercise and Sport*, 1980, **51**, 77-90.

LANDERS, D.M. Reflections on sport psychology and the Olympic athlete. In J. Seagrave & D. Chu (Eds.), *Olympism*. Champaign, IL: Human Kinetics, 1981.

LANDERS, D., Furst, D., & Daniels, F. Anxiety/attention and shooting ability: Testing the predictive validity of the Test of Attentional and Interpersonal Style (TAIS). *Psychology of Motor Behavior and Sport—1981* (Abstracts), NASPSA. Davis, CA: University of California, 1981.

LANGER, P. Varsity football performance. *Perceptual and Motor Skills*, 1966, **23**, 1191-1199.

LAYMAN, E.M. Meditation and sports performance. In W.F. Straub (Ed.), *Sport psychology*. Ithaca, NY: Mouvement, 1978.

LEWIS, S. A comparison of behavior-therapy techniques in the reduction of fearful avoidance behavior. *Behavior Therapy*, 1974, **5**, 648-655.

MAHONEY, M.J. Cognitive skills and athletic performance. In P.C. Kendall & S.D. Hollon (Eds.), *Cognitive-behavioral interventions: Theory, research and procedures*. New York: Academic Press, 1979.

MAHONEY, M.J., & Avener, M. Psychology of the elite athlete: An exploratory study. *Cognitive Therapy and Research*, 1977, **1**, 135-141.

MARTENS, R. Trait and state anxiety. In W.P. Morgan (Ed.), *Ergogenic aids and muscular performance*. New York: Academic Press, 1972.

MARTENS, R. Arousal and motor performance. In J.H. Wilmore (Ed.), *Exercise and sport science reviews* (Vol. 2). New York: Academic Press, 1974.

MARTENS, R. *Sport Competition Anxiety Test*. Champaign, IL: Human Kinetics, 1977.

MARTENS, R. How sport psychology can help Olympians. In J. Seagrave & D. Chu (Eds.), *Olympism*. Champaign, IL: Human Kinetics, 1981.

MCGEER, P.L., & McGeer, E.G. Chemistry of mood and emotion. *Annual Review of Psychology*, 1980, **31**, 273-307.

MEICHENBAUM, D.H. *Cognitive-behavior modification*. New York: Plenum, 1977.

MESSICK, S. Constructs and their vicissitudes in educational and psychological measurement. *Psychological Bulletin*, 1981, **89**, 575-588.

MEYERS, A.W., Cooke, C., Cullen, J., & Liles, L. Psychological aspects of athletic competitors: A replication across sports. *Cognitive Therapy and Research*, 1979, **3**, 361-366.

MEYERS, A.W., & Schleser, R. A cognitive behavioral intervention for improving basketball performance. *Journal of Sport Psychology*, 1980, **2**, 69-73.

MEYERS, A.W., Schleser, R., Cooke, C., & Cuvillier, C. Cognitive contributions to the development of gymnastic skills. *Cognitive Therapy and Research*, 1979, **3**, 75-85.

MEYERS, A.W., Schleser, R., & Okwumabua, T. A cognitive behavioral intervention for improving basketball performance. *Research Quarterly for Exercise and Sport*, 1982, **53**, 344-347.

MILLER, N. Biofeedback and visceral learning. *Annual Review of Psychology*, 1978, **29**, 373-404.

MORGAN, W.P. Pre-match anxiety in a group of college wrestlers. *International Journal of Sport Psychology*, 1970, **1**, 7-13.

MORGAN, W.P. Basic considerations. In W.P. Morgan (Ed.), *Ergogenic aids and muscular performance*. New York: Academic Press, 1972.

MORGAN, W.P. Prediction of performance in athletics. In P. Klavora & J.V. Daniel (Eds.), *Coach, athlete and the sport psychologist*. Champaign, IL: Human Kinetics, 1979.

MORGAN, W.P. Trait psychology controversy. *Research Quarterly for Exercise and Sport*, 1980, **51**, 50-76.

MORGAN, W.P. Psychological benefits of physical activity. In F.J. Nagle & H.J. Montoye (Eds.), *Exercise in health and disease*. Springfield, IL: Charles C. Thomas, 1981. (a)

MORGAN, W.P. Psychophysiology of self-awareness during vigorous physical activity. *Research Quarterly for Exercise and Sport*, 1981, **52**, 315-340. (b)

MORGAN, W.P., & Horstman, E.H. Psychometric correlates of pain perception. *Perceptual and Motor Skills*, 1978, **47**, 27-39.

MORGAN, W.P., Horstman, D.H., Cymerman, A., & Stokes, J. Facilitation of endurance performance by means of a cognitive strategy. *Cognitive therapy and research*, in press.

MORGAN, W.P., & Pollock, M.L. Psychologic characterization of the elite distance runner. *Annals of the New York Academy of Sciences*, 1977, **301**, 382-403.

NELSON, J. Investigation of effects of hypnosis, relaxation, and mental rehearsal on performance scores of golfers and runners (Doctoral dissertation, Louisiana State University and Agricultural and Mechanical College). *Dissertation Abstracts International*, 1980, **41**(4-B), 1484.

NIDEFFER, R.M. Test of attentional and interpersonal style. *Journal of Personality and Social Psychology*, 1976, **34**, 394-404.

NIDEFFER, R.M. *The ethics and practice of applied sport psychology*. Ithaca, NY: Mouvement, 1981.

NIDEFFER, R., Dufresne, P., Nesvig, D., & Selder, D. The future of applied sport psychology. *Journal of Sport Psychology*, 1980, **2**, 170-174.

NOEL, R.C. The effect of visuo-motor behavioral rehearsal on tennis performance. *Journal of Sport Psychology*, 1980, **2**, 221-226.

NUNNALLY, J. *Psychometric theory*, New York: McGraw-Hill, 1978.

ORNE, M., & Paskewitz, D. Aversive situational effects on alpha feed-back training. *Science*, 1974, **186**, 458-460.

PEELE, S. Reductionism in the psychology of the eighties: Can biochemistry eliminate addiction, mental illness and pain? *American Psychologist*, 1981, **36**, 807-818.

PINEL, J., & Schultz, T. Effect of antecedent muscle tension levels on motor behavior, *Medicine and Science in Sports*, 1978, **10**, 177-182.

POLLOCK, M., Jackson, A.J., & Pate, R. Discriminant analysis of physiological differences between good and elite distance runners. *Research Quarterly for Exercise and Sport*, 1980, **51**, 521-532.

RICHARDS, E.D., & Landers, D.M. Test of attentional and interpersonal style scores of shooters. In G.C. Roberts & D.M. Landers (Eds.), *Psychology of motor behavior and sport—1980*. Champaign, IL: Human Kinetics, 1981.

RUSHALL, B.S. Applied behavior analysis for sports and physical education. *International Journal of Sport Psychology*, 1975, **6**, 75-88.

RYAN, E.D., & Foster, R. Athletic participation and perceptual augmentation and reduction. *Journal of Personality and Social Psychology*, 1967, **6**, 472-476.

RYAN, E.D., & Kovacic, C.R. Pain tolerance and athletic participation. *Perceptual and Motor Skills*, 1966, **22**, 383-390.

SCANLAN, T.K., & Passer, M.W. Factors influencing the competitive performance expectancies of young female athletes. *Journal of Sport Psychology*, 1979, **1**, 212-220.

SCHULTZ, J.H., & Luthe, W. *Autogenic training: A psychophysiological approach in psychotherapy*. New York: Grune and Stratton, 1959.

SCHWARTZ, G.E., Davidson, R.J., & Goleman, D. Patterning of cognitive and somatic processes in the self-regulation of anxiety: Effects of meditation versus exercise. *Psychosomatic Medicine*, 1978, **40**, 321-328.

SELYE, H. *The stress of life*, New York: McGraw-Hill, 1976.

SHELTON, T.O., & Mahoney, M.J. The content and effect of "psyching-up" strategies in weight lifters. *Cognitive Therapy and Research*, 1978, **2**, 275-284.

SILVA, J.M. Behavioral and situational factors affecting concentration. *Journal of Sport Psychology*, 1979, **1**, 221-227.

SIME, W.E. A comparison of exercise and meditation in reducing physiological response to stress. *Medicine and Science in Sports*, 1977, **9**, 55.

SIME, W., & Zaichkowsky, L. (Eds.). *Stress management in sport*. Reston, VA: AAHPERD Publications, 1982.

SJOBERG, L., Svensson, E., & Persson, L.O. The measurement of mood. *Scandinavian Journal of Psychology*, 1979, **20**, 1-18.

SMITH, R.E. A cognitive-affective approach to stress management training for athletes. In C. Nadeau, W. Halliwell, K. Newell, & G.C. Roberts (Eds.), *Psychology of Motor Behavior and Sport—1979*. Champaign, IL: Human Kinetics, 1980.

STEVENS, S.S. *Psychophysics*. New York: Wiley & Sons, 1975.

SUINN, R. Behavior rehearsal training for ski racers. *Behavior Therapy*, 1972, **3**, 519-520.

SUINN, R. Stress management for elite athletes. In Y. Hanin (Ed.), *Stress and anxiety in sport*. Moscow: Physical Culture and Sport Publishers, 1981.

SUINN, R. Imagery and sports. In A. Sheikh (Ed.), *Imagery: Current theory, research and application*. New York: Wiley and Sons, 1982.

SUINN, R., & Deffenbacher, J. The behavioral approach. In I. Kutash & L. Schlesinger (Eds.), *Handbook on stress and anxiety: Contemporary knowledge, theory and treatment*. San Francisco: Jossey-Bass, 1980.

TARTER-BENLOLO, L. The role of relaxation in biofeedback training: A critical review of literature. *Psychological Bulletin*, 1978, **85**, 727-755.

TEAGUE, M.L. A combined systematic desensitization and electromyographic biofeedback technique for controlling state anxiety and improving gross motor skill performance (Doctoral dissertation, University of Northern Colorado, 1976). *Dissertation Abstracts International*, 1977, **37-04**, 2062-A.

TITLEY, R. The loneliness of a long distance kicker. *The Athletic Journal*, 1976, **57**, 74-80.

TSUKAMOTO, S. *The effects of EMG biofeedback-assisted relaxation as a self-control strategy for sport competition anxiety*. Unpublished master's thesis, University of Western Ontario, London, Ontario, 1979.

VANEK, M., & Cratty, B.J. *Psychology and the superior athlete*. New York: Macmillan, 1970.

VAN SCHOYCK, S., & Grasha, A.F. Attentional style variations and athletic ability: The advantages of a sports-specific test. *Journal of Sport Psychology*, 1981, **3**, 149-165.

WEINBERG, R.S. The effects of success and failure on the patterning of neuromuscular energy. *Journal of Motor Behavior*, 1978, **10**, 53-61.

WEINBERG, R.S., & Genuchi, M. Relationship between competitive trait anxiety, state anxiety and golf performance: A field study. *Journal of Sport Psychology*, 1980, **2**, 148-154.

WEINBERG, R.S., Gould, D., & Jackson, A.W. Expectations and performance: An empirical test of Bandura's self-efficacy theory. *Journal of Sport Psychology*, 1979, **1**, 320-331.

WEINBERG, R.S., Gould, D., & Jackson, A.W. Cognition and motor performance: Effect of psyching-up strategies on three motor tasks. *Cognitive Therapy and Research*, 1980, **4**, 239-246.

WEINBERG, R.S., Gould, D., & Jackson, A.W. Relationship between the duration of the psych-up interval and strength performance. *Journal of Sport Psychology*, 1981, **3**, 166-170.

WEINBERG, R.S., & Ragan, J. Motor performance under three levels of trait anxiety and stress. *Journal of Motor Behavior*, 1978, **10**, 169-176.

WEINBERG, R.S., Seabourne, T., & Jackson, A.W. Effects of visuo-motor behavior rehearsal, relaxation and imagery on karate performance. *Journal of Sport Psychology*, 1981, **3**, 228-238.

WEINBERG, R.S., Yukelson, D., & Jackson, A.W. Effect of public and private efficacy expectations on competitive performance. *Journal of Sport Psychology*, 1980, **2**, 340-349.

WEINGARTEN, P. Leistungsverhalten jugendlicher Sportler (unter Berucksichtigung der Ergopsychometrie). Wien: Forschungsauftrag des BMFUK, 1980.

WOLPE, J. *Psychotherapy for reciprocal inhibition*. Stanford: Stanford University Press, 1958.

WOLPE, J. The dichotomy between classical conditioned and cognitively learned anxiety. *Journal of Behavior Therapy and Experimental Psychiatry*, 1981, **12**, 35-42.

ZAICHKOWSKY, L. Biofeedback for self-regulation of stress. In W. Sime & L. Zaichkowsky (Eds.), *Stress management in sport*. Reston, VA: AAHPERD Publications, 1982.

ZAICHKOWSKY, L., Jackson, C., & Aronson, R. Attentional and interpersonal factors as predictors of elite athletic performance. In T. Orlick, J. Partington, & J. Salmela (Eds.), *Mental training for coaches and athletes*. Ottawa, Canada: The Coaching Association of Canada, 1982.

ZAJONC, R. Feeling and thinking: Preferences need no inferences. *American Psychologist*, 1980, **35**, 151-175.

ZIEGLER, S. The application of stress management to sport. In W. Sime & L. Zaichkowsky (Eds.), *Stress management in sport*. Reston, VA: AAHPERD Publications, 1982.

ZUCKERMAN, M., Buchsbaum, M., & Murphy, D. Sensation seeking and its biological correlates. *Psychological Bulletin*, 1980, **88**, 187-214.

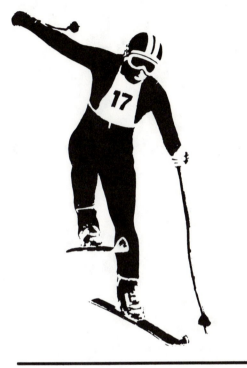

Part 5
Mechanical
Ergogenic Aids

12

Extrinsic Biomechanical Aids

Edward C. Frederick

Many of the constraints on human performance are purely mechanical. Such things as body mass, air resistance, and gravity impose innate limits on performance. In fact, these and other mechanical constraints are so innate that we seldom think of them as being subject to improvement. Many ergogenic aids, however, are biomechanical in nature. They can be divided into two categories: intrinsic and extrinsic.

Intrinsic biomechanical aids improve performance by optimizing body mechanics. For example, changes in body position can significantly influence air resistance in downhill skiing and bicycling, or subtle changes in style can affect the critical transfer of mechanical energy between body segments in high jumping or pole vaulting. This approach to improving performance by using biomechanics to alter intrinsic mechanical constraints is discussed in detail in several excellent texts (e.g., Broer & Zernicke, 1979; Dyson, 1977; Hay, 1978) and so will receive no attention here.

The major concern of this review is extrinsic biomechanical aids to performance. In its broadest definition, an extrinsic biomechani-

Edward C. Frederick, Ph.D., is with NIKE Sports Research Laboratory in Exeter, New Hampshire.

cal aid is anything external to the body that improves performance by favorably altering the influence of a mechanical constraint on performance. Mechanical constraints can be affected by such things as the design of an implement or article of clothing, or the surface on which the activity is performed. Even the selection of the physical environment in which an activity is performed can constitute an ergogenic aid, if the environment is selected to reduce the influence of a mechanical constraint such as air resistance or gravity.

With this definition as a guide, the following review briefly outlines extrinsic mechanical constraints on performance and then looks at examples of how various implements, articles of clothing, and playing surfaces are designed to overcome these constraints and to improve performance.

Theoretical Considerations: Mechanical Constraints on Performance

The physical environment imposes a myriad of limits on human movement. These limits, coupled with the characteristic movements of various sports, produce mechanical constraints on the level of performance that can be attained. The following is a partial list of mechanical constraints on performance:

Forces
- Gravity
- Friction
- Centripetal

Aerodynamics
- Magnus effect
- Lift
- Air resistance

Hydrodynamics
- Water resistance

Even though this list includes most of the major mechanical constraints on performance, it is by no means a complete listing. It includes only those items with which this review is concerned. Most of these constraints will be explained as they are introduced in the discussion, but a few are discussed in this section either because the potential benefits that result from overcoming these constraints are primarily theoretical or they need a more thorough introduction.

Gravitational force, according to Newton, is directly proportional to the product of two interacting masses and inversely proportional to the square of the distance between them.

$$F_g \propto m_1 \cdot m_2/d^2$$

This gravitational force provides a constraining influence on every type of sport in which humans engage; that will continue to be the case until humans begin playing sports in the zero gravity of space. The influence of gravity is exerted directly on the body and on the various implements used in sport and indirectly as a component of most of the other constraints listed above.

Although the acceleration due to gravity is essentially constant in the temperate latitudes, where most sporting events occur, it varies to a slight but potentially significant extent with latitude and to a lesser, negligible degree with altitude above sea level.

Because the acceleration due to gravity (g) is inversely proportional to the square of the distance between interacting masses and because the distance from the center of the earth is about 13 miles greater at the equator than at the poles, g is lower at the equator than it is at higher latitudes:

Latitude	g, in m $\cdot$ sec^{-2}
90° (North Pole)	9.832
60° (e.g., Oslo)	9.819
45° (e.g., Minneapolis)	9.806
0° (equator)	9.780

This difference in g means that work done against gravity such as throwing a shot or jumping would be less at the equator than at high latitudes. For example, if we assume that all but a negligible portion of the work done in putting the shot is work against gravity, then that work would be about 0.4% less at the equator than at the moderately high latitude of 60°. This reduction in g alone would allow a 16-pound shot thrown 21 m in Oslo to travel an additional 8 cm if it were thrown in Nairobi or Quito near the equator. Most scientists might consider such a small percentage improvement insignificant, but world records in the shot put have been improved by as little as 2 cm. This means that the selection of a low latitude as the site of certain athletic competitions can be an aid to performance.

Overcoming air resistance is a major source of energy expenditure in many sports, particularly in skiing, speed skating, and cycling, where high velocities are reached. The importance of velocity as a factor in determining air resistance is emphasized by the fact that air resistance is proportional to velocity cubed (Pugh, 1971).

There is little an athlete can do to overcome the exponential effect of velocity on air resistance short of slowing down. But another important factor in the air resistance equation, namely, air density, can be reduced by selecting appropriate conditions and a high altitude location for competition.

Air resistance or drag (*D*), a similar measure of the force exerted by the air on a moving body, is a function of a drag coefficient (C_D), the density of the air (*d*), the wind velocity (*v*), and the projected area of the body (*Ap*).

$$D \propto C_D \cdot d \cdot Ap \cdot v^2$$

Athletes can adjust body position to reduce *Ap* and, as will be discussed later, they can use streamlining to reduce C_D. Velocity normally cannot be reduced without having an adverse effect on performance, so that leaves *d*, the density of the air.

At sea level and under normal climatic conditions, air density is about 1.22 kg/m^3. At an altitude of 2,000 m, that value is reduced to 1.00 kg/m^3. This constitutes a decrease of 18%, and if all other factors were unchanged, this would mean an 18% decrease in drag. In sports activities where the majority of energy expenditure is allocated to overcoming air resistance, this can have a significant effect on performance.

It is argued that the many world record performances achieved in the 1968 Olympic Games were due in large part to the reduced air density at the altitude of Mexico City (2,206 m), where the games were held. One author has even proposed a time penalty for "altitude aided" sprint marks. Nelson (1979) has proposed adjusting the race times of sprinters by assessing a penalty based on the altitude at which the race was run. For example, the penalty for running 100 m at the altitude of Mexico City would be 0.17 seconds. Nelson bases this adjustment on unspecified sources, but the number seems to be a reasonable approximation.

If air density, and thus drag, are reduced by 18% at a 2,000-m altitude and if, as Pugh (1971) has determined, about 13% of power is being expended to overcome air resistance in sprinting, then speed should increase 2.3%. When assessing a penalty for the increased drag due to increasing speed, the actual improvement in race time should be near 2%, or about 0.2 sec in a 100-m dash.

Altitude is not the only factor that influences air density; higher temperature and, to a lesser extent, humidity can also reduce air density. Air density at 20° C is 1.205 kg/m^3 and 1.128 kg/m^3 at 40° C. Dry air at 30° C and 760 mmHg atmospheric pressure has a density of 1.165 kg/m^3. If air were completely saturated with water vapor, density would be lowered to 1.146 kg/m^3, much less of an effect than either altitude or temperature.

Selecting a high altitude location in conjunction with appropriate climatic conditions can have an appreciable effect on performance in sprint running and proportionately greater effects in events like speed skating or cycling, where drag effects are even greater.

Clothing

A custom-fitted wind suit similar to those used by speed skaters has been worn recently by a U.S. champion female sprinter, presumably to lower the drag encountered in a race. Can such a suit provide significant benefit in sprint running, where top speeds are much lower than they are in speed skating? Despite the lower running speeds in sprinting, there may be a marginal advantage to wearing a drag-minimizing suit, particularly when there is a head wind.

According to Pugh (1971), 13.6% of a sprinter's total energy cost is expended to overcome air resistance while running at 10 m/sec through still air.[1] Running into a head wind increases that cost of overcoming air resistance exponentially. For example, according to Pugh's data, a runner sprinting at 10 m/sec in still air uses the equivalent of 1.7 LO$_2$/min to overcome air resistance, whereas the same runner sprinting at 10 m/sec into a 5 m/sec headwind would use an estimated 3.8 LO$_2$/min to overcome air resistance, an increase of more than 120%.

Considering the high energy cost of overcoming air resistance while running into a headwind, wearing a tight-fitting suit may well have a significant effect on performance. Both form drag and surface drag would be reduced by wearing such a garment rather than the loose fitting singlet and shorts normally worn. Loose garments can increase the projected area of the body by as much as 30% in racing cyclists; a proportional increase in form drag results (Nonweiler, Note 1). It is presumed that similar increases in projected area would occur in sprint running.

---

[1]According to Pugh (1971), under standard conditions and at sea level the O$_2$ cost of overcoming air resistance in LO$_2$/min can be estimated by VO$_2$ = 0.00757v^2 for a runner traveling at 4.47 m/sec. In this equation, v is the relative velocity with respect to the air. The quantity v would be equal to running speed plus head wind speed when running into a wind. The constant 0.00757 was adjusted to 0.0169 to make the equation appropriate for a running speed of 10 m/sec, resulting in the new equation $\dot{V}O_2$ = 0.0169v^2. At 10 m/sec running in still air, $\dot{V}O_2$ = 1.7 LO$_2$/min [0.0169(10)^2]. At the same speed with a 5 m/sec headwind $\dot{V}O_2$ = 3.8 LO$_2$/min [0.0169(15)^2].

The surface drag should also be increased. The flapping of loose clothing and the hair projecting from the scalp, normally covered in a speed skating suit, should produce considerably greater turbulence and a concomitant increase in surface drag.

The actual potential for improvement resulting from wearing a wind suit for sprint running is difficult to estimate because the actual reduction in drag that occurs has never been measured. Given a few assumptions, however, we can attempt a crude estimation of such a potential for improvemement.

Raine (1970) measured the effect that clothing has on the surface drag of skiers in a wind tunnel. At wind speeds of 80 km/hour (22.2 m/sec) Raine was able to show that the increased surface drag produced by large boot buckles alone would add 0.03 seconds per minute to a downhill racer's performance. This time decrement would be proportional to speed squared, so if speed were reduced to 15 m/sec (10 m/sec sprint plus 5 m/sec headwind), the speed decrement would be reduced to 0.014 seconds/minute. In a 10-second, 100-meter race, the time loss produced by an equivalent increase in surface drag to that produced by the skiers in the Raine study would be 0.002 seconds. Considering that the added surface drag produced by loose clothing and a thick head of hair would certainly be several times that produced by ski boot buckles alone, it seems likely that the actual time lost in a 100-meter race might be as much as .01-.02 seconds, a significant amount of time in an event that is often won by that small a margin.

The additional time decrement caused by an increase in projected area and hence an increase in form drag should be directly proportional to the increased energy required to overcome air resistance. For example, an athlete with a projected area of 0.5 m^2 who wears clothing that expands the projected area 10% or 0.05 m^2 should suffer a 10% increase in the time decrement caused by overcoming air resistance. There is no accurate way to estimate what this loss in race time might be, but it is likely to be even larger than that caused by increased surface drag, because form drag is regarded as the more detrimental.

Except for studies by Raine (1970) on the effects of ski boot buckles on drag, any appreciable effect of shoes on performance has been largely ignored. Spiked or cleated shoes have been used for many years because of the added traction they provide, but nothing has been published on how well they work. The other features of athletic shoes have received a small measure of attention.

The weight of a shoe alone can significantly affect running economy and, by inference, performance as well. Adding weight to the feet increases the amount of work that must be performed as they are lifted and accelerated forward in each stride cycle. Running at a speed of 4.5 m/sec (6-minute mile pace) for example, each foot undergoes roughly 90 cycles/minute where it is lifted more than a half meter, accelerated to more than twice the average velocity of the body, and then decelerated to zero velocity again. Choosing values for the average horizontal velocity of the foot of 6.5 m/sec at this speed and for average vertical displacement of the foot of 0.6 meters, it is possible to calculate the theoretical increase in energy expenditure while running at 4.5 m/sec caused by adding weight to the feet. These values for horizontal velocity and vertical displacement were measured from high speed film taken of a typical subject running at the prescribed speed.

The additional work done in lifting 0.100 kg added to each foot is computed as follows:

$$dW = dm \cdot g \cdot h,$$

where dW is the additional work done in joules, dm is the additional mass in kg added to each foot, g is the acceleration due to gravity (9.8 m $\cdot$ sec^{-2}) and h is the height to which the foot is lifted in meters.

Using the values mentioned above,

$$dW = (0.1)(9.8)(0.6) = 0.588 \text{ joules/stride cycle/foot.}$$

For both feet and for the 90 cycles occurring in each minute the result would be:

$$(2)(90)(0.588) = 52.9 \text{ joules/minute.}$$

The additional work done in accelerating the foot forward in each stride cycle is calculated using:

$$dW = \tfrac{1}{2} dM \cdot v_f^2,$$

where v_f is the average velocity of the foot in meters/second. Using the values mentioned above,

$$dW = \frac{(0.1)(6.5)^2}{2} = 2.11 \text{ joules/cycle.}$$

Again, computing the additional work/minute for both feet:

$$(2)(90)(2.11) = 379.8 \text{ joules/minute.}$$

The total increase in work due to the heavier shoes is

$$52.9 + 379.8 = 432.7 \text{ joules/minute.}$$

Assuming an apparent efficiency of 0.5, the theoretical additional energy expended would be 865.4 joules/minute. Converting to calories, the value becomes 206.8 calories/minute. At a speed of 4.5 m/sec, total energy expenditure would be about 17 Kcal/minute. This puts the additional energy cost of carrying 0.1 kg on each foot at about 1.2% of total energy expenditure. This is a small but potentially significant difference.

These theoretical values are close to actual measurements. Catlin and Dressendorfer (1979) compared the energy utilization of runners wearing two different models of shoe, one model with an average weight of 0.87 kg per pair and the other 0.52 kg per pair. There was a statistically significant difference between the energy demands of running in the two models. Mean energy cost was 0.51 Kcal/minute higher while wearing the heavier shoe. The difference between the two models was equivalent to 3.3% of the total energy expenditure. Theory predicts a difference of 2.1% when the estimate of 1.2% given above is adjusted for the greater difference in weight of the shoes in the Catlin and Dressendorfer study.

These results mean that an average runner who would normally run in the heavier model would be able to run as much as 3.3% faster in the lighter model with the same physiological effort. This difference is certainly significant. All else being equal, it should account for several minutes in race time in longer races such as the marathon.

In addition to the advantage of wearing shoes which are light in weight, athletes may also benefit from shoes with appropriate mechanical characteristics. Frederick, Howley, and Powers (1980) compared the oxygen cost of running in two shoes: a conventional training flat with an ethyl vinyl acetate foam midsole and a training flat of similar weight but constructed with a highly resilient inflated air-soled type of midsole. The air-soled type of midsole is similar in appearance to a small air mattress; it is inflated with a pressurized gas and encapsulated in a polymeric foam.

Subjects in this study were asked to run three trials in each type of shoe while oxygen uptake was measured. The subjects ran at speeds that corresponded to their marathon race pace (average speed was 245 m/min; range, 215-273 m/min) and all data were normalized to units of oxygen cost (ml O_2/kg/km).

The mean oxygen cost was 205.7 ml O_2/kg/km in the conventional shoe and 200.0 in the air-soled shoe. This difference of 2.8%

was statistically significant ($p < .001$) and it represents a physiologically significant ergogenic effect as well.

All other factors being held constant, a 2.8% average improvement in running economy should allow the average subject to increase running speed by 2.8% using the same physiological effort. This should result in 2.8% reduction in race time, and in longer distance races such as the marathon this can mean improvements of several minutes. Of course, the shoes used in this study were heavy training shoes (mean wt/pair 678 g) and their extra weight would cancel out any benefits they might offer if they were compared to a lightweight racing shoe (see Catlin & Dressendorfer, 1979).

Because both types of shoe used in the above comparison were heavy training shoes and the subjects were well trained but not elite runners, the question was raised whether the same advantages to running economy would be found with elite-class athletes running at much faster racing speeds. This question was answered by Frederick, Sharkey, and Larsen (Note 2) in a study of seven elite runners. Six of the seven were marathoners with personal bests of under 2 hours, 13 minutes. The seventh is the holder of two American records and championships for distance road races.

While running at 322 m/min (5 min/mile pace), these subjects used an average of 62.5 ml O_2/kg/minute while running in a lightweight racing shoe (average 320 g/pair) and 61.7 ml O_2/kg/min in a heavier but air-soled prototype racing shoe (average 455 g/pair). This 1.3% difference was significant ($p < .05$) largely due to the remarkable repeatability of measurements made on these exceptional subjects. An example of this repeatability is shown in Table 1. The

Table 1
Oxygen Uptake Measurements (ml O_2/kg/min) for an Elite Class Marathoner Running at 322 m/min in an Air-soled vs. a Lighter, Conventionally Soled Shoe

Air-soled	Conventionally Soled
60.7	62.3
60.8	62.1
60.8	61.8
	62.1
x = 60.8	x = 62.1

Subject: m-2: wt = 71.4 kg: Ht = 1.92 m. Weight of air shoe = 467 g/pr. Weight of conventional shoe = 331 g/pr.

measurements were made in a staggered sequence in both morning and afternoon sessions on 2 days.

These results show a smaller difference between air-soled and non-air-soled shoes than was shown in the previously cited study, but at least part of this discrepancy can be explained by the greater weight of the air-soled shoes. Extrapolating from the data of Catlin and Dressendorfer (1979), a 120-g/pair difference in shoe weight should produce a 1.1% difference in oxygen uptake. Adding this to the existing difference between air-soled and non-air-soled racing shoes would result in a 2.4% difference if the shoes were of equal weight, quite close to the 2.8% difference found by Frederick, Howley, and Powers (1980).

Recent studies by Daniels, Larsen, Frederick, and Scardina (Note 3) have shown a statistically significant 1.6% difference between a production, air-soled racing shoe and a special control shoe that was identical to the air-soled shoe except for the substitution of a standard polymeric foam midsole for the air sole. This study answered a criticism of the design of earlier experiments, namely, that the other variables in the design of the shoe besides the midsole composition were not being controlled. The results of these experiments have laid to rest those criticisms and have raised an interesting question about the relationship between speed and the ergogenic effect of air-soled shoes.

In this experiment Daniels et al. took their measurements at four different speeds: two speeds that were used by all subjects—230 m/minute (7:00/mile pace) and 268 m/min (6:00/mile pace)—and two speeds that were near each subject's average training pace and 10,000-meter race pace. The data revealed a significant difference ($p < .01$) between shoes only at speeds near 268 m/minute. At the faster or slower speeds significance was no longer found.

This is a somewhat contradictory finding because significant differences were found at 322 m/min and at an average speed for all subjects of 245 m/min in previous comparisons with other air-soled shoes (Frederick, Howley, & Powers, 1980; Frederick, Sharkey, & Larsen, Note 2). One explanation is that the air-soled shoes used in these three studies each differed in weight, design of the air sole, and the pressure to which the air sole was inflated. This explanation implies that there may have been some coincidental "tuning" of the shoes for particular speeds.

Another explanation is that in each case the speed at which significance was found was near the subjects' marathon race pace, a speed at which they can most easily take advantage of whatever mechanical aid the shoe is providing.

Implements

In the 1950s much attention was paid to the development of javelins that were more aerodynamic in design. These aerodynamic javelins were thought to be responsible for at least part of the rapid improvement in the world record in the javelin event during that time. New regulations have changed the design of the modern javelin from that of the "aerodynamic javelin" of the 1950s, but many of the design features, such as improved surface characteristics and variations in the center of mass, have been retained. Terauds (1974) has estimated, using wind tunnel measurements, that the improved flight characteristics of modern javelins result in a gain of 35 feet or more in the distance of the throw.

The hydrodynamics of the vessels used in rowing competition can have a pronounced effect on performance. Wellicome (1967) has produced data to show that a 1-pound increase in water resistance to a racing shell means a half length in a race over 2,000 meters, and a roughening of the surface of the shell can cost as much as three lengths in a race over the same distance. His data show that the ratio between hull length and beam width can influence water resistance by as much as 12 pounds when comparing possible shell dimensions. Obviously the selection of an appropriately designed racing shell can have a powerful effect on performance.

A given force applied to a golf ball by a driver can produce considerably different results depending on the design of the ball. In fact, the dimples on a golf ball alone account for as much as 75% of the length of a drive (Bade, 1952), and other design features result in additional improvements in the flight characteristics of a golf ball. The historical evolution of the golf ball's design helps demonstrate the mechanical advantages incorporated in the design of the modern ball. The first balls were made of carved boxwood and, due to their poor coefficient of restitution, they did not fly very far. The first major improvement was in the production of the "featherie," a hard leather ball densely packed with feathers, which, due primarily to its greater coefficient of restitution, could be driven much farther than its boxwood predecessor. The next generation of golf balls were made of gutta-percha, a hard rubbery resin that was first molded with a smooth surface. It was soon discovered that when these new balls were nicked they traveled farther, and before long the nicks were being molded into the balls (Chase, 1981). Nicks or dents in the skin of the ball tend to hold a layer of air next to the ball as it spins through the air. This layer of air has the effect of enhancing the Magnus effect and increasing lift, thereby extending the flight of the ball.

In modern golf balls, which consist of a core of rubber with rubber tread wound about it and a hard plastic cover, the nicks have given way to usually round dimples that sometimes vary in shape and depth. Studies of the effect of the depth of the dimples on the length of the drive have been summarized by Bade (1952). Table 2 contains some of these data, and the results are quite surprising. Increasing the depth of the dimple from 0.002 inches to 0.010 inches increases the flight distance by 121 yards, but making the dimple deeper than 0.010 inches seems to have a negative effect.

Recent designs have taken into account the data on optimum dimple depth and added to it the variables of dimple shape and alignment, presumably to further enhance lift. Pie-shaped, hexagonal, and even a nipple-within-a-dimple design have been introduced with claims of greater driving length. One new design has caused a stir because it seems to cure most of the hook and slice problems that plague some players. The USGA is so convinced it works that they have changed their rules on ball design to make this new ball, the "Polara," illegal. The Polara, or as it is commonly known, the "Happy Non-Hooker," works by producing a gyroscopic effect that stabilizes the ball in flight. Deeper dimples are found in a band around the equivalent of the ball's meridian. The ball is teed up with the band of deeper dimples oriented vertically and in the direction of the drive. As the ball is driven the normal backspin produces a thicker band of air over the dimpled meridian than at its equator, and the resulting gyroscopic effect maintains the ball in a straighter course. According to one of its inventors, it can reduce a curved shot by as much as 75% (Chase, 1981), but as yet no carefully controlled studies of this new design have been reported.

Table 2
Depth of Dimples on Golf Balls,
Flight Distance, and Total Length of Drive

Depth of dimple (in)	Flight distance (yd)	Total length of drive (yd)
.002	117	146
.004	187	212
.006	212	232
.008	223	238
.010	238	261
.012	225	240

Note: Data from Bade, 1952.

The design of golf clubs can also have a significant effect on the flight of the ball. The upward tilt and texture of the club face produces a backspin of as much as 8,000 rpm, which causes lift on the ball because of the Magnus effect. That is, the top surface of the ball is moving slower, relative to the wind, than the bottom surface; this produces a negative pressure above and positive pressure below, imparting lift to the ball. Backspin alone can increase the distance of a drive by as much as 80 feet (Chase, 1981).

The Dunlop Sports Company has published an extensive study of the effectiveness of various design features of golf clubs (Note 4). By redesigning the shaft and club head to reduce the twisting movements about the shaft, they were able to produce an average of 2% greater distance with a three iron and greater consistency in length.

Soong (1973) has published a fascinating analysis of the geometry of archery. Using a series of nonlinear equations resulting from the minimization of total strain energy, he was able to come up with theoretically optimum values for the initial curvature of the bow, its stiffness distribution, its centerline length, the length of the bow handle, and the optimum length of the bow string. Soong's recommended bow geometry should maximize the terminal velocity of the arrow for a given draw force and bow opening produced by an archer, and he proposes using a computer program based on his calculations to custom-fit archers with optimum bows for their particular maximum draw force and adjust the opening length of the bow for each archer's physical limitations.

From 1940 to 1962 the world record for the pole vault improved only 9¼ inches. In the 20 years since 1962 the improvement has been over 3 feet, largely due to the introduction of the fiberglass vaulting pole. The obvious ergogenic effect provided by the fiberglass pole is due to two biomechanical advantages: greater conversion of kinetic to potential energy and the possibility of a higher grip on the pole. According to Dillman and Nelson (1968) as much as half of the kinetic energy developed during the run can be stored in the bending of the pole and recovered for conversion into potential energy at the most appropriate times during the vault. As Hay (1978) has pointed out, the greater bend of the fiberglass pole also allows the vaulter to grip the pole much higher than was possible with earlier poles. This is an important factor in determining vault height.

Whitt and Wilson (1974) have reviewed the many ergogenic aids produced by modifying the design of bicycles, so that discussion need not be repeated here.

Playing Surfaces

Centripetal and centrifugal forces come into play when rotational movements are used. This includes running or cycling around an oval as well as the various spinning movements used in other sports movements, such as the hammer and discus throws. Centripetal force acts toward the axis of the rotation; centrifugal force acts in the opposite direction, away from the axis of rotation. In the example of the hammer throw, the spinning thrower is applying a centripetal force to the hammer and the spinning hammer is exerting an equal and opposite centrifugal force on the athlete.

We will be primarily concerned with the effect of the design of oval tracks on the force required to keep a runner moving in a circular path. This force depends on the mass (m) and the velocity (v) of the runner and the radius (r) of the motion:

$$F_c = mv^2/r$$

The allocation of muscular force to the production of the force needed to keep the runner traveling in an arc reduces speed. It has been estimated, by comparing times for a 200-m race on the straightaway with the same race with the usual one turn, that 0.4 seconds or 2% is added to total time as a consequence of negotiating the turn.

The runner uses the surface of the track to provide the centripetal force needed to run in an arc. This force, which is primarily frictional, pushes sideways against the feet towards the center of the track. To prevent this force from knocking their feet out from under them, runners lean into the turn. Banked turns reduce the need for this sideways force because a tilted surface can push more in line with the center of mass of the athlete's body. Indoor tracks are frequently banked, although seldom to an adequate degree, and outdoor tracks are rarely banked.

This lack of banking on outdoor tracks and the fact that the radius of the curve varies with the lane result in an apparent discrepancy in sprint race performances when athletes are forced to run in lanes around a curve. Jain (1980) has produced calculations to show that an athlete running a 200-meter race in the tighter-radius, inside lane suffers a 0.069-second penalty in a 20.0-second race over an opponent who runs in the wider-radius, outside lane. To overcome this discrepancy, Jain suggests changing the dimensions of the track to allow each runner to run a different distance proportional to the radius of the turn.

Greene and McMahon (1979) have proposed a solution to another basic problem inherent in running in a closed circuit, that is, what is the optimum shape of such a circuit? Citing a series of simple experiments in which subjects were asked to run along a straight track and then around arcs varying in radius, they came to the surprising conclusion that tracks should be circular in shape rather than a combination of straightaways and curves. The reason is that the decrement in total running speed that occurs when running two tight curves along with two straightaways is greater than the decrement incurred when running one large circle with a more gradual radius. Greene and McMahon estimate that total running speed would be 3% faster on the circular track.

McMahon (Note 5) has also suggested that to minimize the perturbing forces on the foot necessary to negotiate turns with a minimum loss of speed the banking angle of turns of a track should approximate arctan (v^2/gr). Using a top speed of 8.9 m/sec (average speed for a 45-second 400 meters) and a radius of 13 meters, a reasonable radius for an indoor track, this equation suggests a nearly 32° banking of the turns. Of course, that angle would be much less for slower speeds, e.g., 20° for 6.7 m/sec (4-minute-mile speed) and much greater for smaller radii. Perhaps in the future we will see hydraulically controlled banking of the turns of running tracks with the precise angle determined by the radius and running speed.

McMahon and Greene have also proposed that not only should tracks be banked appropriately to maximize performance but that by using an appropriate compliance the surface may be "tuned" to the harmonics of the runner and provide an additional ergogenic effect. Using surfaces with various degrees of compliance, they were able to show that running across surfaces with spring stiffnesses about three times the spring stiffness of the runners actually enhances speed by decreasing contact time and increasing step length. They have predicted up to 3% increases in running speed as a result of this tuning effect (McMahon & Greene, 1979).

Such a track has been constructed at Harvard University, and the authors point to a 2% improvement in performances during the first season of competition on the new track as evidence in support of its ergogenic properties. However, it is difficult to control for such an effect and there is no way of knowing whether these improvements are due to other factors, such as improved training techniques, or whether they are simply part of the normal progression of improvements in performance.

Nigg and Denoth (1980) have taken a similar but much simpler approach. They have analyzed the relationship between cushioning and resilience of a number of track surfaces and found that certain materials offer excellent shock attenuation properties as well as being highly resilient. This information was used to select the surface for a new track in Zürich on which two world records have since been set. Recalling the effect that wearing a highly resilient shoe had on the energy demands of running, it is possible that a resilient track surface might also provide an ergogenic effect, but, as mentioned above, it is all but impossible to separate this effect from other factors when performances alone are used to quantify potential ergogenic benefits.

Summary and Conclusions

There are a number of mechanical constraints on performance that can be partially overcome by using extrinsic biomechanical aids and by selecting environmental conditions that minimize these constraints. These extrinsic biomechanical aids include wearing aerodynamically designed clothing, lightweight shoes, and shoes with resilient cushioning systems. A number of the implements used in competition can also be designed to aid performance. Aerodynamic javelins, energy-storing fiberglass pole-vault poles, golf balls with improved aerodynamics, archery with a biomechanically optimum geometry, and smooth-surfaced racing shells designed in shapes that reduce drag are among the implements that have ergogenic effects. Running tracks can also aid performance by being banked appropriately and by being resilient and tuned for the harmonic characteristics of runners. These and other extrinsic biomechanical aids can improve performance by a factor of from less than 1% to more than 15% in some cases.

Reference Notes

1. Nonweiler, T. *Air resistance of racing cyclists* (Report No. 106). Cranfield, England: College of Aeronautics, 1956.
2. Frederick, E.C., Sharkey, B.J., & Larsen, J.L. *Running economy of elite runners wearing air-soled and non-air-soled racing flats.* Unpublished report, University of Montana, 1980.
3. Daniels, J.T., Larsen, J.L., Frederick, E.C., & Scardina, N. *Aerobic demands of running: Modified magnum vs. mariah* (Research Report No. 3). Exeter, NH: NIKE Sport Research Laboratory, 1981.
4. Dunlop Sports Co., *Hitting golf balls*, Technical Presentation, Marketing Division. Marketing Division Serial no. 1480. London, 1969.
5. McMahon, T.H. Personal communication, Spring 1981.

References

BADE, E. *The mechanics of sport*, Kingswood, Surrey, U.K.: Andrew George Eliot, 1952.

BROER, M.R., & Zernicke, R.F. *Efficiency of human movement*. Philadelphia: W.B. Saunders, 1979.

CATLIN, M.H., & Dressendorfer, R.H. Effect of shoe weight on the energy cost of running. *Medicine and Science in Sports*, 1979, **11**, 80.

CHASE, A. A slice of golf. *Science 81*, 1981, **2**(6), 90-91.

DILLMAN, C.J., & Nelson, R.C. The mechanical energy transformations of pole vaulting with a fiberglass pole. *Journal of Biomechanics*, 1968, **1**, 175-183.

DYSON, G.H.G. *The mechanics of athletics*. New York: Holmes and Meier, 1977.

FREDERICK, E.C., Howley, E.T., & Powers, S.K. Lower O_2 cost while running in air cushion type shoe. *Medicine and Science in Sport and Exercise*, 1980, **12**, 81-82.

GREENE, P.R., & McMahon, T.A. Running in circles. *The Physiologist*, 1979, **6**, 35-36.

HAY, J.G. *The biomechanics of sports techniques*. Englewood Cliffs, NJ: Prentice-Hall, 1978.

JAIN, P.C. On a discrepancy in track races. *Research Quarterly*, 1980, **51**, 432-436.

MCMAHON, T.A., & Greene, P.R. The influence of track compliance on running. *Journal of Biomechanics*, 1979, **12**, 893-904.

NELSON, B. Of people and things. *Track and Field News*, 1979, **32**, 50.

NIGG, B.M., & Denoth, J. (Eds.). *Sportplatzbeläge*. Zürich: Juris Druck und Verlag, 1980.

PUGH, L.G.C.E. The influence of wind resistance in running and walking and the mechanical efficiency of work against horizontal or vertical forces. *Journal of Physiology*, 1971, **213**, 255-276.

RAINE, A.E. Aerodynamics of skiing. *Science Journal*, 1970, **6**(3), 26-30.

SOONG, T-C. An optimally designed archery. In J.L. Bleustein (Ed.), *Mechanics and sport*. New York: ASME, United Engineering Center, 1973.

TERAUDS, J. Wind tunnel tests of competition javelins. *Track and Field Quarterly Review*, 1974, **74**, 88.

WELLICOME, J.F. Some Hydrodynamic Aspects of Rowing. In J.G.P. Williams & A.C. Scott (Eds.), *Rowing: a scientific approach*. London: Kaye and Ward, 1967.

WHITT, F.R., & Wilson, D.G. *Bicycling science: Ergonomics and mechanics*. Cambridge, MA: MIT Press, 1974.

13

Physical Warm-up

B. Don Franks

Physical activity prior to muscular performance has been widely practiced and accepted for many years as a potential ergogenic aid. It was recognized early that both warm-up and fatigue are related to prior activity (Wells, 1908). The main goal for a participant was enough activity for an effective warm-up without causing fatigue (Robinson & Heron, 1924). A number of studies were conducted on warm-up in the 1950s, 1960s, and 1970s. About 55% found some types of warm-up to be superior to rest, about 5% found rest to be superior, and about 40% found no significant difference between different kinds of warm-up and rest. These studies used a wide variety of warm-ups, usually not carefully quantified in terms of intensity, and many different criterion tasks on subjects of different ages and levels of conditioning. It was difficult to clearly differentiate between the types of warm-ups that were beneficial for different types of performance in particular kinds of people. In the late

B. Don Franks, Ph.D., F.A.C.S.M., is with the School of Health, Physical Education and Recreation at the University of Tennessee in Knoxville.

Thanks to Wendy Bubb, Bob Gutin, Nancy Phillips, and Dick Schmidt for assistance with the chapter.

1970s and early 1980s, there appeared to be increased awareness of the beneficial effect of warm-up for many types of performance. The more recent research studies have more carefully quantified the warm-up to determine optimal levels for different populations for specific tasks. The current attitude seems to be an awareness that warm-up is beneficial for many performances by conditioned persons. Studies are increasingly being designed to determine the optimal warm-up for tasks and to clarify the underlying physiological and psychological causes for the changes in performance due to prior physical activity.

This chapter will review studies concerned with different types of warm-up on different kinds of physical performance. It will emphasize the effects of the use of physical activities as warm-ups, particularly the acute effects of warm-up. These short-term effects are temporary and related only to the immediate performance. Further, this chapter will primarily review studies that used actual performance in large muscle activities as the criterion task. Studies reflecting the effects of warm-up on metabolic changes are included to aid in interpretation of the physiological bases for the changes seen in performance. Some studies using fine motor tasks are included to aid in the interpretation of warm-up in these types of tasks.

Type of Warm-up

Several authors prefer to use terms such as "prior exercise" rather than "warm-up," since some of the prior activities used do not actually increase muscle or core temperature (i.e., warm up). Warm-up will be used in this chapter because of its wider recognition, even though something like "prior physical activities" would technically be more appropriate.

Many types of physical activities have been used prior to performance and can be called "physical" or "active" warm-up. Classification of the type of activity used in warm-up is based on its relationship to the task to be performed. The three types of physical warm-up are activities that are *identical* to the performance, *directly* or *indirectly* related to the performance.

One form of preperformance activity almost universally used in activities of short duration is the exact activity to be performed. Identical warm-up has been one of the activities listed under "formal" or "related" warm-up. For example, a softball or baseball pitcher will normally attempt several pitches using the same position, distance from home plate, form, and velocity to be used during the game as part of the pregame warm-up.

Another type of preperformance activity used widely includes activities that use similar but not identical skills (e.g., distance or speed may vary from those used in the task). Direct warm-up also includes components of the performance done separately. An example of direct warm-up is a discus thrower's working only on the release or going through the entire motion at 75% of the velocity to be used in a meet.

Indirect warm-up activities are different from the task to be performed but are aimed at making changes that will influence the performance, such as increased temperature in the blood or muscles and increased arousal.

Indirect warm-up would attempt to raise the temperature with running or other vigorous activity unrelated to the actual performance. Passive warm-up would attempt to accomplish the same goal as indirect warm-up activities, but with hot baths, showers, diathermy, or massage as the medium.

Although it is necessary to separate the types of warm-up to understand more fully their relative effects on performance, most performers recommend and use a combination of warm-ups. The following example of a tennis serve will illustrate the differentiation made among the different types of warm-up. Identical warm-up would involve serving the ball under the same conditions as found in the match (stance, position, number of balls being held in the hand, and serving with the same velocity to be used in the match). Direct warm-up would consist of serving with less velocity or doing one aspect of the serve, such as tossing the ball to the desired height without hitting it. Indirect warm-up would involve activities such as running, flexibility, and strength exercises. A hot shower, or massage, is an example of passive warm-up.

Theoretical Benefits

Three general types of theoretical benefits for warm-up have been found in the literature. Physiological changes occurring as a result of warming up, psychological sets of the individual engaged in prior activity, and the potential lessening of the stress of strenuous activity have all been proposed as bases for the beneficial effects of warm-up. The detrimental effects of physiological and psychological fatigue and exhaustion are discussed from similar perspectives.

Physiological Bases for Warm-up

The physiological bases for increased performance as a result of warming up have primarily dealt with increased temperature within the body. Increased muscle temperature is associated with less intramuscular resistance, thereby leaving more energy for external work (Astrand & Rodahl, 1977). Increased blood temperature has been associated with enhanced dissociation of oxygen from hemoglobin (Barcroft & King, 1909), thus facilitating aerobic metabolism essential for endurance. Warm-up might reduce the time for initial metabolic adjustment to heavy work, resulting in a lower oxygen deficit (Gutin, Stewart, Lewis, & Kruper, 1976). Warm-up has also been reported to increase velocity of nerve conduction (Ruch, Patton, Woodbury, & Towe, 1966) and to open up more capillaries in the muscles (Cureton, 1947). For an expanded discussion of the physiological aspects of warm-up, see deVries (1980). For detailed analysis of the physiological bases for fatigue, see Dill (1974) or Simonson (1971).

In general, research studies using warm-up routines to increase muscle and/or core temperature have found improvement in performance. However, precise definition of how much temperature increase will cause optimal performance in varying tasks awaits more systematic study. Progress has been made indirectly by using different intensities of warm-up to study physiological responses, as well as performances (Bonner, 1974; Dickenson, Medhurst, & Whittingham, 1979; Gutin, Fogle, Meyer, & Jaeger, 1974; Gutin, Wilkerson, Horvath, & Rochelle, 1981).

Psychological Bases for Prior Activity

Prior physical activity has also been found to assist performance from a psychological viewpoint. Skilled performance is normally better after identical or direct warm-up. Indirect warm-up sometimes facilitates performance. In addition to the physiological bases for increased performance, there appears also to be a mental set that enhances performance. Prior physical activity is one of the ways to provide the optimal mental set. It appears to be better in similar activities (Schmidt, 1975), and in tasks not requiring a lot of inhibition (Gutin, 1973). The relationship of arousal to performance (Martens, 1974) has a link to warm-up, because physical activity causes an increased arousal. Womack (1979) suggested that one of the potential benefits of pre-activity rituals, such as dribbling the ball before a free throw, is to help the athlete selectively attend to appropriate cues in the performance.

Several of these psychological aspects of warm-up are found in the study by Dickenson et al. (1979), which showed that warm-up in which the arm was used in the tapping task (criterion task) had an inverted U effect; that is, warm-up increased performance up to a point, and then performance decreased. However, warm-up without using the arm in the task had a linear relationship with the increased performance. Thus, in this one study, general arousal, in the same activity set, continued to cause improved performance even at high intensities in the opposite arm, but fatigue diminished the performance when using the same arm. For an expanded discussion of the psychological aspects of warm-up, see Martens (1974 [arousal and motor performance]), Schmidt (1975 [type of prior activity]), and Gutin (1973 [type of criterion task]).

Safety Aspects of Warm-up

The safety aspects of warm-up have been discussed in two primary areas—prevention of injury and decreasing the stress of vigorous activity. There is strong clinical support for including warm-up to prevent injuries (Mellerowicz & Hansen, 1971). However, there is little experimental evidence to support the claim that warm-up prevents injury (Start, 1962).

There is some evidence that warm-up can reduce the stressfulness of activity to the heart. For example, Barnard, Gardner, Diaro, MacAlpin, and Kattus (1973), found that the same level of work caused an ischemic response (depressed ST segment of ECG) without warm-up in 6 out of 10 fire fighters who had a normal response to the work following a warm-up. Naughton and Leach (1971) found that there were no reasons not to warm up in terms of left ventricular function.

Research Findings of Increased Performance

Table 1 summarizes the studies finding increased performance as a result of warm-up compared with no warm-up (rest). The table includes information about the subjects, the different types of warm-up (independent variable), the criterion tasks (dependent variable), the results, and authors.

Participants

Many of the studies finding beneficial effects of warm-up used fit subjects, although favorable results were found in some studies with untrained individuals. Significant improvement in performance due to warm-up was found in females and males ranging in age from 7 to 45. As many investigators have pointed out, too much prior activity may cause fatigue, thus causing a decrease in

Table 1
Beneficial Effects of Warm-up

Subjects (Ages)	Warm-up	Criterion	Findings[a]	Investigator
Cycling endurance				
4 male (25-31) athletes	1. 30-min bike, 660 mkg/min 2. 10-min shower, 47 C 3. Short-wave diathermy 4. 15-min massage 5. Rest	Bike, time for 35 and for 450 revolutions	1,2,3 > 4,5	Asmussen & Boje (1945)
60 male (21) students	1. 10-min bike, 350-kpm/min 2. Same, 500 3. Same, 650 4. Same, 800 5. Same, 950 6. Rest	Number of revolutions in 10 min, 1,632 kpm/min	1,2,3 > 4,6 4,6 > 5	Bonner (1974)
8 males (22), fit	1. 50% HR-Max plus 5 min rest 2. Same, 60% 3. Same, 85% 4. Rest	10-min bike, at 1,632 kpm	2,3 > 1,4	Lopez & Ebel (1974)

Table 1 (Continued)
Beneficial Effects of Warm-up

5 male & female athletes & nonathletes	1. 12-15-min run-walk 2. Massage 3. Hot bath 4. Rest	All-out bike ride	1,2,3 > 4	Schmid (1947)
Running endurance				
20 female (21) P.E. majors	1. 1 min, 2 mph plus 1 mph each min to HR = 140, then 2 min plus 30 sec rest 2. Same, 60 sec rest 3. Same, 90 sec rest 4. Same, 120 sec rest 5. Rest	Treadmill run to exhaustion at 95% HR-max	1,2 > 3,4,5	Andzel (1978)
12 female (21) P.E. majors	1. Step up to HR = 140, then 1 min, 0 rest 2. Same, 30 sec rest 3. Same, 60 sec rest 4. Rest	9-min step, 15-inch bench, 54 steps/min, 1 min as fast as possible	2,3 > 1,4	Andzel & Gutin (1976)
13 male college nonathletes & athletes	1. 5-min jog plus calisthenics 2. Same, plus .1 mile sprints 3. Rest	1 mile run time	2 > 1,3	Grodjinovsky & Magel (1970)

Athletes	Warm-up procedures	Test	Results	Source
Athletes	1. 5-30-min jog, calisthenics; rest periods—0, 15, 30, 45 min 2. Sauna bath 3. Rest	100-, 400-, 800-m runs	1 > 2,3 0,15 rest > 30,45	Hogberg & Ljunggren (cited in Astrand & Rodahl, 1977)
12 males (7-9)	1. Intermittent 30-sec run, 30-sec rest 2. Rest	30-sec all-out ride, 4-min bike ride—3 min, 50 rpm 1 min, all out	1 > 2	Inbar & Bar-Or (1975)
15 males, high school track	1. 4-min jog, calisthenics, sprints 2. Same, plus 16-min rest, legs elevated 3. Rest	Drop off in 300-yd runs, 3 trials	2 > 3	Kaufman & Ware (1977)
Running sprints				
54 male track athletes & nonathletes	1. Walk, run, calisthenics 2. Walk, stretch	120 yd time	1 > 2	Blank (1955)
9 male college students	1. Sprint 2. Stretch 3. Calisthenics 4. Rest	100 m time	1,2,3 > 4	Malan (1960)
14 male & female athletes & nonathletes	1. 12-15-min walk/run 2. Massage 3. Hot bath 4. Rest	100 m time	1,2,3 > 4	Schmid (1947)

Table 1 (Continued)
Beneficial Effects of Warm-up

7 male & female athletes	1. 12-14-min run plus calisthenics 2. Breathe 50% oxygen 3. Rest	100 m time	1 > 2,3	Simonson et al. (cited in Astrand & Rodahl, 1977)
Metabolic responses				
5 male (21-34) graduate students	1. Exercise 2. Hot shower 3. Cold shower 4. Rest	5-min bike, HR & $\dot{V}O2$	1,2 > 3,4	Falls & Weibers (1965)
6 males (22-45)	1. 10-min bike at HR = 140, plus 30-sec rest 2. Rest	2-min bike, 1,632 kpm/min, HR, core temp, $\dot{V}O_2$	1 > 2	Gutin, et al. (1976)
12 males (7-9)	1. 15 min intermittent run—30-sec on, 30-sec rest—60% max 2. Rest	4-min bike, 30 sec—HR, core temp, VO_2	1 > 2	Inbar & Bar-Or (1975)
6 males (23-29), trained	1. Run at 60% max $\dot{V}O_2$ until increased core temp 2. Immersed in hot water, 40° C, until increased core temp 3. Rest	4-min treadmill run at 100% max $\dot{V}O_2$ level—VO_2, lactate	1 > 2,3	Ingjer & Stromme (1979)

Group	Warm-up protocol	Measure	Results	Reference
2 males, trained	1. 15-min treadmill run, 10 km/hr, 2% 2. Same, plus 3 min rest 3. Rest	90-sec run, 23.6 km/hr, 2%, muscle temp, HR, lactate, $\dot{V}O_2$	1,2 > 3	Martin, Robinson, Wiegman, & Aulick (1975)
8 males, active	1. 10-min walk 5.6 kpm, 10% plus 4-5-min rest 2. Rest	Run to exhaustion, HR, $\dot{V}O_2$	1 > 2	Watt & Hodgson (1975)
Swimming 13 male college swimmers	1. 500-yd swim 2. Calisthenics, 300 movements 3. 10-min massage 4. 6-min hot shower 5. Rest	100 yd time	1 > 2,3,4,5	deVries (1959)
3 male (30-32) athletes	1. 10-min jog 2. 10-min bike, 1,080 kgm/min 3. 15-min hot shower 4. Diathermy 5. 15-min cold bath 6. Rest	50, 200, & 400 m	1,2,3,4 > 5 > 6	Muido (1946)
14 male & female athletes & nonathletes	1. 20-min swim 2. Massage 3. 15-min hot bath 4. Rest	50 m (breast)	1,2,3 > 4	Schmid (1947)

Table 1 (Continued)
Beneficial Effects of Warm-up

60 male (17-28) students	1. 2-min hot shower, calisthenics, & swimming 2. Calisthenics 3. Rest	30 yd	1 > 2,3	Thompson (1958)
Jumping 10 male & 1 female college students	1. Stretch 2. Deep knee bends 3. Run in place 4. Rest	Vertical jump, 6 trials, 5 days	1,2,3 > 4 NS trials NS days	Pacheco (1957)
166 female junior high school students	1. 3-min run in place 2. Rest	Vertical jump, 5 trials, 2 days	1 > 2; 2nd day > 1st day; 5th trial > 1st trial	Pacheco (1959)
80 female high school students	1. 1-min step, 25 steps/min, 15-inch bench 2. Same, 2 min 3. Same, 4 min 4. Same, 6 min 5. Rest	Vertical jump	1,2 > 3, 5 > 4	Richards (1968)
Sports skills 77 males (17-20)	1. Play catch 2. Run plus calisthenics 3. Rest	Softball throw/ distance, 3 trials	1,2 > 3 NS trials	Michael, Skubic, & Rochelle (1957)

Subjects	Treatment	Task	Results	Source
46 males (18-22)	1. 5-min catch 2. Rest	Softball throw/distance, 3 trials	1 > 2	Rochelle, Skubic, & Michael (1960)
132 male college students	1-10 frames 1-3 games	Number of pins down	Frame 5,10 > 1 game 3 > 1	Singer & Beaver (1969)
20 male college freshmen basketball players	1. Shooting, passing, free throws 2. Rest	Free throws 20 trials	1 > 2	Thompson (1958)

Part of body

Subjects	Treatment	Task	Results	Source
45 male & female college students	1. Practice nonpreferred hand 2. Rest	Rotary pursuit, preferred hand	1 > 2	Barch (1963)
64 male & female nonathletes	1. Trace pattern with load, preferred hand 2. Load, nonpreferred hand 3. Load, preferred hand, opposite direction 4. No load	Rotary pursuit	1,2,3 > 4	Catalano & Whalen (1967)
13 males	1. Calisthenics 2. Static stretch 3. Ballistic stretch 4. Hot shower 5. Rest	Flexion—trunk, shoulder, thigh, ankle	1,2,3 > 4,5	Cotten & Waters (1970)

Table 1 (Continued)
Beneficial Effects of Warm-up

Subjects	Warm-up	Task	Results	Reference
8 males & 2 females	Arm crank at 20, 40, 80% max preferred & nonpreferred hand	Tapping task	Linear increase with nonpreferred; inverted U with preferred hand	Dickenson et al. (1979)
15 males & 7 females	1. Treadmill graded test—100% max 2. Same, 81% max 3. Rest	Tapping task	1 > 2 > 3	Dickenson et al. (1979)
129 male college athletes & nonathletes	1. Bench step plus max push-ups 2. 1.5 hr, basketball 3. Fencing 4. Rest	Finger reaction Palm reaction Body reaction Fencing lunge Matching task	NS 2 > 1,4 2 > 1,4 3 > 4 2 > 4	Elbel (1940)
33 male college students	1. 1 practice trial 2. 4 related calisthenics 3. 6 related calisthenics 4. 8 related calisthenics 5. Rest	Toe touch distance from floor	2,3,4 > 1,5	Fieldman (1968)

Subjects	Warm-up conditions	Task	Results	Author

17 male college students	1. Intensity
	  a. Low
	  b. High
	2. Warm-up type
	  a. Related
	  b. Not related
	3. 7-min hot shower
	4. Rest
		Speed, 1,2 feet tapping, leg circles	1b, 2b best
			1b > 1a
				McGavin (1968)

75 male college students	1. 2.5-min arm calisthenics 2. 10-min heavy stepping 3. Rest	Reaction time Movement time 60 trials	NS 2 > 1,3 NS	Phillips (1963)
28 female junior high school unskilled throwers	1. Jumping jacks & laps, 5 times 2. Same, 10 3. Same, 20 4. Rest	Throw for accuracy	1,2,3 > 4	Witte (1962)

[a]">" indicates better performance; "," indicates nonsignificant difference. Thus, 1 > 2,3 means Warm-up 1 caused a better performance than 2 or 3, and that Warm-ups 2 and 3 were not different from each other.

performance. It would appear that many of the warm-ups that help athletes, or trained individuals, might be too vigorous for untrained persons. Thus, it is not surprising to find that many of the studies showing increased performance with quite vigorous warmups used trained subjects. Although most of the warm-up studies have been done on college students, a few of the studies showing improved performance with warm-up did use younger subjects (Inbar & Bar-Or, 1975; Pacheco, 1959; Witte, 1962). There is no reason to believe that the physiological and psychological bases for warm-up would be different for men and women. None of the studies reviewed suggested a different warm-up effect based on sex. There have been several studies using women, or men and women together, that have found increased performance with warm-up (Andzel, 1978; Andzel & Gutin, 1976; Dickenson et al., 1979; Pacheco, 1957, 1959; Richards, 1968; Schmid, 1947).

One aspect of warm-up that has received some attention is the subjects' attitudes toward warm-up. Most adults apparently believe that warm-up is beneficial to performance. It is difficult to determine how much this attitude toward warm-up affects performance. Some studies (e.g., Asmussen & Boje, 1945) have attempted to "control" this variable by keeping the subjects naive concerning the purpose of the study. They found increased performance with warm-up. Massey, Johnson, and Kramer (1961) administered either indirect warm-up or no warm-up while the subjects were under hypnotic trance. The subjects performed not knowing whether they had warm-up or rest. They found nonsignificant differences. Inbar and Bar-Or (1975) selected subjects who had no understanding or bias about warm-up and found that warm-up still had a beneficial effect. It is, of course, still possible that in those adult subjects who believe in the importance of warm-up, subsequent performance is enhanced simply on that basis. It is also possible that some subjects will not go "all out" without a warm-up because of fear of injury. Although granting that a person's attitude toward an "aid" to performance can itself affect the performance, there is sufficient evidence that attitude toward warm-up cannot completely explain all of the beneficial results found in warm-up studies.

Warm-up

There seem to be some trends in the types of warm-up that benefit performance. Most of the warm-up routines that enhanced performance lasted at least 10 minutes. It is interesting to note that Saltin, Gagge, and Stolwijk (1968) found that muscle temperature reaches relative equilibrium after 10-20 minutes of exercise. Most of the beneficial warm-up routines were at a moderate intensity (60-80% of maximal capacity). In some of the studies that quantified the warm-ups, beneficial, detrimental, and/or no difference from rest were found in the same study, with low levels of warm-up not different from rest, moderate levels better than rest, and/or strenuous warm-up being worse than rest (Bonner, 1974; Gutin et al., 1981; Richards, 1968; Witte, 1962). The beneficial warm-ups are primarily direct warm-ups, although several successful warm-up routines combine both direct and indirect warm-ups.

Criterion Tasks

Most of the criterion tasks that have been used in studies showing increased performance with warm-up have been of the short, explosive, anaerobic type. Very few of the studies using a progressive test, or long endurance tasks, have shown warm-up to be beneficial. One possible reason would be that the progressive test protocols have a built-in warm-up already; therefore, additional prior activity either produces fatigue or adds no additional benefit to the performance.

Summary

Direct warm-ups of moderate intensity and duration prior to explosive tasks would appear to enhance performance in trained individuals. Some of the studies finding beneficial effects of warm-up have used indirect warm-up, other types of tasks (e.g., 4-5 minute bike rides and flexibility), and/or untrained subjects.

Research Findings of Detrimental Effects

There have been relatively few studies (Table 2) that have found rest better than warm-up. Several of the studies presented in Table 2 used different levels of the independent variable and found some of the warm-ups to be beneficial, some detrimental, and some not different from rest (Bonner, 1974; Gutin et al., 1974; Gutin et al., 1981; Richards, 1968; Stewart, Gutin, & Lewis, 1973; Witte, 1962).

Participants

In nearly every study showing detrimental effects of warm-up, the subjects used were untrained. Contrast the type of subjects in

Table 2
Detrimental Effects of Warm-up

Subjects (Ages)	Warm-up	Criterion	Findings[a]	Investigator
Cycling endurance				
60 male (21) P.E. students	1. 10-min bike, 350 kpm/min 2. Same, 500 3. Same, 650 4. Same, 800 5. Same, 950 6. Rest	Number of revolutions in 10 min at 1,632 kpm/min	1,2,3 > 4,6 4,6 > 5	Bonner (1974)
12 male (22-50) prisoners	1. 15-min bike ride, 0 load 2. Rest	Time for all-out ride, mod intensity	2 > 1	Karpovich & Pestrecov (1941)
12 male (22-45) graduate students	1. 10-min bike ride at 110 HR 2. Same, 140 HR 3. Same, 170 HR 4. Rest	Number of revolutions in 10 min on bike, 3 kg (68 rpm)	1,2,4 > 3	Stewart, Gutin & Lewis (1973)
Running endurance				
4 male Army volunteers	1. Hot bath at 46° C to raise core temp > 37.2 2. Rest	Graded treadmill walk, 46° C temp	2 > 1	Craig & Froehlich (1968)

Subjects	Warm-up	Task	Results	Reference
5 males (22-34)	1. 20 min, 30% max $\dot{V}O_2$ plus 1 min rest 2. Same, 45% max 3. Same, 60% 4. Same, 75% 5. Rest	10 min at 75% max, then plus 10 m/min to exhaustion	5 > 3,4	Gutin et al. (1981)
Running speed				
10 males (12-13)	1-5. Trials, 50 yd dash	50 yd dash time	1,2,3 > 4,5	Hipple (1955)
Jumping				
80 female high school students	1. 1 min step 25 s/min 2. Same, 2' 3. Same, 4' 4. Same, 6' 5. Rest	Vertical jump	1,2 > 3,5 > 4	Richards (1968)
Part of body				
120 undergraduates	1. 10 min arm crank 2. Rest	Pursuit rotor & movement time—perf. & learning	2 > 1 on performance	Alderman (1965)
10 male (34) end runners	1. Treadmill anaerobic run to exhaustion (< 3 min) plus 1 min rest 2. Same, repeated with 2 min rest between bouts 3. Aerobic run to exhaustion (> 25 min) plus 1 min rest	Foot reaction time	All caused worse time 3 > 1	Crews (1979)

Table 2 (Continued)
Detrimental Effects of Warm-up

18 male (22) P.E. majors & instructors	1. 5-min bike, HR = 100 2. Same, 130 HR 3. Same, 160 HR 4. Rest	Steadiness test— 40 sec	1,2 > 3	Gutin et al. (1974)
14 male undergraduate & graduate students	1. 7-min bike, HR = 160, 0 rest 2. Same, 30 sec rest 3. Same, 60 sec rest 4. Same, 120 sec 5. Same, 240 sec	Steadiness test— 40 sec	4,5 > 1,2,3	Gutin et al. (1974)
20 male (20) students	1. Short wave diathermy 2. Rest	Elbow flexion strength	2 > 1	Sedgwick & Whalen (1964)
128 female junior high school skilled throwers	1. Jumping jacks & laps, 5 times 2. Same, 10 3. Same, 20 4. Rest	Throw for accuracy	4 > 3	Witte (1962)

[a]">" indicates better performance; "," indicates nonsignificant difference. Thus, 1 > 2,3 means Warm-up 1 caused a better performance than Warm-up 2 or 3, and Warm-ups 2 and 3 were not different from each other.

Table 2 with the type of subjects in Table 1. In Table 1 (beneficial effects), there were many trained subjects as well as some untrained subjects. However, in Table 2 (detrimental effects), nearly all the subjects were untrained. The logical explanation would be that one has to have a certain level of conditioning to benefit from warm-up. When a subject is untrained, the warm-up may fatigue to the extent of decreasing the performance.

Warm-up

Another element of the studies finding detrimental effects of warm-up is that many of the warm-ups were at a very high intensity. Subjects were riding bikes at 950 kpm/min (Bonner, 1974) or working at heart rates of 160-170 for 5-10 minutes (Stewart et al., 1973; Gutin et al., 1974). Untrained subjects simply could not tolerate this level of warm-up and then perform on all-out tasks or on tasks requiring a lot of control. Many of the warm-ups were indirect, especially in the fine motor tasks. Although indirect warm-ups have been found to aid performance in some studies, the direct and identical warm-ups, or a combination of direct and indirect, are normally more effective.

Criterion Tasks

In addition to the pre-task warm-up, several of the criterion tasks had a built-in warm-up in terms of a test consisting of several levels of work or working for several minutes at a submaximal level (Craig & Froehlich, 1968; Gutin et al., 1981; Karpovich & Pestrecov, 1941). In effect, the studies found that two warm-ups were too much for the subjects. In other studies, the criterion task required a great deal of what Gutin (1973) has called inhibition. Subjects were asked to keep a stylus on a rotating target (Alderman, 1965), throw for accuracy (not speed) (Witte, 1962), or hold a stylus steady (Gutin et al., 1974). In these fine-motor-skill type of tasks, the intensive indirect warm-ups decreased the performance.

Summary

Untrained persons cannot tolerate high intensity warm-ups. Warm-ups prior to progressive tests may decrease the test performance. Heavy, indirect warm-up appears to interfere with one's ability to perform fine motor tasks requiring careful control.

Indefinite Research Results

Table 3 summarizes studies that have found nonsignificant results comparing warm-up with rest. One hypothesis for these results is that the warm-up used and rest had the same effect on performance. That is quite likely the appropriate explanation for the results in some of the studies. However, it must be pointed out that there are other reasons for nonsignificant differences that cannot be ignored. Small numbers of subjects, large variance, and/or unreliable tests can also cause nonsignificant results. If a significant difference is found between warm-up and rest (either positive or negative), there is a high probability that similar warm-ups would produce similar differences from rest on the same type of tasks and subjects. However, if nonsignificant differences are found between warm-up and rest, predictions that similar warm-ups would not produce any difference from rest in the same type of tasks are much more precarious. Thus, the comparison of Tables 1 and 2 provides the major information concerning the general question, Is warm-up helpful? One must be careful in drawing conclusions from the studies in Table 3.

Participants

It is difficult to characterize the subjects used in studies finding nonsignificant results. Most were untrained, but several studies did use athletes. Most had a substantial number of persons participating in the study, but a few had less than 10 (Gutin et al., 1981; Howard, Blyth, & Thornton, 1966; Karpovich & Hale, 1956; Knowlton, Miles, & Sawka, 1978; Stamford, Rowland, & Moffatt, 1978).

Warm-up

Several points were revealed when evaluating the studies finding nonsignificant results. Many of the warm-ups were light in intensity (less than 50% max) (Gutin et al., 1981; Knowlton et al., 1978; Skubic & Hodgkins, 1957; Stewart et al., 1973); many were of relatively short duration (5 minutes or less) (Aronchick & Burke, 1977; Busuttil & Ruhling, 1977; Grodjinovsky & Magel, 1970; Knowlton et al., 1978; Lotter, 1959; Phillips, 1963; Skubic & Hodgkins, 1957; Thompson, 1958); and some had little activity (e.g., eight revolutions on the bike, a few throws) (Pyke, 1968; Skubic & Hodgkins, 1957).

Table 3
Nonsignificant Warm-up Results

Subjects (Ages)	Warm-up	Criterion	Findings[a]	Investigator
Cycling endurance				
16 males (22)	1. 3-min bike, at 98 w plus 2-min rest 2. Rest	8-min bike test— HR, BP, temp, VO_2	NS, except + HR, work − HR, rec	Busuttil & Ruhling (1977)
15 male college athletes & P.E. majors	1. 10-min jog plus calisthenics 2. Rest	Time for 100 revolutions	NS	Massey, Johnson, & Kramer (1961)
12 male (22-45) graduate students	1. 10-min bike ride at HR = 110 2. Same, 140 HR 3. Same, 170 HR 4. Rest	Number of revolutions, bike, 3 kg (68 rpm)	1,2,4 > 3	Stewart, Gutin, & Lewis (1973)
Cycling speed				
3 male college experienced bike riders	1. 5-min bike, 5.5 lb, 60 rpm 2. Rest	Time for 35 revolutions	NS	Karpovich & Hale (1956)
20 males (19-34)	1. 2-min run with arm movement 2. Same, 4 min	Rate of arm crank, 2 days	NS	Lotter (1959)

Table 3 (Continued)
Nonsignificant Warm-up Results

Subjects	Treatments	Task	Results	Reference
45 males (15-17)	1. Trials on criterion tasks 2. Strength 3. Flexibility 4. Rest	Bike speed	NS	Pyke (1968)
13 female college P.E. majors	1. 8 revolutions on bike 2. Rest	Bike, 0.1 mile	NS	Skubic & Hodgkins (1957)
Running endurance				
5 males (22-34)	1. 20 min, 30% max oxygen uptake, plus 1-min rest 2. Same, 45% 3. Rest	10 min at 75% max, then increase 10 m/min until exhaustion	NS	Gutin et al. (1981)
8 females & 10 males (11-33) with exer-induced asthma	1. 3 min, 60% max HR 2. Rest	5-min treadmill run, 85% max HR	NS	Morton, Fitch, & Davis (1979)
Running sprints				
7 male college freshmen & varsity track runners	1. 10-min jog, calisthenics, sprints 2. 10-min massage 3. 10-min digital stroking	440 yd	NS	Karpovich & Hale (1956)

Subjects	Warm-up conditions	Task/Measure	Results	Reference
50 male high school nonathletes	1. Jog, sprints, calisthenics 2. Rest	440 yd	NS	Mathews & Snyder (1959)
45 males (15-17)	1. Trials on criterion task 2. Strength 3. Flexibility 4. Rest	60 yd	NS	Pyke (1968)
18 males (19-28)	1. 10-min walk-jog 2. Cold spray 3. Rest	Number steps, 10 sec run in place	2 > 1,3	Sills & O'Riley (1956)
Metabolic responses				
16 males (21), moderately fit	1. 5 min, 75% max HR, 0 rest 2. Same, 1 min rest 3. Same, 5 min 4. Same, 10 min	8-min bike—HR, State anxiety, Perceived exertion	NS	Aronchick & Burke (1977)
13 college nonathletes	1. 5-min jog plus calisthenics 2. Same plus 0.1 mile sprints 3. Rest	Max $\dot{V}O_2$	NS	Grodjinovsky & Magel (1970)
8 male college track runners	1. Track warm-up 2. Rest	HR before, during, & after 15 100 yd; 1 440 yd, & Harvard step	NS	Howard, Blyth, & Thornton (1966)

Table 3 (Continued)
Nonsignificant Warm-up Results

7 males, untrained	1. 2 min at 20% max $\dot{V}O_2$, 2 min at 40% 2. Rest	5-min bike at 75% max $\dot{V}O_2$ — HR, vent, lactate, $\dot{V}O_2$	NS	Knowlton, Miles, & Sawka (1978)
5 males, moderately fit	3 max tests/day separated by 10-, 20-, 30-, 40-min rest	Max $\dot{V}O_2$ Performance	NS 1st trial better	Stamford, Rowland, & Moffatt (1978)
Jumping				
45 males (15-17)	1. Trials on criterion task 2. Strength 3. Flexibility 4. Rest	Jump & reach	NS	Pyke (1968)
Sports skills				
45 males (15-17)	1. Trials on criterion task 2. Strength 3. Flexibility 4. Rest	Cricket ball throw/distance	NS	Pyke (1968)
13 female P.E. majors	1. Bike, 8 revolutions 2. 5 softball throws 3. Free throws 4. 12 jumping jacks 5. Rest	Softball throw basketball free throws	NS	Skubic & Hodgkins (1957)

Subjects	Treatments	Task	Result	Reference
60 male college students	1. 20 throws, 15-oz ball 2. Same, 20-oz 3. Same, regular ball	Baseball throw for velocity & accuracy	NS	Straub (1968)
Part of body				
129 male college athletes & nonathletes	1. Bench step plus max push-ups 2. 1.5 hr basketball 3. Fencing 4. Rest	Finger reaction	NS	Elbel (1940)
75 male college students	1. 2.5-min arm calisthenics 2. 10-min step 3. Rest	Reaction time	NS	Phillips (1963)
21 male college students	1. 9-min arm and hand calisthenics 2. Rest	Grip end	NS	Sedgwick (1964)
20 males (18-48)	1. Short-wave diathermy 2. Rest	Grip end	NS	Sedgwick & Whalen (1964)
20 male (18-23) P.E. majors	Calisthenics plus 2 min run in place	Leg extension strength	NS	Thompson (1958)
70 male undergraduate students	1. 10-min heavy stepping 2. Rest	Pursuit rotor Reaction time	NS	Welch (1969)

[a]NS means nonsignificant differences among warm-up treatments.

Criterion Tasks

Several of the criterion tasks had the same characteristics of the studies where warm-up was found to be detrimental; namely, a progressive test or a fine motor task. In addition, a few of the tasks finding nonsignificant differences were submaximal tasks (i.e., working for a set time below maximal level) (Aronchick & Burke, 1977; Busuttil & Ruhling, 1977; Knowlton et al., 1978; Morton, Fitch, & Davis, 1979).

Summary

Studies finding nonsignificant differences between warm-up and rest included a wide variety of numbers of subjects, types of warm-up, and criterion tasks. Some possible reasons for the nonsignificant findings would include small number of subjects, low intensity warm-ups, warm-ups of short duration or of little activity, and criterion tasks that were fine motor, submaximal, or had progressive workload protocols. In addition, other factors in the design and conduct of research studies produce nonsignificant results and warrant caution in accepting the null hypothesis.

Some of the studies that found detrimental and/or nonsignificant effects of warm-up were designed to determine the optimal levels for warm-up. In order to accomplish this goal, it was necessary to include levels of warm-up that one would hypothesize were better than, not different from, and worse than rest. Studies such as these will more clearly define optimal warm-up. The fact that they found nonsignificant or fatigue effects is a tribute to their pre-planned design. Some of the earlier studies that used only one type of warm-up and found nonsignificant differences may have simply had insufficient information concerning adequate levels of warm-up.

Injury

Clinical Opinion

Numerous coaches, trainers, and performers have observed that lack of warm-up leads to increased risk of injury (Mellerowicz & Hansen, 1971). These observations have led to increased emphasis on warming up and additional observations that incidents of injury have decreased.

Safety

In addition to prevention of injury during sporting events, there has been concern about the stressfulness of vigorous activity without any prior activity. The study by Barnard et al. (1973) illustrates the stress that sudden activity can have on the heart when not preceded by lighter activity. The ischemic response to hard work without warm-up was not found in response to the same hard work preceded by a progressive test protocol (warm-up).

Experimental Evidence

In light of the clinical opinion about injury and concern for stress to the heart, one might expect that research studies that ask subjects to go "all out" with and without warm-up would report numbers of injuries and perhaps some myocardial infarctions as a result of the "no warm-up" condition. In fact, the literature is almost without reference to injury resulting from these studies. In the rare instances where injuries have been reported, it was almost always a recurrence of an early injury.

Summary

The testimony and opinions of professionals in the field cannot be completely ignored. There is some theoretical basis (e.g., loosen connective tissue, decrease muscle viscosity), but there is little experimental evidence to justify warm-up on the basis of prevention of injury. There is some evidence that warm-up would cause less stress to the heart. The effect of warm-up on injury may simply be an academic question, since there does appear to be substantial evidence supporting warm-up for many explosive activities in trained persons, and almost no evidence supporting no warm-up being superior to warm-up.

Summary and Conclusions

In summarizing the evidence concerning the effects of warm-up on performance, a *tentative* model is presented dealing with the conditions necessary for the optimal effects of warm-up on performance. Table 4 lists the hypothesized elements of optimal warm-up in terms of the participant, the nature of the warm-up, and the performance task.

Table 4
Proposed Model for Optimal Warm-up Effects

Desired warm-up component	Physiological aspects	Psychological aspects
Direct warm-up	Increase muscle temperature	Focus on task
Indirect warm-up Large muscle groups	Increase core temperature without local fatigue	Increase arousal
Similar activities		Readiness for activity set
Moderate intensity (60-80% max)	Increase temperature; minimize time to reach desired intensity	Increase arousal
Moderate duration (>10 min)	Does not use anaerobic energy reserves	
Short rest interval (<60 sec)	Retain effects of warm-up	Retain effects of warm-up
Conditioned participant	Can increase temperature without fatigue	Can increase arousal without fatigue
Skilled player	Utilizes physiological processes efficiently	Can increase arousal and focus on task without fatigue
Short explosive, uninhibited task	Most likely to be improved by physiological changes	Most likely to be improved with high levels of arousal

Participant

The participant must be well conditioned to be able to obtain the maximal physiological effects of warm-up. The well trained person can work hard enough to increase the muscle and core temperature without fatigue. To the extent that persons are not at peak condition, they may need to use a shorter and/or less intense warm-up. Future research will have to determine whether less fit subjects using lighter warm-ups can make proportionally similar improvement in performances. Based on current evidence concerning desired levels of warm-up, it would appear that untrained subjects cannot receive maximal benefit from warm-up due to earlier onset of fatigue.

It is also important for the participant to be at a high level of conditioning from a psychological perspective in order to engage in prior activity that will raise the arousal level without fatigue. Optimal warm-up effects are also related to skill level. One of the effects of arousal is to enlist the person's dominant responses, which are more likely to be correct responses in the skilled player. Finally, the skilled participant has a better understanding of the appropriate cues as warm-up assists in selectively attending to stimuli.

Warm-up

Both physiological and psychological evidence support the use of direct and indirect warm-up. Direct warm-up increases the temperature of the muscles being used. It also helps the person focus on the specific task and its components. Indirect warm-up using large muscle groups is recommended to increase the core temperature and to minimize the time it takes to attain the desired intensity level of the performance. Indirect warm-up using the same type(s) of activities in muscles that are not being used in the task also increases the arousal level and assists mental preparation for the related task. Identical warm-up should be used sparingly in explosive tasks because the anaerobic reserves would be diminished in that type of all-out effort. In submaximal tasks (e.g., bowling), identical warm-up would be recommended.

It appears that warm-up routines in the intensity range of 60-80 percent of maximal functional capacity increase the body temperature and can be sustained for an extended period of time without fatigue. In addition, most of the evidence indicates that the warm-up should last at least 10 minutes with a relatively short rest period (0-60 seconds) between the warm-up and the performance. It is possible that the warm-up should increase aerobic metabolism (beyond the "aerobic" threshold) to increase heat production, but be at intensities below the "anaerobic" threshold, which would begin to utilize energy reserves needed for the performance. Additional research would be necessary to confirm or reject this suggestion.

If direct and indirect warm-ups are not possible, passive warm-ups are recommended. These are clearly a second choice because most studies find the direct and indirect warm-ups superior to passive. However, a number of studies find some forms of passive warm-up to be better than rest.

Performance

Warm-up appears to have the most consistent effect on tasks that are of short duration, high intensity, and do not require fine motor control. In general, one would suggest that the warm-up be less intense for submaximal tasks and/or skills that require inhibition of various movements. The light intensity warm-up can still minimize the time necessary to reach the desired metabolic intensity while keeping the arousal level at a more moderate level. In fine motor control tasks, a lower arousal level apparently is more appropriate for optimal performance.

Although no evidence is available dealing directly with the content of mental activities during warm-up, it would appear plausible that one should alternate general arousing thoughts (e.g., the importance of playing well) with attention to specific aspects of the performance in the uninhibited, explosive tasks. On the other hand, in activities requiring more control, one might alternate thinking about the specific aspects of the skill, and relaxation (e.g., having the mind go "blank"). These mental activities would help focus on the task at higher or lower arousal levels appropriate to the different types of performance.

Next Steps

The hypothesized conditions for optimal warm-up effects are certainly tentative positions. Although there is some evidence to support the model, many of the recommendations have not been tested directly. A more definite model awaits systematic research that will test the hypotheses concerning optimal warm-ups. Future research should include several levels of the independent variables, and different kinds of subjects and tasks, as well as different mental activities. In addition, joint psychological-physiological studies based on the best information available in both fields is essential before a complete understanding will be possible.

References

ALDERMAN, R.B. Influence of local fatigue on speed and accuracy in motor learning. *Research Quarterly*, 1965, **36**, 131-140.

ANDZEL, W.D. The effects of moderate prior exercise and various rest intervals upon cardiorespiratory endurance performance. *Journal of Sports Medicine and Physical Fitness*, 1978, **18**, 245-252.

ANDZEL, W.D., & Gutin, B. Prior exercise and endurance performance: A test of the mobilization hypothesis. *Research Quarterly*, 1976, **47**, 269-276.

ARONCHICK, J., & Burke, E.J. Psycho-physical effects of varied rest intervals following warm-up. *Research Quarterly*, 1977, **48**, 260-264.

ASMUSSEN, E., & Boje, O. Body temperature and capacity for work. *Acta Physiologica Scandinavica*, 1945, **10**, 1-22.

ASTRAND, P.O., & Rodahl, K. *Textbook of work physiology* (2nd ed.). New York: McGraw-Hill, 1977.

BARCH, A.M. Bilateral transfer of warm-up in rotary pursuit. *Perceptual and Motor Skills*, 1963, **17**, 723-726.

BARCROFT, J., & King, W. The effect of temperature on the dissociation curve of blood. *Journal of Physiology*, 1909, **39**, 374-384.

BARNARD, R.J., Gardner, G.W., Diaro, W.V., MacAlpin, R.N., & Kattus, A.A. Cardiovascular responses to sudden strenuous exercise—heart rate, blood pressure, and ECG. *Journal of Applied Physiology*, 1973, **34**, 833-837.

BLANK, L.B. Effects of warm-up on speed. *Athletic Journal*, 1955, **35**, 10.

BONNER, H.W. Preliminary exercise: A two-factor theory. *Research Quarterly*, 1974, **45**, 138-147.

BUSUTTIL, C.P., & Ruhling, R.O. Warm-up and circulo-respiratory adaptations. *Journal of Sports Medicine and Physical Fitness*, 1977, **17**, 69-74.

CATALANO, J.F., & Whalen, P.M. Factors in recovery from performance decrement: Activation, inhibition and warm-up. *Perceptual and Motor Skills*, 1967, **24**, 1223-1231.

COTTEN, D.J., & Waters, J.S. Immediate effect of four types of warm-up activities upon static flexibility of four selected joints. *American Corrective Therapy Journal*, 1970, **24**, 133-136.

CRAIG, F.N., & Froehlich, H.L. Endurance of preheated men in exhausting work. *Journal of Applied Physiology*, 1968, **24**, 636-639.

CREWS, R. The influence of exhaustive exercise on reaction time of conditioned adult men. *American Corrective Therapy Journal*, 1979, **33**, 127-130.

CURETON, T.K. *Physical fitness appraisal and guidance*. St. Louis: C.V. Mosby, 1947.

DEVRIES, H.A. Effects of various warm-up procedures on 100-yard times of competitive swimmers. *Research Quarterly*, 1959, **30**, 11-20.

DEVRIES, H.A. *Physiology of exercise in physical education and athletics* (3rd ed.). Dubuque: W.C. Brown, 1980.

DICKENSON, J., Medhurst, C., & Whittingham, N. Warm-up and fatigue in skill acquisition and performance. *Journal of Motor Behavior*, 1979, **11**, 81-86.

DILL, D.B. Fatigue and physical fitness. In W.R. Johnson & E.R. Buskirk (Eds.), *Science and medicine of exercise and sport* (2nd ed.). New York: Harper & Row, 1974.

ELBEL, E.R. A study of the response time before and after strenuous exercise. *Research Quarterly*, 1940, **11**, 86-95.

FALLS, H.B., & Weibers, J.E. The effects of pre-exercise conditions on heart rate and oxygen uptake during exercise and recovery. *Research Quarterly*, 1965, **36**, 243-252.

FIELDMAN, H. Relative contribution of the back and hamstring muscles in the performance of the toe-touch test after selected extensibility exercises. *Research Quarterly*, 1968, **39**, 518-523.

GRODJINOVSKY, A., & Magel, J.R. Effects of warm-up on running performance. *Research Quarterly*, 1970, **41**, 116-119.

GUTIN, B. Exercise-induced activation and human performance: A review. *Research Quarterly*, 1973, **44**, 256-267.

GUTIN, B., Fogle, R.K., Meyer, J., & Jaeger, M. Steadiness as a function of prior exercise. *Journal of Motor Behavior*, 1974, **6**, 69-76.

GUTIN, B., Stewart, K., Lewis, S., & Kruper, J. Oxygen consumption in the first stages of strenuous work as a function of prior exercise. *Journal of Sports Medicine and Physical Fitness*, 1976, **16**, 60-65.

GUTIN, B., Wilkerson, J.E., Horvath, S.M., & Rochelle, R.D. Physiological response to endurance work as a function of prior exercise. *International Journal of Sports Medicine*, 1981, **2**, 87-91.

HIPPLE, J. Warm-up and fatigue in junior high school sprints. *Research Quarterly*, 1955, **26**, 246-247.

HOWARD, G.E., Blyth, C.S., & Thornton, W.E. Effects of warm-up on the heart rate during exercise. *Research Quarterly*, 1966, **37**, 360-367.

INBAR, O., & Bar-Or, O. The effects of intermittent warm-up on 7-9 year old boys. *European Journal of Applied Physiology and Occupational Physiology*, 1975, **34**, 81-89.

INGJER, F., & Stromme, S.B. Effects of active, passive, or no warm-up on the physiological response to heavy work. *European Journal of Applied Physiology and Occupational Physiology*, 1979, **40**, 273-282.

KARPOVICH, P.V., & Hale, C. Effects of warming-up upon physical performance. *Journal of the American Medical Association*, 1956, **162**, 1117-1119.

KARPOVICH, P.V., & Pestrecov, K. Effect of gelatin upon muscular work in man. *American Journal of Physiology*, 1941, **134**, 300-309.

KAUFMAN, D.A., & Ware, W.B. Effect of warm-up and recovery techniques on repeated running endurance. *Research Quarterly*, 1977, **48**, 328-332.

KNOWLTON, R.G., Miles, D.S., & Sawka, M.N. Metabolic responses of untrained individuals to warm-up. *European Journal of Applied Physiology and Occupational Physiology*, 1978, **40**, 1-5.

LOPEZ, R., & Ebel, H. Endurance performance as a function of prior-exercise heart rate. *Journal of Sports Medicine*, 1974, **2**, 291-294.

LOTTER, W.S. Effects of fatigue and warm-up on speed of arm movements. *Research Quarterly*, 1959, **30**, 57-65.

MALAN, E. The effects of rest following warm-up upon physical performance. *Proceedings of the College Physical Education Association*, 1960, **36**, 45-48.

MARTENS, R. Arousal and motor performance. In J. Wilmore (Ed.), *Exercise and sport sciences reviews* (Vol. 2). New York: Academic Press, 1974.

MARTIN, B.J., Robinson, S., Wiegman, D., & Aulick, L.H. Effect of warm-up on metabolic responses to strenuous exercise. *Medicine and Science in Sports*, 1975, **7**, 146-149.

MASSEY, B., Johnson, W.R., & Kramer, G.F. Effect of warm-up exercise upon muscular performance using hypnosis to control the psychological variable. *Research Quarterly*, 1961, **32**, 63-71.

MATHEWS, D.K., & Snyder, H.A. Effect of warm-up on the 440-yard dash. *Research Quarterly*, 1959, **30**, 446-451.

MCGAVIN, R.J. Effect of different warm-up exercises of varying intensities on speed of leg movement. *Research Quarterly*, 1968, **39**, 125-130.

MELLEROWICZ, H., & Hansen, G. Conditioning. In L. Larson (Ed.), *Encyclopedia of sport sciences and medicine*. New York: Macmillan, 1971.

MICHAEL, E., Skubic, V., & Rochelle, R. Effect of warm-up on softball throw for distance. *Research Quarterly*, 1957, **28**, 357-363.

MORTON, A.R., Fitch, K.D., & Davis, T. The effect of "warm-up" on exercise-induced asthma. *Annals of Allergy*, 1979, **42**, 257-260.

MUIDO, L. The influence of body temperature on performances in swimming. *Acta Physiologica Scandinavica*, 1946, **12**, 102-109.

NAUGHTON, J., & Leach, W. The effect of a simulated warm-up on ventricular performance. *Medicine and Science in Sports*, 1971, **3**, 169-171.

PACHECO, B.A. Improvement in jumping performance due to preliminary exercise. *Research Quarterly*, 1957, **28**, 55-63.

PACHECO, B.A. Effectiveness of warm-up exercise in junior high school girls. *Research Quarterly*, 1959, **30**, 202-213.

PHILLIPS, W.H. Influence of fatiguing warm-up exercises on speed of movement and reaction latency. *Research Quarterly*, 1963, **34**, 370-378.

PYKE, F.S. The effect of preliminary activity on maximal performance. *Research Quarterly*, 1968, **39**, 1069-1075.

RICHARDS, D.K. A two-factor theory of the warm-up effect in jumping performance. *Research Quarterly*, 1968, **39**, 668-673.

ROBINSON, E.S., & Heron, W.T. The warming-up effect. *Journal of Experimental Psychology*, 1924, **7**, 81-97.

ROCHELLE, R.H., Skubic, V., & Michael, E. Performance as affected by incentive and preliminary warm-up. *Research Quarterly*, 1960, **31**, 499-504.

RUCH, T., Patton, H., Woodbury, J., & Towe, A. *Neurophysiology*. Philadelphia: Saunders, 1966.

SALTIN, B., Gagge, A.P., & Stolwijk, J.A. Muscle temperature during submaximal exercise in man. *Journal of Applied Physiology*, 1968, **25**, 679-688.

SCHMID, L. Increasing the bodily output by warming-up. *Casopis Lekaru Ceskych*, 1947, **86**, 950-958.

SCHMIDT, R.A. *Motor skills*. New York: Harper and Row, 1975.

SEDGWICK, A.W. Effect of actively increased muscle temperature on local muscular endurance. *Research Quarterly*, 1964, **35**, 532-538.

SEDGWICK, A.W., & Whalen, H.R. Effect of passive warm-up on muscular strength and endurance. *Research Quarterly*, 1964, **35**, 45-59.

SILLS, F.D., & O'Riley, V.E. Comparative effect of rest, exercise, and cold spray upon performance in spot running. *Research Quarterly*, 1956, **27**, 217-219.

SIMONSON, E. (Ed.). *Physiology of work capacity and fatigue*. Springfield, IL: Charles C. Thomas, 1971.

SINGER, R.N., & Beaver, R. Bowling and the warm-up effect. *Research Quarterly*, 1969, **40**, 372-375.

SKUBIC, V., & Hodgkins, J. Effect of warm-up activities on speed, strength, and accuracy. *Research Quarterly*, 1957, **28**, 147.

STAMFORD, B., Rowland, R., & Moffatt, R. Effects of severe prior exercise on assessment of maximal oxygen uptake. *Journal of Applied Physiology: Respiratory, Environmental, and Exercise Physiology*, 1978, **44**, 559-563.

START, K.B. Incidence of injury in muscles undergoing maximum isometric contraction without warm-up. *Archives of Physical Medicine & Rehabilitation*, 1962, **43**, 284-286.

STEWART, K., Gutin, B., & Lewis, S. Prior exercise and circulorespiratory endurance. *Research Quarterly*, 1973, **44**, 169-177.

STRAUB, W.F. Effect of overload training procedures upon velocity and accuracy of the overarm throw. *Research Quarterly*, 1968, **39**, 370-379.

THOMPSON, H. Effect of warm-up upon physical performance in selected activities. *Research Quarterly*, 1958, **29**, 231-246.

WATT, E.W., & Hodgson, J.L. The effect of warm-up on total oxygen cost of a short treadmill run to exhaustion. *Ergonomics*, 1975, **18**, 397-401.

WELCH, M. Specificity of heavy work fatigue: Absence of transfer from heavy leg work to coordination tasks using the arms. *Research Quarterly*, 1969, **40**, 402-406.

WELLS, F.L. Normal performance in the tapping test, before and during practice with special reference to fatigue phenomena. *American Journal of Psychology*, 1908, **19**, 437-483.

WITTE, F. Effect of participation in light, medium, and heavy exercise upon accuracy in motor performance of junior high school girls. *Research Quarterly*, 1962, **33**, 308-312.

WOMACK, M. Why athletes need ritual: A study of magic among professional athletes. In W.J. Morgan (Ed.), *Sport and the Humanities*. Knoxville, TN: College of Education, 1979.

Index ―――――――――

A

Acid base balance, 66-68
Acidosis, lactate
  and blood doping, 204-205
Acid-citrate-dextrose, 206
Air resistance
  effects on performance, 326-327
Alcohol
  disinhibition effect, 226-227
Alpha-tocopherol (see Vitamin E)
Altitude
  and air resistance, 326
  effect on oxygen pressure, 189
  performance, and Vitamine E, 42-43
  training, effect on
    hematocrit, 209
    hemoglobin, 202
Amphetamines, 101-120
  addiction, 120
  athletes, use by, 101-102
  blood levels after intake, 102-103
  disinhibition effect, 226-227
  effects of
    high dosages, 118-120
  effects on
    aerobic endurance, 105-107,
    112-114, 117-119
  body function
    central effects, 103-104
    peripheral effects, 104-105
  local muscular endurance, 107-109,
  113-115, 119
  power, 116, 119
  reaction time, 110-111, 116-117,
  119-120
  speed, 111-112, 116-117, 120
  strength, 109-110, 115-116, 119-120
  elimination of, 102
  theoretical benefits of, 103-105
Anabolic steroids, 164-177
  athletics and, 164-177
  diet and, 165, 171-173, 174
  dosage, 164-165, 170-171, 172-175,
  176
  effects on
    appetite, 165-166
    body weight, 164-167, 170,
    172-173, 173-174, 176
    erythropoiesis (see "red blood
    cells")
    erythropoietin, 167
    lean body mass, 164-166, 170, 171,

oxygen transport, 206-207, 211
perceived exertion, 209-214
respiratory rate, 209-210
running speed, 211-212
stroke volume, 209
swimming performance, 207-208
ventilation, 209-210
ethical concerns, 215-216
legal concerns, 215-216
medical concerns, 215-216
research methodology problems, 206
storage techniques, 206
Blood pressure
and caffeine, 134-135
Blood volume, effect of
sweat loss on, 69
training on, 202-203
Body fluids
description, 59
Body temperature
and warm-up, 343
effect of
hyperhydration, 81
hypohydration, 71-72
high
effect on physical performance, 78
Body water (also see water), 58-59
control mechanisms, 65-66
losses (also see sweat)
and physical performance, 75-77
prevention of, 74-75
Body weight
effects of anabolic steroids, 164-167,
170-174, 176

C

Caffeine, 128-153
absorption, 132
as doping agent, 128
content in
chocolate, 130
coffee, 130
colas, 130
over-the-counter drugs, 130
tea, 130
effects on
blood lipids, 141-148
blood vessels, 134-137
calcium, muscle, 137-140
central nervous system, 133-134
endurance, 148-153
free fatty acids, blood, 141-148
use during exercise, 144-146,
151-152

fuels for exercise, 140-148
general body, 128
glucose utilization, 140-141,
143-144
glycogen metabolism, 147-148
during exercise, 144-146
heart, 134-137
muscle contraction, 136-140
nervous stimulation, 133-134
oxygen uptake, 151-152
physical performance, 148-153
reaction time, 149-151
skeletal muscle, 136-137
glycogen sparing effect, 151-152
mechanism of action, 131
possible health effects, 129, 131
research methodology problems,
128-132, 148-149, 152-153
structure, 129
Calcium (also see electrolytes)
effect on temperature set point,
82-83
role in body, 64-65
Carbohydrates, 3-21
Carbohydrate loading (also see glycogen), 3-21
and liver glycogen stores, 10-11, 20
depletion stage, problems in, 11-13
effects on physical performance,
16-20
aerobic events, 19
anaerobic events, 18
regimens, analysis of, 11-13
Carbohydrate metabolism
and oxygen supplementation,
194-195
and Vitamin B, 35-39
Cardiovascular system
and caffeine, 134-137
Centripetal force, 324, 336
Citrate - phosphate dextrose, 206
Coffee, 129, 131. 148-149
Cognition, 304-305
Cognitive behavior modification,
262-264
Cognitive psyching, effect on
anxiety, 291-292
central arousal, 290
confidence, 291
gymnastic performance, 292
muscular endurance, 291
strength, 291-292
treadmill endurance, 292

172-174, 176
limb girth, 171, 172, 174
liver function, 175, 176
maximal oxygen uptake, 168, 173,
175-176
menstruation, 176
muscle, 165-168, 170-171, 172,
173-174, 176-177
protein synthesis, 164-165
red blood cells, 167-168, 176
reproductive system, 175
salt retention, 166-167
strength, 164, 166, 170, 171, 173,
175, 176
experimental difficulties, 170-171
females and, 164, 165-167, 168, 170,
175, 176
medical ethics and, 170-171, 176-177
harmful side effects, 175-177
placebo effect, 170-171
properties of, 164
theoretical benefits, 165-169
Anaerobic capacity
and Vitamin C, 40-41
Androgenic-anabolic steroids (see
anabolic steroids)
Androgens (also see anabolic steroids)
endogenous, effects of
acute exercise on, 168-169
chronic exercise on, 169-170
Anemia
iron deficiency, 45
sports (see sports anemia)
Anxiety (see also state anxiety and
trait anxiety)
weight loss, effects on, 72
Appetite
effect of anabolic steroids, 165-166
Arousal, 343-344
Arousal response, 277-282
Ascorbic acid (see Vitamin C)
Aspartates, 83-84
Athletes
psychological characteristics of,
296-297
Attention control training, 284-285

B
Behavioral modeling and
anxiety, 289-291
confidence, 292
diving performance, 289
muscular endurance, 290-291

Behaviorism, 255
Biofeedback, 284-285, 299
effect on
anxiety, 287-289
archery, 287
balance, 287-289
basketball performance, 288
football performance, 288
gymnastic performance, 288-289
muscular tension, 299
rifle shooting, 287
tension, 287-288
Biomechanical aids, 323-338
air resistance, reduction of, 327-328
archery, 335
bicycles, 335
clothing, 327-332
shoes, 328-332
wind suits, 327-328
definition, 323-324
drag, reduction of, 327-328
extrinsic, 323-338
fiberglass pole, 335
golf balls, 333-335
golf clubs, 335
implements, 333-336
intrinsic, 323
javelins, aerodynamic, 333
mechanical constraints, 324
playing surfaces, 336-338
racing shell, 333
shoes, racing
composition, 330-332
weight, 328-330
tracks, 336-338
wind suits, 327-328
Blood doping, 202-216
and 2, 3 DPG, 206
benefits, theoretical, 203-207
critical factors, 214-216
disadvantages, theoretical, 205
effects on
arterial oxygen content, 211
cardiac output, 208-211
heart rate, 206-207, 209-210,
213-214
hematocrit, 208-209
hemoglobin levels, 207-210,
211-214
lactic acid, 209-211
maximal oxygen uptake, 207-215
maximal work time, 207-208,
210-215

Continuity assumption, 255
Covert rehearsal, 253-271
  anticipatory conditions, 254-255
  and altitude performance, 256-257
  audio modality, 259
  behavioral boundaries, 264
  coping strategy, 256, 261, 262, 264, 267
  definition, 253-254
  high caliber athletes, 256-257
  intervention strategies, 260, 263-264
  long distance running, 253
  methodological approaches, 269-270
  physical practice, 253, 258-260, 264, 265-268
  progressive relaxation, 260, 264, 270
  research needs, 270-271
  retention, 9
  theoretical considerations, 254-255
Covert rehearsal, effects on
  ball and socket task, 265
  basketball skills, 258, 261
  dart throwing, 262-265, 268-269
  football performance, 263
  gymnastic skills, 267
  heart rate, 258
  hockey performance, 264-265
  juggling, 266
  karate performance, 262
  manual dexterity, 258
  motor skills, 257-270
  Olympic skiers, 260-261
  overt behavior, 256-257
  place kicking, 260-262
  psychomotor tasks, 260, 267
  respiratory rate, 258
  swimming start, 259
  strength, 270-271
  tennis skills, 259, 261, 262
  trait anxiety, 262
  volleyball skills, 259
Cycling
  effect of warm-up, 345-347, 356, 361-362

D

Dehydration (see hypohydration)
Dianabol, 170-174
2, 3 - diphosphoglycerate, and blood doping, 206
Drag, 326-328
Drive theory, 283-284
Drugs
  amphetamines, 101-120

anabolic steroids, 164-177
and stress reduction, 298
caffeine, 128-153

E

Electrolytes, 56-92
  and acid base balance, 66-68
  calcium, 59, 64-65, 68, 73-74, 83
  chloride, 59, 70, 72-73, 77, 87, 88-89
  distribution in body fluids, 59-68
  effect on
    fluid absorption, 73-74
    physical performance, 73, 81-84, 87-89, 90-92
  imbalance of, 61
  losses in sweat, 57, 62
  potassium, 59, 62-63, 68, 70, 72-74, 82-83, 87-89
  replacement of, 56-92
  roles in body, 89
  sodium, 59-63, 68, 70, 71-72, 72-74, 77, 82-83, 88-89
Endorphins, 303
Ephedrine, 101
Epinephrine, 303
Erythrocythemia (see blood doping)
Estradiol, 164-165
Estrogenic compounds, 165-166
Exercise
  and body water control, 65-66
  and muscle pH, 66-67
  and sweat losses, 57
  for stress reduction, 285
Extrinsic biomechanical aids, 323-328

F

Fat
  energy source during exercise, 5, 16
  metabolism
    and niacin, 38
Fatigue (also see local muscular endurance), 5-7
  and muscle pH, 66-67
  effect of amphetamines on, 105-109
Females
  and iron status, 23-24
  effects of anabolic steroids, 164-167, 168, 170, 175-176
FFA (see free fatty acids)
Fluid replacement (see also water, rehydration), 56-92
  and absorption rate, 73-74
  body temperature effects, 77-80
  cardiovascular effects, 75-78

during exercise, 73-80
in wrestlers, 74-77
Free fatty acids
and amphetamines, 105, 118-119
and caffeine, 134
and oxygen supplementation, 195

G

Glucose (also see glycogen and carbohydrate), 75
effect on fluid absorption, 73-74
Glucose-alanine cycle, 29
Glucose electrolyte solutions, 58,
76-78, 81-83, 88-89
absorption rate, 73-74
Glutamine, 29
Glycogen (also see carbohydrate), 3-21
depletion
and amphetamines, 105
and protein use, 29-30
and oxygen supplementation,
194-195
loading (also see carbohydrate loading), 3-21
and types of carbohydrate, 11
upper limits, 9-11
metabolism
effects of caffeine, 147-148
muscle, 3-21
content, 7-8, 29-30
effect of diet, 8
effect of exercise, 8
effect of training, 7-8
dehydration effects, 72
depletion, 5, 8
factors affecting use of, 4
fatigue, 4-5, 7
fiber type utilization, 6-8
niacin, 38
resynthesis patterns, 8-9
supercompensation, 3-21
mechanisms of, 8, 13-16
regimens, 11-12, 15-16
water retention, 17
work intensity, 4-5, 8, 11-12, 17-19
sparing effect of
amphetamines, 118
caffeine, 143-146
training, 14-15
synthase, 8, 11
role in supercompensation, 13-16
utilization during exercise, 3-21
effect of caffeine, 141, 144-146

glycolysis
and potassium release, 70
gravity
effects on performance, 324-325

H

Hallucinated exercise
physiological effects of, 239-241
Hawthorne effect, 227-228
Health risk
anabolic steroids, 165-175
Heat distress
potassium depletion, 72-73, 87-89
Heat injury, 71-72
Hematocrit
and altitude training, 209
and blood doping, 204-205
effect of exercise on, 204-205
Hemoglobin, 46-47
affinity for oxygen, 206
and acid-base balance, 66-67
effect of
altitude training on, 202-203
blood doping on, 204-205
exercise on, 204-205
iron deficiency on, 43
loss
effects on maximal oxygen uptake,
202-203
protein intake, 30, 32-34
saturation at altitude, 189
status in athletes, 44-45
Heparin, 144
Hydrogen ion
and acid-base balance, 66-68
Hyperhydration, 80-82, 86-87
and sweat rates, 87
effects on physical performance,
80-82
Hyperthermia (also see body temperature)
and amphetamines, 120
Hypnosis, 223-246
and altered states of consciousness,
245
and application to athletics, 241-246
and endurance, 238-239
and motor performance, 241
and muscular performance, 237-238
and optimal performance, 245
and sports medicine research,
234-235
and strength, 238-239

and warm-up, 354
clinical applications, 241-246
effects on
  anxiety, 244-246
  arousal level, 244-245
  athletic injuries, 243, 246
  athletic performance, 231-233,
  234-235
  dynamic performance, 240
  endurance, 233-235, 237-239
  heart rate, 236, 246
  isometric strength, 239
  lactate production, 246
  muscular performance, 231-232
  perceived exertion, 237-238, 246
  performance slump, 242
  power, 233, 237-238
  psychomotor traits, 240-241
  reaction time, 240
  running, 239
  staleness, 240
  strength, 231, 233, 237-239, 246
  treadmill running performance,
  238
  ventilation, 236
  vertical jump, 239
  weight lifting, 239
qualifications of practitioners,
224-226
research
  applications, 235-242
  methodology problems, 227-230,
  232
  roles of suggestion, 226-229
  theoretical considerations, 226-230
Hypnotist
  qualifications of, 224
Hypoglycemia, 20
Hypohydration
  and anaerobic exercise, 70-72
  and blood volume, 69-70
  and body temperature in exercise,
  70-72
  and electrolyte levels, 70
  and state anxiety, 72
  effects on
    physical performance, 57, 70-72,
    84-85, 90
    heat injury, 71-72
Hypothalamus
  effects of amphetamines on, 103-104

I

Imagery, 254-255, 259-264, 270-271,

284-285
Inner mental training, 245
Insulin, 11, 15
  effect of caffeine, 141-142
International Olympic Committee, 129,
131
Inverted U-model, 282, 343-344
Iron, 43-47
  deficiency, 43-44
  functions in the body, 43-44
  RDA, 43
  status in athletes, 43-44
  supplements and physical performance, 45-47
  theoretical benefits, 43-44
  use by athletes, 27-28

J

Jumping
  effects of warm-up, 349-350, 356-357,
  363-364

L

Lactic acid
  and caffeine, 145
  and supplemental oxygen, 189-190
Liver function
  effects of anabolic steroids, 175-176

M

Magnesium, 59-60, 64
  role in the body, 64-65
Marathon running
  and androgens, 168
  and carbohydrate loading, 5, 7, 12
  and fluid replacement, 77-78
Maximal oxygen uptake, 188
  effect of
    amphetamines, 108
    anabolic steroids, 168, 173, 175-176
    blood doping, 207-215
    caffeine, 149
    hypohydration, 70-71
    Vitamin C, 40-41
    Vitamin E, 42-43
  limiting factors, 203-204
  role of the blood, 202-203
Mechanical aids (also see biomechanical aids, extrinsic), 323-328
Menstruation
  effects of anabolic steroids, 176
Mental practice (also see covert rehearsal), 259-262, 264-265, 267-270
Methandrostenolone (see Dianabol)

Methyltestosterone (see Dianabol)
Muscle
  glycogen (see glycogen, muscle)
  hypertrophy
    and protein supplements, 33-34
  soreness,
    and Vitamin C, 41
  tissue
    effects of anabolic steroids,
    165-174, 176-177

N

Niacin (also see Vitamin B complex)
  effects on
    free fatty acids, 38-39
    glycogen utilization, 38-39
Nicotinic acid (see Vitamin B complex
and niacin)
Nitrogen
  balance, 29, 31-34
  excretion, 29, 31-34
  in oxygen supplementation, 186
  sweat losses of, 29
Norepinephrine, 303

O

Overtraining
  and stress, 305-306
Oxygen
  as ergogenic aid
    methodological approaches,
    187-188
  cost
    to overcome air resistance, 327-328
  deficit
    and warm-up, 343
  supplemental
    effects of administration
      after exercise, 197-198
      before exercise, 196-197
      during exercise, 189-196
    effects on
      aerobic metabolism, 186-187, 189,
      191-192
      anaerobic metabolism, 186-187,
      189, 191
      blood flow, 195
      blood lactate, 189-191, 194,
      196-197
      blood pressure, 195-197
      carbohydrate metabolism, 195
      cardiac output, 186-187, 189-191
      central mechanisms, 189-190
      endurance, 189-197
      fatty acid metabolism, 195
      glycogen depletion, 194-195
      heart rate, 189-191, 193-194, 196
      maximal oxygen uptake, 189,
      192-195
      oxygen consumption, 195
      oxygen debt, 191
      peripheral mechanisms, 194-196
      psychomotor performance,
      197-198
      pulmonary diffusing capacity,
      188-189
      recovery from exercise, 197
      running speed, 196
      ventilation, 189, 191, 193
    research methodology problems,
    185-187
    theoretical considerations, 188-190
  uptake
    effect of running shoes on, 330-331

P

Perceived exertion, 303
  and blood doping, 209, 211-213
  and hypnosis, 236-238
Perception, 304-305
Perceptual-motor skills, 254
Physical performance
  limiting factors, 185-186, 226
  mechanical constraints, 324-328
Physical warm-up (see warm-up)
Placebo effect, 228-229, 234-235
  and anabolic steroids, 170-171
Polycythemia (see blood doping)
Potassium (also see electrolytes), 59-60
  and cardiac problems, 87-89
  and physical performance, 72-73,
  87-88
  body stores, 62-63
  deficiency, 62
  excess, 63
  excretion, 63
  in sweat, 63
Progressive relaxation, 281, 287-289
  effects on
    anxiety, 287-289
    baseball performance, 288
    gymnastic performance, 287-289
Protein, 27-34
  and acid-base balance, 66-67
  and muscle tissue synthesis, 28-29
  and sports anemia, 29
  as energy source during exercise,
  29-31

deficiency
  and physical performance, 32-34
degradation, 27-28
effect of training on requirement,
  28-29
intake
  and energy, 32
  effect on performance, 29-34
  nitrogen balance, 29, 31-34
  nitrogen excretion, 29, 31-34
RDA, 27-29
requirements during exercise, 29-34
synthesis
  effect of anabolic steroids, 164-165
supplementation
  and hemoglobin, 33-34
  and performance, 29-34
theoretical benefits to athletes, 28-29
Psyching (see cognitive psyching)
Psychological aids
  covert rehearsal strategies, 253-271
  hypnosis, 223-246
  stress management, 275-310
Psychomotor tasks
  effect of covert rehearsal, 257-271
  effect of hypnosis, 239-240
  effect of stress management, 287-295
  effect of warm-up, 350-353, 357-358,
  365
Pyridoxine (see Vitamin B complex)

R

Reaction time
  and amphetamines, 110-111, 116
  and caffeine, 149
Red blood cells (also see blood doping)
  effect of anabolic steroids, 167-168,
  176
Rehydration (also see fluid replacement)
  before exercise, 74-75, 84-85
  during exercise, 76-80, 85-86
  effect on
    physical performance, 84-86, 91-92
    temperature regulation, 84-85
Research methodology problems
  anabolic steroids, 164-168, 170,
  175-176
  blood doping, 206
  caffeine, 128-132, 148-149, 152-153
  hypnosis, 227-230, 232
  oxygen, 185-187
  stress management procedures, 286,

296, 300-301, 309-310
  warm-up, 355, 359, 366
Riboflavin (see Vitamin B complex)
Running
  effect of warm-up, 345-347, 356-357,
  362-363

S

Salt (also see electrolytes; sodium)
  intake, 87-89
    and physical performance, 87-88
    and resources during exercise,
    82-83
  retention
    effect of anabolic steroids, 166-167
  tablets, 87-89
    and potassium depletion, 87-89
Scaling, 301
Shoes, running
  as biomechanical aid, 328-332
Skiing
  drag effects, 327-328
Sleep loss
  effects of amphetamines, 110-111
Sodium (also see electrolytes; salt)
  daily intake, 64
  effect on temperature set point,
  82-83
  in body fluids, 61
  in sweat, 61
Sports anemia, 29, 44-45
  and protein needs, 30-31
Sports management procedures
  effectiveness of, 287-295
Staleness in athletes, 305-306
State anxiety, 244-246, 304-306
Strength
  effect of
    amphetamines, 109-110, 115-116
    anabolic steroids, 164, 166, 170-176
    hypnosis, 227-229
    hypohydration, 71-72
    placebos, 229
    protein supplements, 33-34
    warm-up, 358, 365
  psychological aspects, 226
Stress
  acute (also see state anxiety), 304-306
  adaptations to training, 305-306
  and learning, 306-307
  and arousal, 277-282
  as a sports predictor, 304-306
  behavioral measures of, 302

biological nature of, 277-282
chronic model of, 305-307
coping with, 306-307
definition, 276-277
drug effects, 298
effects on
  heart rate, 298
  strength, 296-297
intervention specificity, 298-299
levels, and prediction of athletic performance, 302-303
measurement of, 277-278
muscular tension in, 281
physiological indicators of, 301-302
responses to, 277-282
reduction by exercise, 285-286
Selye's theory of, 277-278
sport specificity of, 299-300
theoretical benefits to physical performance, 282-284
theory of, 276-278
Stress management procedures, 275-310
  application to the sport, 307-308
  clinical intervention, 283
    adjunctive procedures, 285
    attention control training, 284-285
    biofeedback, 283-285
    visual-motor behavior rehearsal, 285-286
  effects on physical performance, 287-295
  learning, 306-307
  research methodology problems, 286, 296, 300-301, 309-310
  theories, recent, 275-276
Stress response, 276-277
  in athletes, 296-298
  individual differences, 286, 296-298
Stressors, 276-277
  abstract, 277-278
  concrete, 277-278
Sweat losses (also see hypohydration)
  and electrolyte supplementation, 89
  and plasma volume, 69
  during exercise, 57
  effect on performance, 69
  iron content, 43-44
  replacement, 74-75
    during exercise, 76-80, 85-86
    effect on performance, 84-86
Sweat rate
  and glucose-electrolyte solutions, 30

effect of hyperhydration, 81
Swimming
  and amphetamines, 111-112, 116-117
  and warm-up, 349-350
Systematic desensitization, 255

                    T
Testosterone (also see anabolic steroids; androgens), 164, 168-170
Thiamin (see Vitamin B complex)
Trait anxiety, 296-297

                    U
Urea, 27, 29-30

                    V
Visual-motor behavior rehearsal, 260-262, 285
  effects on
    anxiety, 293-294
    athletic performance, 293-294
    attention, 293-294
    basketball performance, 294-295
    confidence, 294
    cross-country skiing, 294
    golf performance, 294
    karate, 295
    motivation, 295
    tennis performance, 293, 295
    tension, 293-295
    wrestling performance, 293
Vitamins, 27-28, 34-43
  B complex, 34-39
  C, 39-41
  E, 41-43
  RDA, 35
  supplements, multiple, 37-38
  use by athletes, 27-28
VMBR (see visual-motor behavior rehearsal)
$\dot{V}O_2$ max (see maximal oxygen uptake)

                    W
Warm-up, 340-370
  effect of
    attitude towards, 344, 354
    criterion tasks, 355, 359, 366, 370
    subject's fitness level, 344, 355, 360, 367-369
    types of, 354-355, 359-360, 366, 369
  effects on
    anaerobic performance, 355
    cycling
      endurance, 345-347, 356, 361
      speed, 361-362

EKG, 344, 367
fine motor skills, 359
injury prevention, 344, 366
jumping performance, 349-351,
356-357, 363-364
long endurance tasks, 355
metabolic responses, 348-349,
363-364
physiological responses, 348-349,
363-364
psychomotor tasks, 350-351,
357-358, 365
running
endurance, 345-347, 356-357
speed, 347, 356-357, 362-363
step test performance, 346-347
sports skills, 350-351, 364
strength, 358, 365
swimming, 349-350
model for research, proposed,
367-370
passive, 342, 369
physiological bases for, 342-343
psychological basis for, 343-344
research methodology problems,
355, 359, 366
safety aspects, 344, 366-368
theoretical benefits to physical performance, 342-344
types of
direct, 341-342

identical, 341-342
indirect, 341-342
passive, 342
Water (also see fluids), 56-92
body
and acid-base balance, 66-68
and carbohydrate loading, 17
compartments, 58-59
functions of, 58-59
intake
absorption rate, 73-74
effects on physical performance,
90-92
losses
and physical performance, 69-72
diuretics, 69-70
rehydration
effects on physical performance,
75-77
roles in the body, 89
Weight lifting
and protein intake, 31
Wheat germ oil, 42
Wrestling
performance, effects of
hypohydration, 71-72
rehydration, 84-86
weight losses, 56-57

X
Xanthine (see caffeine)